W WHA 2015
009461

RESEARCH METHODS IN HEALTH COMMUNICATION

This volume provides an essential roster of primary research methods as they apply to health communication inquiry. Editor Bryan B. Whaley brings together key health communication researchers to write about their primary methodological areas. Their chapters offer guidance and insights for a variety of approaches to answering research questions. The methods included here cover:

- **Exploration and Description:** interview/focus groups, case study, ethnography, and surveys;
- **Examining Messages and Interpersonal Exchanges:** narrative analysis, conversational analysis, analyzing physician–patient interactions, social network analysis, and content analysis;
- **Causal Explication:** experimental research, meta-analysis, and meta-synthesis; and
- **Cultural, Population, and Critical Concerns:** rhetorical methods and criticism, and methodological issues when investigating stigmatized populations and groups with health disparities.

Chapters cite or use examples from allied health areas—nursing, public health, sociology, medicine—to demonstrate the breadth of health communication studies.

This work highlights the importance of methodology in health communication research in multiple contexts. Developed to provide a fundamental reference for investigating health communication, this volume will serve as an invaluable tool for researchers and students across the social science and health disciplines.

Bryan B. Whaley is Professor of Communication at University of San Francisco. His research concerns linguistic factors related to explaining illness and complex health-related information, the function and design of interpersonal messages to patients, and language/message variables in social influence.

RESEARCH METHODS IN HEALTH COMMUNICATION

Papworth Hospital NHS Foundation Trust O12
Library and Knowledge Services
For renewals contact:
library@papworth.nhs.uk or ring 01480 364245
This book is due for return on or before the last date shown below.

31 MAR 2015
15 APR 2023
15 APR 2019

First published 2014
by Routledge
711 Third Avenue, New York, NY 10017

and by Routledge
2 Park Square, Milton Park, Abingdon, Oxon OX14 4RN

Routledge is an imprint of the Taylor & Francis Group, an informa business

© 2014 Taylor & Francis

The right of the editor to be identified as the author of the editorial material, and of the authors for their individual chapters, has been asserted in accordance with sections 77 and 78 of the Copyright, Designs and Patents Act 1988.

All rights reserved. No part of this book may be reprinted or reproduced or utilized in any form or by any electronic, mechanical, or other means, now known or hereafter invented, including photocopying and recording, or in any information storage or retrieval system, without permission in writing from the publishers.

Trademark notice: Product or corporate names may be trademarks or registered trademarks, and are used only for identification and explanation without intent to infringe.

Library of Congress Cataloging in Publication Data
Research methods in health communication : principles and application / edited by Bryan B. Whaley.
pages cm
1. Communication in medicine. 2. Communication in medicine—Research—Methodology. I. Whaley, Bryan B.
R118.R46 2014
610.72—dc23 2013048961

ISBN: 978-0-415-53185-6 (hbk)
ISBN: 978-0-415-53186-3 (pbk)
ISBN: 978-0-203-11529-9 (ebk)

Typeset in Bembo
by RefineCatch Limited, Bungay, Suffolk

Printed and bound by CPI Group (UK) Ltd, Croydon, CR0 4YY

Dedicated to

Dr. James M. Betts, MD

and

the incredible medical, nursing, and support staff

of

Children's Hospital and Research Center
Oakland

for saving my daughter . . . . . . THANK YOU!

CONTENTS

Meta-Synthesis

FIGURES

TABLES

CONTRIBUTORS

Austin S. Babrow (PhD, University of Illinois at Urbana–Champaign) is Professor of Communication Studies at Ohio University. His teaching and research focus on the intersection of communication, uncertainty, and values, and particularly the social construction of the uncertainty and the profound values associated with health, illness, and risk. He has also begun to explore environmental communication, as well as spiritual and ethical wisdom, communication, and human suffering.

Robert A. Bell (PhD, University of Texas at Austin) is Professor in the Departments of Communication and Public Health Sciences at the University of California, Davis. He has a long-standing interest in communication and social influence processes, and has applied this interest in the domains of prescription drug advertising, media and health, and physician–patient interaction. His current research focuses on health information-seeking, linguistic agency and health promotion, and physician–patient interactions regarding genetic screening for inheritable disease.

Nick L. Carcioppolo (PhD, Purdue University) is Assistant Professor in the Communication Studies Department at the University of Miami. His research focuses on the development and assessment of persuasive messages for health communication campaigns and interventions, with an emphasis on cancer prevention and screening behaviors, as well as the persuasive effects of entertainment media on health-related attitudes, beliefs, and behaviors.

Louis P. Cusella (PhD, Purdue University) is Professor of Communication at the University of Dayton. His research focuses on organizational communication issues, including feedback and loose versus tight coupling in health organizations.

Erin E. Donovan (PhD, University of Illinois at Urbana–Champaign) is Assistant Professor of Communication Studies at the University of Texas at Austin. She specializes in how people exchange information while coping with times characterized by stress, illness, and uncertainty. Her scholarship addresses topics ranging from antecedents and consequences of conversations about cancer and HIV to strategies for improving communication during the informed consent process before medical procedures.

Laura L. Ellingson (PhD, University of South Florida) is Professor of Communication and Women's & Gender Studies at Santa Clara University. Her research focuses on gender in extended families, feminist and qualitative methodologies, and interdisciplinary teamwork in healthcare organizations. She teaches courses in qualitative methods, feminist methods, and gendered communication as it intersects with health, sexuality, and family.

Leigh Arden Ford (PhD, Purdue University) is Professor and Director of the School of Communication at Western Michigan University. Dr. Ford's research interests emphasize supportive communication, the communication of health messages within disenfranchised communities, and contextualized understandings of health communication practices.

Mindi A. Golden (PhD, University of Utah) is Associate Professor in the Department of Communication Studies at San Francisco State University. Her research focuses on social support and relational issues in dementia caregiving and communication at the end of life.

Daena J. Goldsmith (PhD, University of Washington) is Professor of Rhetoric and Media Studies at Lewis & Clark College. She studies how we enact identities and relationships in everyday interactions, including conversations between spouses or partners, advice-giving among friends and family, and storytelling face to face and online. In addition, her recent research efforts have focused on how couples or families talk about illnesses, including heart disease, cancer, HIV/AIDS, and autism.

Kathryn Greene (PhD, University of Georgia) is Professor in the Department of Communication at Rutgers, The State University of New Jersey.

Her teaching and research interests include persuasion, health communication, and interpersonal communication. She explores decision making related to various health risks. Her research foci are increasing involvement in message processing and exploring message features in prevention, especially with adolescent risk-taking; and how people choose to share or conceal health diagnoses, medical updates, or other information in relationships.

Lynn M. Harter (PhD, University of Nebraska) is Professor of Communication Studies at Ohio University. Her research focuses on discourses of health and healing and organizing processes, narrative and feminist theory–praxis. Her work has encompassed a range of issues, including disability-related concerns, pediatric cancer care, and organizing healthcare resources for underserved populations. She has taught narrative theory courses at both the undergraduate and doctoral levels.

Joan A. Jurich (PhD, Purdue University) is Associate Professor of Social and Public Health at Ohio University. She teaches courses in middle childhood and adolescent development as well as advanced family development. Her research interests are in the areas of sexuality and reproductive health among adolescents and young adults, including child–parent communication about sexuality.

Christopher J. Koenig (PhD, University of California, Los Angeles) is Adjunct Assistant Professor of Medicine at the San Francisco Veterans Affairs Medical Center and at the Philip R. Lee Institute for Health Policy Studies at University of California, San Francisco. His research focuses on the social dimensions of health and illness, and emphasizes the mediating role of communication on the social, organizational, and cultural contexts of providing patient-centered healthcare and policy.

Richard L. Kravitz (MD, University of California, San Francisco) is Professor in the Department of Internal Medicine at the University of California, Davis. His research interests center on the causes and consequences of physician behavior.

Kate Magsamen-Conrad (PhD, Rutgers, The State University of New Jersey) is Assistant Professor in the Department of Communication at Bowling Green State University. Her teaching and research interests include health communication, relational communication, and aging and communication.

Laura E. Miller (PhD, University of Illinois at Urbana–Champaign) is Assistant Professor in the School of Communication Studies at the University of Tennessee. She studies communication about cancer between patients, partners, and social networks and the implications such conversations may have on uncertainty and identity management.

Michelle Miller-Day (PhD, Arizona State University) is Professor of Communication Studies at Chapman University. She addresses issues at the intersection of health and communication, specifically substance abuse prevention, obesity, and diabetes prevention. Her cross-disciplinary work spans family, medicine, health, communication, and sociology.

Susan E. Morgan (PhD, University of Arizona) is Professor in the Brian Lamb School of Communication at Purdue University. Her research focuses on message design as well as the development and evaluation of health communication campaigns.

Christopher R. Morse (PhD, The Pennsylvania State University) is Assistant Professor in the Department of Communication at Bryant University. His research focuses on uncertainty management in health and relational contexts, as well as examining the role that mood and emotion have on individuals' decision making.

Seth M. Noar (PhD, University of Rhode Island) is Associate Professor in the School of Journalism and Mass Communication at the University of North Carolina, Chapel Hill, and a member of its Lineberger Comprehensive Cancer Center. His work addresses health behavior theories, message design and mass media campaigns, and eHealth applications.

Spencer D. Patterson (PhD, Ohio University) is Adjunct Professor of Communication at Utah Valley University. His research focuses on organizing healthcare and communication training for providers, patients, and caregivers.

Brian L. Quick (PhD, Texas A&M University) is Associate Professor in the Department of Communication and in the College of Medicine at the University of Illinois at Urbana–Champaign. His work examines various strategies to create, disseminate, and evaluate organ and tissue donation campaigns.

William K. Rawlins (PhD, Temple University) is Professor of Communication Studies at Ohio University. His research draws on theories of narrative and dialogue to investigate how communicating as friends facilitates the well-lived life, including health, for persons and societies.

Eileen Berlin Ray (PhD, University of Washington) is Professor in the School of Communication at Cleveland State University in Ohio. Her research interests include communication related to chronic health disabilities, adult survivors of sexual abuse, and communication and mental health.

James D. Robinson (PhD, Purdue University) is Professor of Communication at the University of Dayton. His research focuses on health communication, media use, and media effects.

Jeffrey D. Robinson (PhD, University of California, Los Angeles) is Professor in the Department of Communi-cation at Portland State University. His research concerns how face-to-face communication between healthcare providers and patients affects healthcare delivery and health promotion.

Lindsey M. Rose (PhD, Ohio University) is an online Adjunct Professor for Ohio University. She employs qualitative research methods to explore issues in health communication, community organizing, and pedagogy.

Aaron T. Seaman (MA, University of Illinois at Urbana–Champaign) is a doctoral candidate in the Department of Comparative Human Development at the University of Chicago. His dissertation research focuses on families and caregiving in the context of young-onset dementia.

Barbara F. Sharf (PhD, University of Minnesota) is an independent scholar and Professor Emerita, Department of Communication, Texas A&M University. Her research in health communication spans more than 35 years, encompassing topics such as patients' experiences with serious illness, practitioner–patient communication, cross-cultural communication in healthcare settings, and food insecurity as a community health focus. A current research interest is the practice and institutionalization of integrative medicine in the United States.

Rachel A. Smith (PhD, Michigan State University) is Associate Professor of Communication Arts & Sciences and Human Development & Family Studies, and an Investigator in the Center for Infectious Disease Dynamics and the Methodology Center at The Pennsylvania State University. Her research program focuses on how social identities, social interactions, social memberships, and patterns of relationships shape and are shaped by communication, as well as interpersonal or intergroup influences in persuasion and compliance. Recently, her research has centered on building and testing theories focusing on the relationships and dynamics among stigmas, communication, and health.

Leslie B. Snyder (PhD, Stanford University) is Professor of Communication and Director of the Center for Health Communication & Marketing at the University of Connecticut. Her research focuses on the intended and unintended consequences of media use, including design and evaluation of communication-based interventions.

Brian G. Southwell (PhD, University of Pennsylvania) is a Senior Research Scientist with RTI International and holds faculty appointments at the University of North Carolina at Chapel Hill and Duke University. His research involves public understanding of health and science, including assessment of information diffusion via mass communication and social networks and factors affecting human interaction with risk information.

Lisa Sparks (PhD, University of Oklahoma) is Professor of Communication at Chapman University. Her research concerns issues of health promotion, disease prevention, survivorship, and health disparities and literacy, risk, crisis communication, and public health campaigns.

Ashli Q. Stokes (PhD, University of Georgia) is Associate Professor in the Department of Communication Studies at the University of North Carolina at Charlotte. She pursues a wide variety of research in public relations and public communication, specializing in rhetorical approaches to analyzing public relations and health controversies.

Anne M. Stone (PhD, University of Illinois at Urbana–Champaign) is Assistant Professor of Communication at Rollins College. Her recent research has focused on the role of communication in improving experiences for persons with Alzheimer's disease and those of their families.

Teresa L. Thompson (PhD, Temple University) is Professor of Communication at the University of Dayton. Her research focuses on concerns related to provider–patient interaction, organ donation, disability and communication, and gender issues.

Yan Tian (PhD, Temple University) is Associate Professor in Communication at the University of Missouri–St. Louis. Her research concerns health communication, new communication technologies, and media effects.

Julie E. Volkman (PhD, The Pennsylvania State University) is a Research Health Scientist with the U.S. Department of Veterans Affairs' eHealth Quality Enhancement Research Initiative (eHealth-QUERI) and the Center for Healthcare Organization and Implementation Research (CHOIR) at the Edith Nourse Rogers Memorial Veterans Hospital in Massachusetts. She is also an Assistant Professor in the Department of Quantitative Health Sciences and the Division of Health Informatics and Implementation Science at the University of Massachusetts Medical School. Dr. Volkman's research focuses on the intersections of health communication and health services research for patient-centered care and self-management of diseases.

Bryan B. Whaley (Ph.D., Purdue University) is Professor of Communication at the University of San Francisco. His research concerns linguistic factors related to explaining illness and complex health-related information, the function and design of interpersonal messages to patients, and language/message variables in social influence.

Jill Yamasaki (PhD, Texas A&M University) is Assistant Professor of Health Communication in the Valenti School of Communication at the University of Houston. Her research focuses on personal and cultural meanings of old age and experiences of aging, particularly in the contexts of community, long-term care, and quality of life. Employing a variety of qualitative approaches, her ongoing research interests include humanizing communication practices and innovative approaches for nurturing biographical continuity, creative engagement, and person-centered care in late life.

PREFACE

I have had this book in mind for close to a decade. The impetus was the experience of my oldest daughter's unexplained perforated colon when she was nine years old. I watched incredibly competent medical personnel—Dr. James Betts (surgery), Dr. Elliott Vichinsky (hematology/oncology), Dr. Beth Gleghorn (gastroenterology)—three of the best in the world, and numerous pathologists and laboratory personnel at the Children's Hospital and Research Center Oakland use *research methods* to help my daughter. With their world-renowned expertise, and the latest knowledge and technology, my daughter's perforated colon is recorded as "unexplained." Life is full of tricky stuff, and health is often the slyest of foes. All this got me thinking about research methods—the tools we employ when trying to understand the world. As the case at hand demonstrates, research methods powerfully constitute and impact what we know and how we communicate about health.

When we use various research methods to investigate health contexts and topics, there are assumptions and procedures involved that affect every aspect of the research process, and, ultimately, the findings. That is, our methods determine what we know. Given the importance of health to every one of us, the more we know, the better. However, there has yet to be a volume that addresses the wide diversity of research methods that can be applied in health communication contexts—a reference title such as this one. Research methods are tools of inquiry. And, like other tools, it is crucial that the right tool is chosen for its intended job. Each tool has its inherent strengths, weaknesses, and concerns, but each creates understandings that have potentially profound impacts for patients, their loved ones, practitioners, and scholars. This volume is a collection of the research methods that can be applied when investigating health and communication for its intended users (i.e., investigators from allied health professions, communication, medicine, nursing, psychology, public health, sociology, and the like).

The organization of this book is dictated by the purpose and nature of the methods discussed. Specifically, even though tools are constitutionally different, they can be grouped given similarities in their general underlying function. The text begins with an introductory chapter—"Method Matters"—concerning the foundational issues of research methods. The first group of methods, "Exploration and Description," contains interview/focus groups, case studies, ethnography, and surveys. Narrative analysis, conversational analysis, analyzing physician–patient interactions, social network analysis, and content analysis comprise the second cluster of tools, "Examining Messages and Interpersonal Exchanges." The third set of methods, "Causal Explication," includes experimental, meta-analysis, and meta-synthesis. The final collection of chapters, "Cultural, Population, and Critical Concerns," addresses rhetorical methods and criticism, as well as methodological issues when investigating stigmatized populations and populations with health disparities. The volume concludes with "Method Reflections," a discussion of meta-theoretical concerns as applied to research methodology and what our tools provide us. Assembled, these chapters fill the void for a single methodological reference for health communication researchers to consult.

ACKNOWLEDGMENTS

Thanks to my contributors to this book. After my last read of the chapters before sending to press, I thought of Steve Jobs' premise: "You can only connect the dots looking back." It then occurred to me that I had asked the right dots … to connect. I am extremely appreciative and proud of the work by my colleagues for this volume. Again, I thank you. Importantly, as well, I thank the anonymous reviewers of this book's proposal for their insightful suggestions. Their comments were seriously considered, and we did our best to address reviewers' concerns within the confines of the initial vision of this project. Finally, much appreciation to Linda Bathgate at Routledge for her insight and support; she gets it done.

B. B. Whaley
San Francisco

Method Matters

METHOD MATTERS

Teresa L. Thompson, Louis P. Cusella, and Brian G. Southwell

A "method" is a technique or specific procedure used to collect and analyze information, frequently referred to as "data," about a particular subject matter (Kaplan, 1964). The title of this chapter, then, has a dual meaning. It can be interpreted as an overview of research methods in the field of health communication, indicating the "stuff" of which method is composed. Our focus here is on the "stuff" of health communication research methods. In a sense, a research method is a lens through which a researcher "sees" what he or she is studying. Beyond that layer of meaning, we also want to suggest that the enactment of a particular method *makes a difference*: method choices matter in distinct ways. We will focus on those ways, then, that methods do matter and the ways in which method makes a difference.

In general, the study of health communication emphasizes the interrelationships between (a) communicative, message-oriented processes and (b) both health and health care delivery. We begin our discussion with a very brief focus on the history of the study of health communication and then move to an examination of some of the reasons that methods matter in this area of inquiry. The remainder of the chapter will focus on such overriding methodological concerns as philosophy of science issues, units of analysis, sampling concerns, measurement innovations, triangulation, and the interrelationships among theory and methods.

As we move ahead in our discussion, a distinction between two oft-misused terms—"method" and "methodology"—is necessary. Methodology refers to the *study* of methods, whereas a particular method is a way of conducting research that is used in a specific study or type of study. This book is a methodological examination of different methods as they apply to investigating health communication. Each of the chapters within this book will focus on a particular type of research method. When you conduct a study, you do not employ a "methodology"—you employ a "method." The distinction is consequential, as it reminds us that there are both choices among methods to consider and a methodological literature from which to draw inspiration.

Beyond grammar, the distinction also helps to underscore the relationship of methods as behavior with an underlying philosophy which originally called for that behavior as a response. We also can draw a distinction between a method and the perspective, philosophy, or presuppositions underlying the method. For instance, as we think about qualitative research methods, we focus on such data collection approaches as focus groups, unstructured in-depth interviews, observation, introspection, recording, or studying conversation. Although it is possible to quantify data from such approaches as focus groups or interviews, these methods are more commonly used qualitatively. The *perspectives* underlying the development and employment of such methods, however, might include ethnography, grounded theory, or phenomenology, among others. These issues will be reviewed in subsequent chapters in this volume.

Studying Health Communication

The study of health communication as a distinct phenomenon is a relatively new one, beginning with work by pediatrician Barbara Korsch and colleagues in the late 1960s (e.g., Korsch, Gozzi, & Francis, 1968). Sociological and psychological work on the diffusion of ideas related to health and medicine also appeared throughout the 20th century (e.g., Coleman, Katz, & Menzel, 1966). Korsch and colleagues suggested that health communication might offer a distinct arena for consideration, and assessed healthcare provider–patient interaction. The initial issues of the journal *Health Communication,* which began publication in January of 1989, emphasized such interpersonally oriented scholarship. Within a short period of time, however, more work emerged that focused on the messages of health campaigns and their impact on audience members. Some of this work came from a sociological or public health perspective. Health campaign research has now become a very important area of the field of health communication, especially among those scholars with a background in communication or public health. Those with a background in medicine or nursing are more likely to focus upon provider–patient interaction issues. The newer *Journal of Health Communication* provides a primary focus on campaigns research, much of which takes a social marketing perspective. A social marketing approach applies the traditional methods of commercial marketing to social issues (e.g., Edgar, Volkman, & Logan, 2011). Scholars whose backgrounds are in medicine or nursing are more likely to continue to focus on provider–patient interaction, and, although this kind of research continues to be published in such communication-oriented outlets as *Health Communication*, it is even more commonly disseminated in journals such as *Patient Education and Counseling*. In recent years, two new foci have become pervasive in the area—health content in the media and the role of technology in health communication. The first of these examines how various health and healthcare issues are presented on television, in print, and in various social media forums such as YouTube, Facebook, or Twitter; the second includes not only changes in medical technology within health care but also the role of information technology and social media in this setting.

In addition, a focus on critical/cultural issues also has emerged, in part as a counterweight to administrative evaluation of campaigns as to their success or failure from the perspective of campaign planners. This perspective is concerned, for example, with power relationships in a particular culture that may impact health care processes. Whereas most early health communication research was strongly quantitative in nature, qualitative research is now also common and is providing important contributions. The emergence of more interpretive (meaning-making) perspectives makes evident the recognition of the roles of both determinism and free will in the study of health communication processes. It is no longer assumed that all individuals respond in the same way to messages or communicative processes. Interpretive and more deterministic perspectives go hand in hand, and operate in a complementary fashion to facilitate our understanding of the interrelationships of communication and health. Deterministic research and theorizing is based on the assumption that behavior is caused by such variables as heredity and the environment. It emphasizes objectivity and the generation of universal laws. By contrast, more interpretive approaches emphasize free will, interpretive guides, and emancipation of individuals and larger social collectivities.

Over the last several decades, health communication research has become increasingly sophisticated. More recent research has built upon and extended earlier investigations. Research has become much more strongly based in theory, which we define briefly later in this chapter. Hypotheses—predictions made by a researcher before he or she conducts a research study—have become narrower and more specialized. Whereas some early research investigated a single variable at a time, health communication researchers now often assess variables as they interact with one another. Most importantly, scholars have recognized to an increased extent that the theoretical approach that appears to best explain the processes in question and the variables of research interest should determine the method that is used to test new hypotheses and explore new research questions in health communication research (as it should in any other area of inquiry). Reliance on only one method or a small number of methods for all research in this arena would greatly limit our understanding of health communication and the knowledge claims that would be possible.

Why Methods Matter

Each of the chapters presented within this volume will make clear the uses to which the method presented within that chapter are most appropriate and the kinds of information that method yields. Methods do matter. The method that is used in a particular study constrains our understanding of the process of communication itself. The method that is used in a study essentially is a sense-making tool, in that it helps the researcher determine what data mean in a particular health communication context. Method determines the knowledge claims that are possible; it shapes what we can claim to know. Method determines to what we pay attention by bringing a particular focus to a phenomenon.

Scientific knowledge is always, in every respect, socially situated. It involves people in a particular context. Neither researchers nor the knowledge they produce are or can be impartial or value neutral (Madge, 1965). Interpretive perspectives more explicitly bring the voice of the researcher to bear in the illumination of social phenomena. Researchers, when employing quantitative-oriented tools, attempt to minimize the impact of their personal perspective on the phenomena under investigation, but assumptions underlying the research are nonetheless present. As has been argued in the work of Guttman (2003) and Cho and Salmon (2006; see also Salmon & Cho, 2007), research on health campaigns often is based on a set of values indicating that certain health conditions are to be avoided. Those assumptions may not be consistent with the cultural values of the group on whom the campaign is being imposed. A method-level decision to measure a particular outcome as an indicator of campaign success may mask the idea that success may be defined differently by different groups. For example, research on doctor–patient interaction is frequently based on the assumption that more patient participation is better than less, even though not all patients desire to participate at a high level. Different methods make different assumptions and can yield varying results; understanding that can help to contextualize those results.

Let us imagine a situation where a doctor and one of his/her patients are talking to each other during a medical exam. An example of the focus provided by different methods is evident in Robinson's (2011) summary of health communication research utilizing conversation analysis (CA), which provides a microscopic assessment of the phrasing of particular statements occurring within health provider (doctor)–patient interaction. CA allows the reader to understand the subtle differences between such questions as "is there *anything* else that you want to address in the visit today?" and "is there *something* else that you want to address in the visit today?" (Robinson, 2011, p. 515). Despite the apparent similarity of these questions, the second question results in patients bringing up more issues and leaving the encounter with fewer unmet concerns. This is just one example of the different understandings of the process of communication that a particular method yields. CA leads to an understanding of the organization of medical activities and the sequencing of talk. Robinson contrasts this with the broader categorization of provider–patient communication that would be allowed by interaction analysis (Roter & McNeilis, 2003). In the most commonly used interaction analysis coding scheme, Roter's Interaction Analysis System (RIAS), both questions would fall into the same category, and differences between using the word "anything" versus the word "something" would be lost.

Method also affects data analysis—how a researcher analyzes the information collected in a study—and, thus, the conclusions that data analysis might appear to yield. Continuing with the theme of CA as described by Robinson, for instance, it becomes apparent that data produced through CA cannot be analyzed using many statistical tests, even those that are nonparametric. Even a non-powerful, non-robust statistic such as the chi-squared test requires independence of cells (the assumption that the same person or response does not fall into more than one cell or category), so much conventional statistical analysis is not possible with CA data. This is because in real interaction a statement does not fulfill just one function. Thus, communication interaction data cannot be coded into mutually exclusive categories. If categories are not mutually exclusive, the assumption of independence of cells cannot be met.

Similarly, some methods are more appropriate for understanding the complexity of health communication processes. In their discussion of qualitative health communication research, du Pré and Crandall (2011) note that "the activities of everyday life do not occur as discrete units, but within a sophisticated web of factors" (p. 533). Qualitative methods, in appropriate cases, more adequately allow examination of this web of factors than do many other methods. Again, this is just one example of how method can affect our tendencies toward particular conclusions about health communication processes.

Method also determines the relationships that can be ascertained between health communication processes and various health outcomes. One of the most exciting aspects of the study of health communication is the ability to relate communication processes and variables to real-world, bottom-line, important outcomes, such as mortality, speed of recovery, reliance on medication, or the likelihood of post-operative vomiting. The ability to understand and relate communicative processes to such outcomes, however, is dependent on the methodological approach taken by a researcher. As will be apparent in the chapters that follow, some methods allow such a focus while this is foreign to other approaches. Data generated through an empirical categorization of provider–patient interaction, such as RIAS, can easily be related to health outcome data. Robinson (2011) notes, however, the ways in which CA data also may be related to such medical outcomes as insurance approvals (Boyd, 1998) or antibiotic prescription (Stivers, 2007). Interaction patterns identified through CA are also related to patient post-visit satisfaction, which is associated with numerous health outcomes (Robinson, Raup-Krieger, Burke, Weber, & Oesterling, 2008). Similarly, only some of the methods that are used in health communication allow the generation of causal claims in which a researcher asserts that one variable causes another variable to change in a particular way; experimentation would be the most notable such method. In experimentation, an independent variable (the suspected cause) is manipulated by the researcher and its effect on the dependent variable (the suspected effect) is studied. Many other methods of research lead to claims of relationship or correlation at best. Health campaign research is the area of the field that is most likely to utilize experimental design at the present time.

An essential fundamental finding of health communication research is that neither interpersonal nor mass mediated channels of communication function separately in terms of their impact on health and healthcare delivery (Southwell & Yzer, 2007). Although some methodological approaches are most commonly used to study the interpersonal context, and others to examine various mediated contexts, in actuality, the two types of channels often interact. By "interact," researchers typically mean that two or more independent variables combine to affect a dependent variable, but, in this case, we can see an even more complex chain of relationships and processes at play. A patient acquires information from one source, which he or she then discusses with friends, family members, or health care providers. Alternatively, a patient might be told something about health through an interpersonal source, and he or she then goes to the Internet to acquire more information about that issue. The information that is acquired through a web-based source may then be conveyed to a health care provider, and the provider will then need to respond to that information. So the concern is more than just statistical interactions: it is the interaction of various processes. Methodological approaches such as social network analysis (Smith, this volume), where who communicates with whom and how often are measured (Valente, 2011), are more amenable to looking at the interaction between different sources of information than are some other methods. Valente points out, "Understanding who delivers the message and the context of interpersonal consumption [of] media may be just as important, if not more so, than the message itself" (p. 530).

One foundational purpose of doing research is to build theory. A theory is a set of abstract statements that are considered part of scientific knowledge in that they help explain, predict, or control how something considered important occurs (Reynolds, 1971). All the methods discussed in this book are useful for the generation of theory. For instance, both quantitative and qualitative methods are frequently used for theory generation; however, experimentation might be a better way to test a theory. This is thus another way in which methods differ (and matter!).

Methods also differ in the ethical dilemmas that are inherent within them. Although most discussion of ethics in health communication to date has focused upon the ethics of health campaigns (Guttman, 2003; 2011), recent work has extended this concern to broader aspects of the field (Guttman & Thompson, 2010). Provider–patient interaction is replete with ethical issues that would emerge from a qualitative assessment of dyadic communication, but would not be as apparent utilizing some survey methods. Examples related to end-of-life discussions would be particularly relevant here (Thompson, 2011).

Similarly, methods differ in their effectiveness in helping a researcher understand a patient or provider's experience of a health communication reality. Only a phenomenological perspective, for instance, would allow a researcher "to take into account a person's *experience* of being healthy or unhealthy" (du Pré & Crandall, 2011, p. 539, emphasis original). This is also related to the degree to which various methods involve those stakeholders whose health the researchers desire to impact, as critical/cultural (Gustafson, 2005) and community organizing research approaches (Dearing, Gaglio, & Rabin, 2011) both go well beyond the imposition of the researcher's health goals for the target population and involve members of the population in the research process or in the understanding of health issues.

Perhaps most importantly, the methodological approach taken by a researcher affects the likelihood that the results of a study may be understood and applied by medical practitioners. Few scholars collect data and conduct research just for the sake of doing research. This is particularly true of health communication scholars, who generally do not study esoteric, unimportant topics. Almost all health communication researchers are very concerned about the application or translation of their findings to health policy, health care delivery, and the quality of the health of various populations. Methods differ in the ease with which they can be translated for practitioners and patients. Little research is of value without the ability to translate it into practical applications.

Fundamental to all research is the appropriateness of the match between method and topic/goal/focus. No one method is the be-all and end-all of health communication or any area of study. Even more important is how well the method is applied—how well the research is conducted. Health communication is a methodologically sophisticated and complex area of study. Any researcher must use the right tool for the job. The chapters that follow will provide focus for utilizing each method appropriately and well. The present chapter is not a primer on research methods—but the remainder of this volume is!

Theory—The Beginning of Method

Except for some qualitative approaches, such as grounded theory or ethnography, most good research begins with theoretical assumptions. Research that is atheoretical—without a theoretical base or that does not lead to the generation of theory—generally provides much less of a contribution, ultimately, than does research that is grounded in or helps generate theory. There will be times when one will see a study published that focuses descriptively on just one particular health problem per se (such as research that looks just at HPV), but that type of research rarely makes the level of contribution to our understanding of health communication processes that theoretically framed research is able to provide. Problem-based research typically illuminates only processes that relate to that health problem, and cannot be generalized to broader health communication concerns. A study, however, that examines a particular health issue, such as HPV, or processes, such as communication about medical mistakes, within the frame of a theory may be generalized to other health issues or processes that also relate to that theory. It makes a much broader contribution. Indeed, Robinson and Agne's (2010) analysis of the most common reasons for rejection of articles submitted to the journal *Health Communication* indicated reviewers' recognition of the importance of theory: lack of a theoretical framework for a study was the most pervasive reason for rejection of research submissions to that journal.

Earlier, we shared with you Reynold's (1971) definition of theory. Put most simply, "theory is a way to talk about what we experience and explain things systematically" (Littlejohn, 2007, p. 2). Note the import of the term "systematically" in this definition—a theory looks at the interrelationships among variables, determinants, and outcomes. Importantly, we did not use the term "prove," as proof suggests closure to further empirical evidence in a manner inconsistent with what social science can typically accomplish. In social science, we provide support for a theory or for hypotheses, rather than definitive proof. Don't be misled by the media's use of the term "prove" in their discussions of research, as they will communicate that "research has proven that . . ." Our goal in social science is to be able to generalize to most people most of the time about the way a certain set of things occurs, under certain conditions. To "prove" something would also require a demonstration that the phenomenon will not change across time, which cannot be determined.

A theory then leads to the generation of hypotheses or research questions under investigation in a particular study. Methods can provide support for or against that theoretical proposition. It is the theory and the hypotheses/research questions that should determine the method that is most appropriate for the investigation of a particular phenomenon.

"Useful" research, in addition to being theory-driven, is based upon a suitable match between hypotheses/research questions and research method. To use a rather obvious example, one cannot do a content analysis of a particular communication medium (e.g., television) in an attempt to test hypotheses about the effect of that content on viewers. It is surprising, however, how frequently researchers will attempt to draw conclusions about media effects based upon a content analysis of a medium.

Another example of a mismatch between theory/hypotheses and methods would be a study of the organizational culture of a hospital that attempts to understand the culture through the sole application of a survey using closed survey questions; your authors have seen such attempts. Actually, culture might be better understood through the use of qualitative methods and the examination of stories, rituals, and metaphors that occur or are used in that particular hospital. Similarly, culture cannot be manipulated and studied in an experiment; it is a set of ideas in which people operate routinely. There is sometimes a perception that more traditional methods such as experiments and surveys are always the appropriate methodological tools simply because of the numbers attached to them, but that is just not the case.

Although the example above looked at the use of more traditionally rigorous methods to address a concept that cannot be easily operationalized quantitatively, the opposite problem also occurs. An article was recently rejected from *Health Communication* based on the following concern from a reviewer: "However, I am not sure if the authors actually used appropriate methods to reflect literature review/research questions. In other words, it would have been an important study if the authors had used more rigorous/concrete methods to test the research questions." In this case, the authors had used a very general (not highly quantitative) coding scheme applied to online support group responses to "test" the Theory of Planned Behavior. This theory is more amenable to quantitative assessment, and has been well operationalized in past research in ways that these researchers could have utilized. Again, we see a mismatch between theory/hypotheses and method.

Interrelationships of Theory and Methods

One informative approach to explore the crucial ways theory and research methods work hand in hand is to consider the very important framework developed by Poole, McPhee, and Canary (2002). They developed their framework to explain interpersonal communication theory and research, but it also applies to health communication research and theory. They characterize a researcher much like a detective in a murder mystery, who tries to understand a complex problem with various devices and strategies. In a sense, both a detective and a health communication researcher are seeking to explain and understand something. These techniques can be called methods. If we use an extremely simplified version of the Poole et al. (2002) framework for the student who is new to research and research methods, we can explore the combined nature of theory and methods and how they might work together.

As we noted above, explanation and understanding are the primary goals of social science. These are what it is hoped theories will do. The methods and techniques employed to collect and analyze the reasons for the theory, then, are called research methods. Poole et al. (2002) suggest four types of theoretical explanation available to the researcher: causal, conventional, narrative, and dialectical.

The four types of theoretical explanations available to a researcher can be loosely described in the following manner. Causal explanations consist of interrelated statements of the form "x causes y, under conditions $C_1 \ldots C_n$," where x and y are variables or constructs identified by the researcher and $C_1 \ldots C_n$ are statements that characterize the conditions for the causal relation to hold. For example, in health communication research, most quantitative investigation that looks at the impact of a health campaign on health outcomes would fall into this category (see, for example, Chang, 2010). This type of approach to the study of health communication has traditionally been the dominant one within the field.

Conventional explanations are based on the assumption that the social world is a product of people discussing, deciding, and acting. Conventional theories consist of demonstrating how people act and react in a manner that is meaningful, understandable, or efficacious in a context where actions are usually taken in a certain way. In health communication research, an example of this would be the work of Robinson (2011), noted earlier, and other CA work. This approach to the study of health communication has not been as dominant within the field as causal research, but is making important contributions to the field. This is particularly true in our understanding of provider–patient interaction.

Narrative explanations of a health communication phenomenon are based on stories people tell, whether those stories appear to be truthful, and whether the elements of the story "fit together." This is a type of process theory where things are explained as a sequence of events that develop and change. Some of the early examples of narrative approaches to health communication process include Sharf's (1990) study of a patient narrative and Cherry and Smith's (1993) examination of the loneliness of men living with HIV/AIDS. With the publication of Harter, Japp, and Beck's (2005) volume, *Narratives, Health, and Healing*, a narrative approach has become more common within the field.

Finally, a dialectical explanation pits variables or forces that clash with each other and must be reconciled for health communication to succeed to some degree. Long seen as important in the study of interpersonal communication, a dialectical approach is now increasingly seen in health communication work. Brann, Himes, Dillow, and Weber's (2010) study of dialectical tensions in stroke survivor relationships would be an example of this approach.

In addition to the four types of explanation just presented, Poole et al. (2002) remind us that, as mentioned above, research methods are generally considered to fall into one of two categories: either quantitative methods or qualitative methods. Quantitative methods include all those research techniques that involve the numerical counting or measurement of things the researcher is interested in studying. Qualitative research methods include all those techniques that do not include numerical measurement. Much more research in health communication is conducted using quantitative methods than qualitative approaches, but qualitative methods are increasingly prominent within the field. Mixed method approaches are also being seen more frequently in recent years. In such studies, both qualitative and quantitative research methods are employed.

These basic distinctions of research methods, when considered in terms of the Poole et al. (2002) framework of four different types of theoretical explanation, help us organize the possibilities for health communication research into eight different forms of research (see Table 1.1).

Although not all eight types of research presented within Table 1.1 might actually be observed in current health communication research, all are

TABLE 1.1 Mixes of Theory: Types of Theoretical Explanation

	Causal	*Conventional*	*Process*	*Dialectical*
Quantitative methods	1	2	3	4
Qualitative methods	5	6	7	8

possibilities that the budding researcher should keep in mind as he or she plans research projects. In many of these types of research, there are some additional research considerations that must be addressed: triangulation, units of analysis, and measurement innovations.

Triangulation—Mixed Methods

Up until this point in our conversation, a reader might assume that any particular study uses only one research method, but that is not indeed the case. Frequently, a research study employs triangulation, or the use of more than one research method to study the same thing. The term "triangulation" is borrowed loosely from trigonometry, where it refers to a method for calculating the distance to a point by looking at it from two other points (Vogt, 1993). The value of triangulation in terms of measurement and methods has long been supported in social science and is becoming increasingly common in health communication research. Triangulation refers to measuring variables in more than one way or addressing hypotheses/research questions using more than one method. The goal is twofold: (a) multiple measures/methods allow more confidence in findings if two or more methods provide consistent results, and (b) different methods allow the examination of different aspects of a process. For instance, Thompson, Robinson, and Kenny's (2004) study of family communication about organ donation decisions combined closed questions that could be statistically correlated among themselves with open-ended questions that were nominally coded to yield insight into the reasons for the closed responses. More recently, scholars have applied mixed methods to such issues as nurse–physician communication (Pirnejad, Niazkhani, van der Sijs, Berg, & Bal, 2009), patient care communication in integrated care settings (Gulmans, Vollenbroek-Hutten, Van Gemert-Pijnen, & Van Harten, 2009), and triadic communication involving adolescents with chronic conditions (van Staa, 2011).

Units of Analysis

The special nature of communication as a phenomenon, as a process involving interaction between multiple entities that generates outcomes both in individual minds and bodies and in broad information environments, suggests that communication researchers routinely face fundamental methodological and conceptual challenges. More specifically, communication theory is typically not limited to a single *unit of analysis* that unifies all studies in this domain. In fact, we might go so far as to suggest that much of our communication theory straddles multiple levels of conceptualization, even if we tend to pursue studies that are operationalized at a single level.

A *unit of analysis* can be conceived as the main entity, typically an object or an event, under investigation in a study (Singleton, Straits, & Straits, 1993). A sample or census that has been marshaled to assess a particular research question is comprised of a group of units. A variable, in turn, theoretically describes a unit of analysis. For example, age is a variable that can describe an individual person; so is body mass index or number of hours spent watching television in the past month. At the same time, we might also consider the extent to which blog posts mentioned H1N1 over a 12-month period, which would suggest potential studies of blogs or months as units. Unfortunately, researchers sometimes ignore the importance of assigning appropriate units of analysis in organizing, analyzing, interpreting, and discussing data. The consequent ambiguity can obscure theoretical innovation and hide what should be glaring absences, such as the lack of whole categories of important explanatory variables.

Consider, for example, the simple concept of awareness, a basic goal for many health campaigns. Might we make a case that awareness of campaign messages is a function of forces at multiple levels of analysis? A quick assessment suggests that we can. If on-going awareness depends on memory for campaign material and for the salience of that memory, there are many different factors that likely shape simple awareness. After all, we know that certain people might be more likely to remember campaign messages because they perceived them to be relevant when first encountering them (which demonstrates how individual-level variables matter), but we also know that the sheer prevalence of campaign materials on television or radio matters (which we might understand as a description of an information environment at various points in time), as do other factors that reside at the level of the campaign content itself (such as editing). Discussion of the content in social networks might even matter (see Southwell, 2005, for empirical evidence related to these points). For all of these reasons, we probably cannot say that health communication researchers interested in campaign awareness can fully understand the concept with studies that only focus on self-reported questionnaires among individual people.

All these circumstances suggest that a book such as this one needs to invite consideration of a wide range of units of analysis, potential for cross-level interaction, and the methodological challenges inherent with such work.

Measurement Innovations

An important lesson emergent from recent decades of health communication research is that the classic survey sometimes does not capture all that is relevant to our understanding of the ways in which visual and verbal content affects health beliefs, perceptions, and behaviors. Behavior itself might be best observed in some circumstances rather than reported. Condom sales or distribution may better indicate condom use than self-reported sexual activity, for example. Moreover, consider attention. Eye-tracking equipment may provide a better indicator of visual attention than does self-reported exposure. On a different plane, a wide literature suggests the importance of emotion in understanding media effects. Again, there are alternatives to self-report measures. Physiological measures such as galvanic skin response do not rely on survey participation per se.

Conclusion

As you move ahead with your study of the various methods that are available to you and your research efforts, you will be able to keep in mind the excitement afforded by this area of study as you ponder the difficult choices among methods we have discussed here. We study health communication because of the inherent value of examining how communicative processes impact and interrelate with health and health care delivery. We have an opportunity to make a significant impact on the quality of life of other people. By paying attention to what might seem like mundane details related to methods, you can help to ensure that future health communication research contributes to collective and individual well-being in productive ways.

References

Boyd, E. A. (1998). Bureaucratic authority in the "company of equals": The interactional management of medical peer review. *American Sociological Review, 63*(2), 200–224.

Brann, M., Himes, K. L., Dillow, M. R., & Weber, K. (2010). Dialectical tensions in stroke survivor relationships. *Health Communication, 25*(4), 323–332.

Chang, C. (2010). The effects of retrieval ease on health issue judgments: Implications for campaign strategies. *Health Communication, 25*(8), 670–680.

Cherry, K. & Smith, D. H. (1993). Sometimes I cry: The experience of loneliness for men with AIDS. *Health Communication, 5*(3), 181–208.

Cho, H., & Salmon, C. T. (2006). Fear appeals for individuals in different stages of change: Intended and unintended effects and implications on health communication campaigns. *Health Communication, 20*(1), 91–99.

Coleman, J. S., Katz, E., & Menzel, H. (1966). *Medical innovation: A diffusion study*. Indianapolis, IN: Bobbs-Merrill Co.

Dearing, J. W., Gaglio, B., & Rabin, B. A. (2011). Community organizing research approaches. In T. L. Thompson, R. Parrott, & J. F. Nussbaum (Eds.), *Routledge handbook of health communication* (2nd ed.) (pp. 546–559). New York, NY: Routledge.

Du Pré, A., & Crandall, S. J. (2011). Qualitative methods: Bridging the gap between research and daily practice. In T. L. Thompson, R. Parrott, & J. F. Nussbaum (Eds.), *Routledge handbook of health communication* (2nd ed.) (pp. 532–545). New York, NY: Routledge.

Edgar, T., Volkman, J. E., & Logan, A. M. B. (2011). Social marketing: Its meaning, use, and application for health communication. In T. L. Thompson, R. Parrott, & J. F. Nussbaum (Eds.), *Routledge handbook of health communication* (2nd ed.) (pp. 235–251). New York, NY: Routledge.

Gulmans, J., Vollenbroek-Hutten, M. M., Van Gemert-Pijnen, J. E., & Van Harten, W. H. (2009). Evaluating patient care communication in integrated care settings: Application of a mixed method approach in cerebral palsy programs. *International Journal for Quality in Health Care, 21*(1), 58–65.

Gustafson, D. L. (2005). Transcultural nursing from a critical cultural perspective. *Advances in Nursing Science, 28*(1), 2–16.

Guttman, N. (2003). Ethics in health communication interventions. In T. L. Thompson, A. Dorsey, K. I. Miller, & R. Parrott (Eds.) *Handbook of health communication* (pp. 651–680). Mahwah, NJ: Lawrence Erlbaum Associates.

Guttman, N. (2011). Ethics in communication for health promotion in clinical settings and campaigns. In T. L. Thompson, R. Parrott, & J. F. Nussbaum (Eds.), *Routledge handbook of health communication* (2nd ed.) (pp. 632–646). New York, NY: Routledge.

Guttman, N., & Thompson, T. L. (2010). Ethics in health communication. In G. Cheney, S. May, & D. Munshi (Eds.) *Handbook of communication ethics* (pp. 293–308). New York, NY: Routledge.

Harter, L. M., Japp, P. M., & Beck, C. S. (2005). *Narratives, health, and healing: Communication theory, research, and practice.* Mahwah, NJ: Lawrence Erlbaum Associates.

Kaplan, A. (1964). *The conduct of inquiry: Methodology for behavioral science.* San Francisco, CA: Chandler Pub. Co.

Korsch, B. M., Gozzi, E. K., & Francis, V. (1968). Gaps in doctor–patient communication. 1. Doctor–patient interaction and patient satisfaction. *Pediatrics, 42*(5), 855–871.

Littlejohn, S. W. (2007). The nature and evaluation of theory. In B. B. Whaley & W. Samter (Eds.), *Explaining communication: Contemporary theories and exemplars* (pp. 1–14). Mahwah, NJ: Lawrence Erlbaum Associates.

Madge, J. (1965). *The tools of social science.* Garden City, NY: Anchor Books.

Pirnejad, H., Niazkhani, Z., van der Sijs, H., Berg, M., & Bal, R. A. (2009). Evaluation of the impact of a CPOE system on nurse–physician communication—a mixed method study. *Methods of Information in Medicine, 48*(4), 350–360.

Poole, M. S., McPhee, R., & Canary, D. (2002). Hypothesis testing and modeling perspectives on inquiry. In M. L. Knapp & J. A. Daly (Eds.) *Handbook of interpersonal communication* (pp. 23–72). Thousand Oaks, CA: Sage Publications.

Reynolds, P. D. (1971). *A primer in theory construction.* New York, NY: Macmillan.

Robinson, J. D. (2011). Conversation analysis and health communication. In T. L. Thompson, R. Parrott, & J. F. Nussbaum (Eds.), *Routledge handbook of health communication* (2nd ed.) (pp. 501–518). New York, NY: Routledge.

Robinson, J. D., & Agne, R. R. (2010). Kindness, gentility, and rejection: An analysis of 99 manuscript reviews. *Health Communication, 25*(6–7), 504–511.

Robinson, J. D., Raup-Krieger, J. L., Burke, G., Weber, V., & Oesterling, B. (2008). The relative influence of patients' pre-visit global satisfaction with medical care on patients' post-visit satisfaction with physicians' communication. *Communication Research Reports, 25*(1), 1–9.

Roter, D., & McNeilis, K. S. (2003). The nature of the therapeutic relationship and the assessment of its discourse in routine medical visits. In T. L. Thompson, A. Dorsey, K. I. Miller, & R. Parrott (Eds.) *Handbook of health communication* (pp. 121–140). Mahwah, NJ: Lawrence Erlbaum Associates.

Salmon, C. T., & Cho, H. (2007). Unintended effects of health communication campaigns. *Journal of Communication, 57*(2), 293–317.

Sharf, B. F. (1990). Physician–patient communication as interpersonal rhetoric: A narrative approach. *Health Communication, 2*(4), 217–231.

Singleton, R., Straits, B. C., & Straits, M. M. (1993). *Approaches to social research* (2nd ed.). New York, NY: Oxford University Press.

Southwell, B. G. (2005). Between messages and people: A multilevel model of memory for television content. *Communication Research, 32*(1), 112–140.

Southwell, B. G., & Yzer, M. C. (2007). The roles of interpersonal communication in mass media campaigns. In C. Beck (Ed.), *Communication Yearbook 31* (pp. 420–462). New York, NY: Lawrence Erlbaum Associates.

Stivers, T. (2007). Prescribing under pressure: Parent–physician conversations and antibiotics. Oxford, England: Oxford University Press.

Thompson, T. L. (2011). Hope and the act of informed dialogue: A delicate balance at end of life. *Journal of Language and Social Psychology, 30*(2), 177–192.

Thompson, T. L., Robinson, J. D., & Kenny, R. W. (2004). Family conversations about organ donation. *Progress in Transplantation, 14*(1), 49–55.

Valente, T. W. (2011). Social networks and health communication. In T. L. Thompson, R. Parrott, & J. F. Nussbaum (Eds.), *Routledge handbook of health communication* (2nd ed.) (pp. 519–531). New York, NY: Routledge.

van Staa, A. (2011). Unraveling triadic communication in hospital consultations with adolescents with chronic conditions: The added value of mixed methods research. *Patient Education and Counseling, 82*(3), 455–464.

Vogt, W. P. (1993). *Dictionary of statistics and methodology: A nontechnical guide for the social sciences*. Newbury Park, CA: Sage Publications.

Exploration and Description

"TELL ME ABOUT A TIME WHEN . . ."

Studying Health Communication Through In-Depth Interviews

Erin E. Donovan, Laura E. Miller, and Daena J. Goldsmith

The Nature of Interviews in Health Communication Research

As a communicative act, the interview is a cornerstone of health and medicine. Anyone who has received or provided healthcare has participated in conversations during which important information is exchanged between patient and health professional. Part art, part clinical science, a skillful medical interview reflects the collaboration that is essential to a successful therapeutic relationship, and underscores the fundamental humanity of health and illness (Lichstein, 1990). Clinicians recognize that learning a patient's history is frequently more valuable than physical examinations or "objective" laboratory tests alone (Rich, Crowson, & Harris, 1987). Healing is greatly aided by drawing out and listening to patients' concerns.

Health communication researchers do not conduct interviews to diagnose or remedy individual patient complaints. Yet, by engaging in the interpersonal and analytical processes of interviewing, autobiographical information that answers important questions and that provides a means of improving how people orient toward their health and healthcare is garnered. Interviews capture the voices of participants and go on to tell their stories, creating detailed renderings of what they have lived and what they know. Through the interview process, researchers hear and learn what it is to be healthy, ill, and somewhere in between. Interviewers get to know what it is like to be a patient, survivor, healthcare provider, family caregiver, administrator, or policymaker—all in the distinctive words of the people who have occupied those roles.

Sizable and diverse bodies of literature have flourished over the past few decades as interviews have become an increasingly common method of collecting health-related data (Al-Busaidi, 2008; Liamputtong & Ezzy, 2005). Through interviews, health communication researchers gather depictions of how low-income women perceive messages about cancer prevention (Marshall, Smith, & McKeon, 1995), young people's accounts of what it is like to abstain from alcohol (Romo, 2012) and cancer survivors' reports of the questions that still plague them even after finishing treatment (Miller, 2012). Researchers get a sense of how communication is helpful (or not) for people who are awaiting heart transplants (Scott, Martin, Stone, & Brashers, 2011) and better understand the functions and challenges of medical interpreters (Hsieh & Kramer, 2012), as well as the management of chronic illness and identity challenges therein (Charmaz, 1991; Miller & Caughlin, 2013).

Research interviews have been compared to the process of having "a good conversation" (Liamputtong & Ezzy, 2005, p. 55). In the current chapter, an analysis of what constitutes a good conversation in the context of health communication research is offered. The theoretical underpinnings of interview methodologies and their implications for studying messages about health are discussed. The chapter includes a description of some attributes of research problems for which interviews are an appropriate methodological choice. After providing an overview of some procedural considerations, several of the primary strengths, limitations, and challenges of this type of research strategy are articulated. Throughout the chapter, lessons that we have learned when conducting our research and engaging with others' work are shared. A description of con-temporary scholarship exemplars that, with the help of good interviews, have contributed to health communication theory and practice with findings that may have gone otherwise undetected is provided. There are many resources on the nuts and bolts of how to interview effectively (e.g., McCracken, 1988; Taylor & Bogdan, 1998; Weiss, 1994); our focus will be on the larger rationale for choosing to do interviews and on some of the broad considerations in designing and evaluating studies that utilize interviews.

In this chapter, one style of interviewing in particular that has proven useful for health communication researchers—namely, in-depth interviews—will be the focus. Sometimes also referred to as depth, intensive, or qualitative interviews, in-depth interviews are designed to elicit participants' experiences, perceptions, and narratives in their own words (Noller & Feeney, 2004). Some quantitative studies rely on structured interviews to generate text that can be content analyzed into categories and subjected to various kinds of statistical analyses. In contrast, our focus is on the use of interviews as grist for interpretive analyses. Rather than being concerned with how often categories occur, the researcher is concerned with developing models of what and how participants think, feel, and experience. This form of interview also differs from orally administered surveys or highly structured interviews in its commitment to privileging the participant's meanings and views over an a priori agenda. These are conversations between researchers and participants, steered by open-ended questions that range from loose topical guides to semi-structured protocols from which interviewers may regularly deviate as they follow respondents' trains of thought.

Theoretical Assumptions

Interviewing is a flexible method that can be employed in diverse ways toward diverse ends, from post-positivist to postmodern approaches. Among health communication researchers who utilize interviews, studies have been undertaken from the perspective of narrative theory, grounded theory, phenomenology, ethnography, critical theory (including feminist and queer theory), and autoethnography. These broader methodological commitments shape the types of research questions one pursues as well as many particulars of the interview itself (e.g., how structured a protocol is, what role the interviewer plays, whether and how interviews are recorded, whether interviews are one-time encounters or part of an ongoing relationship). One's interpretive paradigm also suggests analytic strategies and norms for presentation of results. Denzin and Lincoln's (2008) observations about qualitative inquiry apply to researchers using interviews in health communication: Multiple paradigms inform our work and meta-theoretical perspectives continue to develop. Nonetheless, those who interview tend to share a desire to "seek answers to questions that stress how social experience is created and given meaning" (Denzin & Lincoln, 2008, p. 14).

This desire to understand participant experience and meaning is embedded in several broader intellectual currents. We have become an interview society (Silverman, 1997) in which interviews are a common feature of everyday life and public discourse. Individuals are "accepted as significant commentators on their own experience," and are presumed to have "significant views and feelings about life that are accessible to others who undertake to ask about them" (Gubrium & Holstein, 2002, p. 5). In the past 50 years, scholars across disciplines have turned to interviews for thick descriptions (Geertz, 1973) of the meanings and context of action, and for narratives that reveal experience and enact identity. These interpretive and narrative turns across the disciplines coincided with increased attention in health-related fields to patient experience and socio-cultural influences on beliefs and action. Health researchers recognized that health and illness are not merely matters of physiology, but are socially constructed through cultures, communities, and conversations (Kleinman, 1988). The stories we tell about health and illness were identified as sites where doctor–patient relationships (Mishler, 1984) and individual identities (Frank, 1995) were enacted.

Interviews are guided conversations, not interrogations (Lofland & Lofland, 1995). The analogy to conversation suggests several epistemological commitments that underlie practical decisions such as how much interviewees are allowed to guide the direction of the interview or when and to what extent researcher's own experiences are reciprocally disclosed. Although researchers who interview vary considerably in their philosophical commitments, those who use interviews are inclined to recognize that the interview is both a source of information about health communication phenomena in the participants' life worlds but also an instance of communication in its own right, shaped by the particularities of the interviewer, the interviewee, the context for their interaction, and so on. Thus, an *interview about* health communication is also an *instance of* health communication.

When thoughtfully designed, skillfully executed, and reflexively monitored, interviews are an excellent method for finding out how our participants interpret, choose, and evaluate messages and actions related to health. As Vanderford, Jenks, and Sharf (1997) have observed, if we conceptualize patients as active agents in their own health care, interviews are especially useful for revealing how they process health information, reconcile conflicting recommendations, and interpret their participation. If we wish to humanize healthcare providers, interviews can give insight into how they negotiate professional identity, respond to ethical dilemmas, and coordinate team work. If we believe that private interactions with friends and family impact health, then interviews provide accounts of otherwise difficult-to-access private interactions. Interviews are a central part of the audience reception tradition, shedding light on how people interpret health information—in news media, in public health campaigns, and in entertainment.

An assumption of this chapter and of many in-depth interview studies is that "reality can be interpreted in various ways and the understanding is dependent on subjective interpretation" (Graneheim & Lundman, 2004, p. 106). In the style of interviewing we are discussing here, the researcher has an open mind, though not an empty mind (Janesick, 2000). The researcher brings to the interview an interest in particular topics or aspects of participant experience, informed by his or her reading of previous research and theory; however, he or she remains open to seeing phenomena in new ways and allowing the research to proceed in unexpected directions.

Applications

As the theoretical assumptions just outlined suggest, interviews are a productive means of understanding what people think about health and illness as social processes. Health communication research presents many questions about human interaction and interpretation, and the answers to such questions may be useful in improving healthcare policy and patient care. In-depth interviewing allows researchers to access points of view from the patients, professionals, and families affected. Interviews are an excellent choice when one's goal is to achieve deep and detailed data. These data are made possible, in part, by interviewers' opportunities to further probe for clarification and greater depth. According to Baxter and Babbie (2004):

> [I]nterviews are especially appropriate when the researcher wants to understand in a richly detailed manner what an interviewee thinks and feels about some phenomenon. Although thoughts and feelings can be assessed through structured questionnaires and surveys, survey research limits individuals' responses to a selection of a number or a phrase as defined by the researcher.
>
> *(p. 326)*

For example, a survey instrument could reveal important patterns in patients' reasons for medication non-adherence. However, in order to design a useful questionnaire, the researchers would need a relatively comprehensive understanding of the possible reasons. In-depth interviews enable researchers to explain their own reasons for their non-adherence behavior, and well-designed questions would limit the extent to which respondents are constrained by researchers' pre-existing knowledge or led by demand characteristics.

The aim of health communication studies is often to develop and elaborate on concepts and social phenomena, emphasizing the meanings, experiences, and views of the participants. In-depth interviews are a natural fit for exploratory projects. They are particularly well suited for determining the meanings people place on the events, processes, and perceptions of their lives. Health communication scholars may utilize in-depth interviewing to determine specific nuances in various illness contexts. For instance, determining the most salient aspects of an illness experience is a common application of in-depth interviews (du Pré & Crandall, 2011). Participants can speak candidly about personal concerns (e.g., losing autonomy) that may go unacknowledged or unexplored in medical interviews or patient intake surveys. With interview data, researchers can learn about individual cognitions and emotions that are as complex as the biomedical conditions that engender them—identifying the tensions, dilemmas, and ambivalence in people's narratives. We can note what people say, how they say it, what they leave out, and the ostensible reasons for the omissions (Charmaz, 2006).

In-depth interviews are one of the best methods for investigating health communication processes that are not readily observable in other ways. For example, it is challenging to witness private conversations about or experiences with relatively invisible health conditions such as infertility (Bute, 2009) or parental mental illness (Oskouie, Zeighami, & Joolaee, 2011). In addition, like other self-report techniques, interviews allow researchers to study subjective phenomena about which only the participants have access (Clark & Reis, 1988)—including the meanings that people ascribe to each other's communication about health, illness, and lifestyle choices (Goldsmith, Lindholm, & Bute, 2006). Just as physicians must rely on patients' own descriptions of discomfort and quality of life, we depend on people's accounts of events, attitudes, and beliefs.

Interviews are also occasions for performing health narratives and identities (Frank, 1995; Sharf, Harter, Yamasaki, & Haidet, 2011). Narrative is an activity that people employ to help them make sense of their worlds, especially to organize the unexpected (Eggly, 2002); it is "the human way of dealing with disruption" (Leeman, 2011, p. 108). Through their responses to interview questions, participants can construct narratives that are comprehensible representations of their experiences. These narratives not only result in rich data that can be analyzed in their own right, they are socio-cognitive events during which people arrive at better understandings of their own health and illness, and enact identities that have been influenced by the state of their health (Sharf et al., 2011). They create a space in which participants co-construct meaning, perform identity, and weave stories. As such, interviews are not only a window into other phenomena that occur outside the interview, they sometimes constitute the phenomenon we wish to study.

Employing Interviews in Health Communication Research

Procedures

Sampling

Interview studies of health communication are often iterative in nature, as scholars engage in sequences of concurrent sampling, interviewing, analyzing, and theorizing (Strauss & Corbin, 1990). When sampling, interviewers make ongoing determinations about whose point of view matters: Who knows about the process you wish to understand? Quality interviews depend on knowledgeable respondents. Purposive (or theoretical) sampling is often employed by interviewers who wish to selectively recruit individuals who have a specialized understanding or experience of the subject (Mays & Pope, 1995). It is also a strategy for including negative cases (Taylor & Bogdan, 1998), which involves speaking with people who may illuminate exceptions to the themes embedded in the majority of key informants' descriptions.

In identifying potential respondents, it is worthwhile to think through the various stakeholders in the medical hierarchy and in the world of the healthcare consumer—who they are, with whom they interact, and where their communication occurs. In some studies, the value lies in delving deeply into one person's perspective. In other work, divergent or complementary perspectives may be revealed via interviewing multiple members of a family or healthcare organization. For example, Daena (third author of the present chapter) has found that, in some couples, one partner's perception that their communication about cancer is entirely open and unconstrained is sustained by the other partner's skillful withholding and protective buffering (Goldsmith & Domann-Scholz, 2013).

Questions

Interviewers are responsible for making the most of their opportunity to speak with key informants. Physicians' interviews of patients are likely to be most productive when they exert as little control over the medical encounter as possible, while still encouraging the patient to stay on topic (Lichstein, 1990). In a similar vein, research interviews tend to be successful when they are active and structured enough to keep informants focused, but give people plenty of leeway and emphasize that, as participants, they are the experts. Charmaz (2006) and others recommend prompts that are broad, open ended, and encourage narrative, such as, "Tell me the story of how you became a patient advocate."

Interview questions may or may not be the same for every participant; it is advantageous to strike a balance between consistency and flexibility. It makes sense to ask many participants about the same topics so that responses can be compared and contrasted and themes can emerge. Pilot interviews can help with refining research questions and revising the interview protocol (e.g., see Kosenko, 2010). As the study progresses and preliminary observations are made, it may be useful to add and change interview questions in order to develop theoretical hunches and allow the focus of the project and the findings to evolve (Corbin & Strauss, 1990). In general, interviews may last from approximately one hour to several hours, and are likely to be on the longer side if they are conducted in tandem with field observations. Erin (first author of the present chapter) has found it useful to follow up with interviewees for elaboration and confirmation of theoretical development (Donovan-Kicken, Tollison, & Goins, 2011).

Focus groups

Semi-structured interviews can occur as one-on-one conversations between researcher and key informant, and in focus groups of individuals who share a common characteristic, such as a type of illness, a genetic risk factor, or a caregiving role. Focus groups are expedient ways to collect responses from a variety of people, and they can be beneficial instances of small-group health communication in which participants generate discussion among themselves, respond to each other's ideas, and share anecdotes, while simultaneously producing interaction data (Baxter & Babbie, 2004; Brashers et al., 1999). Generally speaking, a good target for focus group interviews is four to five focus groups of six to eight participants each (Kitzinger, 1994). This size is small enough so that each member of the group can contribute regularly and meaningfully, but not so small that people are likely to feel put on the spot during frequent lulls in conversation.

The interview session

One-on-one interviews often follow a recognizable, sequential structure. Building rapport during the early stages of an interview can open the door for a successful interview. As the interview progresses, the researcher should begin with easy, nonthreatening questions, leaving the most difficult questions and probes until rapport has been built (Ulin, Robinson, & Tolley, 2005). It is wise to embed the meatiest questions in the middle of the session, so that interviewees gain confidence with the easy early questions and then wind down into more relaxed questions again. Toward the end of the interview, researchers are encouraged to present grand, imaginative thought exercises: "What advice would you give to people who are starting new jobs as emergency department nurses?"; "If you were put in charge of designing a new rehab program, and had an unlimited budget, what would you do?"

To invoke the medical analogy again, it is common for patients not to mention serious concerns until late in an appointment (a so-called "doorknob question"; White, Levinson, & Roter, 1994). Physicians can glean crucial information by simply asking, "Is there anything else you wanted to discuss today?" when they are still seated and attentive. Researchers can gather some remarkably worthwhile responses with a similar prompt. When closing the interview, researchers should express their gratitude for the participant's time and reiterate confidentiality. Casual conversation often continues after the formal interview has ended, in order to answer participants' questions and to conclude the session on a positive note (Bowling, 2009). It is useful to exchange contact information so that follow-up ideas and updates can be communicated.

Interviewers benefit from training in an array of interpersonal skills, such as listening. Charmaz (1991, p. 275) described this salient skill: "As a researcher, I sought to have people tell me about their lives from their perspectives rather than to force my preconceived interests and categories upon them. So I listened." As such, providing an encouraging and listening ear to participants can heighten comfort levels and facilitate participant disclosure. Interviewers should also be trained to properly handle sensitive questioning (e.g., the financial burdens and psychological effects of diabetes). When sensitive questioning is required, the researcher may need to be trained on how to minimize the emotional impact of the questions and how to respond if a participant becomes visibly upset. For example, acknowledging the sensitivity of the topic can help to soften participants' anxiety (e.g., "I know this is a hard thing to discuss—I really appreciate your sharing," Ulin et al., 2005, p. 87).

Working with data

A whole series of steps occur after conversations have ended, as researchers turn their attention to deriving insights from their data. There are many different types of analysis. Deciding what to do with one's data depends on the purpose of the study and the theoretical framework guiding it, but, in essence, researchers add analytic value while respecting participants' voices. We seek to identify what it is in a particular experience that may have some broader resonance or heuristic power. Sometimes this value might be a taxonomy of categories or a model of concepts and processes; sometimes, it might be evoking appreciation for human values, witnessing suffering, or drawing attention to a structure or performance that embodies some larger principle. In this section, some of the conventions to which health communication scholars tend to adhere are reviewed.

As discussed, analysis is often ongoing with interviews. Immersing oneself in transcripts influences one's choices about the evolution of the interview protocol and informs one's choices about probing and sampling (Charmaz, 1995). A benchmark of interview studies is when a researcher believes he or she has reached saturation (Glaser & Strauss, 1967). This is the point at which virtually no new information is being collected during interviews; instead, themes are being repeated continuously, and conceptual categories and their interrelationships are confirmed multiple times. Negative cases have been included and accounted for within the emerging explanatory structure. At this time, researchers will typically stop conducting interviews, at least temporarily. In our estimation, in the majority of interview studies published in journals dedicated to health communication and allied fields, authors tend to deem that theoretical saturation has occurred after 20 to 40 participants, which is reflected in their sample sizes.

Analyzing interview data is labor intensive, and a detailed tutorial is beyond the scope of this chapter. Fortunately, numerous guides exist for making the most of participants' stories (e.g., McCracken, 1988; Lincoln & Guba, 1985). Many health communication scholars today rely on Strauss and Corbin's (1990) explication of grounded theory methodology, which offers directions for different levels of coding and suggestions for interacting with data in order to distill them into theoretical abstractions. More recently, Charmaz (2006) has written about employing grounded theory techniques in a style that is highly accessible and more social constructivist in nature. Although not specific to health communication scholarship, Riessman (2007) provides an excellent introduction to narrative methods (see also Yamasaki, Sharf, & Harter, this volume, for narrative methods in health communication research).

It is worth mentioning two other types of resources on which interviewers draw when analyzing their data. First, there are collaborators. Thematic analysis and theory development need not be solitary pursuits. Partnering during data analysis can assist with organizing data, corroborating and challenging observations, and selecting exemplars. Quite a bit of health communication research is interdisciplinary, and some communication scholars find it beneficial to build teams that include colleagues from medicine, nursing, and public health (e.g., Wittenberg-Lyles, Goldsmith, Ragan, & Sanchez-Reilly, 2010). Observations from individuals from different specialties may complement each other in important ways. Second, there is technology. Depending on the size and complexity of one's data set, and the utility of visually representing how codes occur, it may be advisable to use qualitative data analysis software, such as Atlas or NVivo. These are generally viewed as organizational tools, and are not a substitute for researchers' own intense involvement with their data or coding of themes.

Ultimately, the interview process is less about "finding results" and more about engaging in sense making, observing positioning, identifying tensions and contradictions in respondents' narratives, and examining how people talk about their lives. It should be emphasized that experienced analysts can draw from various analytic techniques in flexible ways. Even the aforementioned scholars who have codified analytic systems more than anyone else acknowledge that these procedures are not dogma to be slavishly followed, but tools to be used thoughtfully in order to generate knowledge.

Reliability and Validity

Because in-depth interviews can be utilized within multiple paradigms of knowledge, there is variability in how researchers establish reliability and validity and to what extent they agree that these are relevant criteria. For example, some have suggested that qualitative research be assessed by credibility, dependability, confirmability, and transferability instead (Baxter & Babbie, 2002; Lincoln & Guba, 1985). Nonetheless, there are some considerations that are likely to be shared as a means of ensuring excellent scholarship.

The contribution that a study makes is inextricably linked to the quality of the interview responses that a researcher elicits (Charmaz, 2006). Findings from interview studies are given shape in the researcher's mind, but, fundamentally, they emerge from the data themselves. Therefore, one of the most decisive aspects of validity involves demonstrating to reviewers and readers that the conclusions that one has drawn are supported by respondents' words. There is a purpose and virtue behind including participants' direct quotations: "[I]t creates verisimilitude, statements that produce for the readers the feeling that they have experienced, or could experience, the events being described in a study" (Creswell & Miller, 2000, p. 128).

Achieving this level of verisimilitude depends on preparation, creative insight, and a systematic, documentable approach to data collection and analysis (Patton, 1999). The coinciding processes of sampling, reviewing literature, and returning to the interview transcripts constitute the work that helps researchers to identify meaningful patterns, themes, and structures. Standard practices for establishing data credibility include member checking (consulting with members of the sample or population on the veracity of findings), negative case analysis (evaluating exceptions to conclusions), and peer debriefing (having a knowledgeable but dispassionate colleague review the data to check for selective perception; Baxter & Eyles, 1997; Lindlof & Taylor, 2002; Patton, 1999).

On the other hand, Barbour (2001) has warned against reducing rigor in interview (and other qualitative) studies to a mere checklist of tasks. She noted that researchers ought not to feel satisfied simply because they have conducted perfunctory inspections of their data and managed to come up with a tidy descriptive list of themes. Rather, they should embrace the competing viewpoints expressed by respondents for the analytical potential that they offer. Many theorists who rely on interviews contend that what matters most is to demonstrate that one's findings and conclusions are indeed substantiated by the data themselves—that validity means trusting in what truly emerges (Glaser & Strauss, 1967).

As an additional measure of ensuring validity, an interviewer is encouraged to take a reflexive approach to his or her work and contemplate and disclose how her role as the researcher may be influencing the findings (Alvesson & Sköldberg, 2009; Suddaby, 2006). As Patton (1999) put it: "Because the researcher is the instrument in qualitative inquiry, a qualitative report must include information about the researcher" (p. 1198). For example, what skills, special insights, or unique characteristics does the researcher bring to the project? How does his or her own health history, and, perhaps, any outwardly visible elements of it, situate her as a participant in the interview conversation? Scholars have differing positions about the extent to which it is appropriate or even possible to begin a study from a tabula rasa perspective. It makes sense to reflect on one's positioning in relation to the phenomena and participants, whether that be to minimize "bias" in hearing others' experiences or to embrace one's role as a source of understanding and opportunity in the co-constructed process of interpretation.

Strengths and Limitations of Method

Strengths

The topic of validity relates directly to a prominent strength of interviews: Because interviewing is a malleable process, it confers the specific advantage of enabling researchers to make adjustments by observing how questions resonate with participants. With in-person interviews, there are no forced choice survey items, and, rather than simply checking a box labeled "n/a," participants can steer the conversation in directions that allow them to tell the stories that matter to them. If interview questions do not have face validity, so to speak, then candid respondents are likely to redirect the focus of the conversation on the truths that matter to them. Researchers also have the opportunity to observe when respondents interpret their questions in unexpected ways. As such, a recalibration and clarification of what we meant can occur.

An illustration: Erin (first author of the present chapter) began one study of communication about cancer by asking survivors to describe the mainstream resources that they had consulted about interpersonal health communication behaviors—for example, whether certain books or websites offered helpful suggestions for navigating difficult conversations with family members about their cancer. This line of questioning fell flat. Participants in her study had not been purposefully seeking or receiving advice about communication; any resources for this were not on their radar. After the same series of questions garnered confused silences multiple times, she altered her approach by encouraging participants to describe any questions they had about how to talk to people about their cancer. From there, she and her collaborators were able to draw out ideas for how to create their own guide to talking with loved ones about cancer and how to make it available to survivors (Donovan-Kicken, Tollison, & Goins, 2012). Rather than identifying resources that they had used, participants repeatedly expressed the opinion that "No one asked us if we needed advice about how to deal with people, but, yes, that would have been helpful."

The authors have also witnessed how interviews draw out some complexities of health communication that we would not have thought to study or ask about, were it not for participants' earnest narratives and surprising comments. The theories with which researchers work focus their sights on particular phenomena and connections among them. Interviews give people a chance to dialogue about how health is punctuated and is situated among other meaningful marks in a person's life and illness trajectories. With interviews, investigators can follow unexpected leads and report on the creativity that people display in their health communication strategies—behaviors and broader theoretical principles that they might not have thought to include in survey or experimental designs. Unusual cases might be overlooked in a survey interview designed to generalize; however, an interview may be able to uncover from the rare or unusual case a set of broader principles or possibilities that are nonetheless instructive.

When interview questions are tapping into meaningful experiences, they yield evocative and illustrative data from participants. A second strength of the interview method, then, is the vibrant accounts and direct quotations that humanize the findings of one's study. Interview studies are a joy to read (and review) when they incorporate memorable moments from informants' accounts. Brashers and colleagues' (1999) study of persons living with HIV revealed the tensions that people experienced when their health improved with new treatment options, and what had once seemed like an imminent death from AIDS now seemed to have abated. Participants' comments reflected the powerful uncertainties of their new circumstances (e.g., "Do you buy green bananas?"; p. 209). Erin (present chapter) will never forget one participant from a study she conducted with Jennifer Bute and Nicole Martins (Bute, Donovan-Kicken, & Martins, 2007) who, in reflecting upon her mother's life with dementia, assessed her mother's behavior by saying, "I think she thinks she lives in a restaurant." It is difficult to imagine such a unique and personal sentiment being borne out of a different methodology.

Because they are typically designed to feel like pleasant, non-threatening conversations, a third advantage of in-depth interview methods is that they may put participants at ease in ways that other data collection techniques might not. Some potential respondents (e.g., those low in health literacy or struggling with cognitive impairments) may not feel confident in their ability to write down answers to survey items, but can relax into the familiar (if, admittedly, contrived) rhythm of having a chat with a new acquaintance. Interviews may accompany questionnaires, which gives researchers the opportunity to develop rapport and to clarify participants' answers to scaled items. These sorts of relationship-building strategies may aid in the participation of individuals with relatively low education, literacy, and/or income (Bute & Jensen, 2010), particularly if the interview team actively partners with community members to develop interview materials, recruit participants, and conduct interviews.

Fourth, the interview process can be a rewarding and cathartic experience for participants, which is, in turn, gratifying for researchers alike. Scholars like Karp (1996) have noted how interview participants often express appreciation for the opportunity to share their stories. Interviews can help people make sense of their lives (Liamputtong & Ezzy, 2005). Individuals who are coping with the frustrations of managing health may appreciate the release that comes with discussing topics that they have not been invited to talk about before. Furthermore, participants may bring up sentiments that they have been reticent to discuss with even close relational partners, for fear of upsetting them. In one of Daena's interviews, a participant revealed that she had secretly made a tape recording of advice to her then teenaged son about all the things she would want to be able to tell him as he grew up—"marriage and babies and stuff like that"—so that, if her cancer proved terminal, he could still hear her voice as he went through milestones in his life. She had not told anyone about the tape, but it was meaningful to her; a way to cope with her fear of death and her intense sadness when she contemplated the possibility of leaving her son and husband behind. Even if interviews can be intimidating due to the sensitive nature of health-related topics, it is worth noting that at least some participants welcome the opportunity to open up.

Although we certainly do not advocate that researchers misrepresent themselves as therapists, we have recognized in our own work that participants often convey an appreciation for the opportunity to tell their stories to a captive, unbiased listener. In Laura's (second author of the present chapter) research on cancer survivorship, some participants mentioned that they were glad to have the opportunity to talk about issues that they may not have felt comfortable getting into otherwise (Miller, 2013). One participant said that the interview was the most she had ever talked about her cancer experience with anyone. Eliciting and caring about people's stories has a strong ethical dimension. Frank (1995) observed what is at stake:

> As wounded, people may be cared for, but, as storytellers, they care for others. The ill, and all those who suffer, can also be healers . . . Through their stories, the ill create empathic bonds between themselves and their listener. These bonds expand as the stories are retold. Those who listened then tell others, and the circle of shared experience widens.
>
> *(p. xii)*

This form of research participation also lets people contribute in unique ways. Interviews are by no means the only type of research design that can satisfy participants' desire to "pay it forward" by imparting hard-earned wisdom so that others can learn from their experiences. However, there does seem to be something special about the one-on-one session with its open-ended questions. Erin (present chapter) recalls one breast cancer survivor who was pleased to have a chance to "get up on her soapbox" to describe her satisfaction with the alternative and complementary treatment approaches that she pursued in lieu of traditional lumpectomy and radiation. Successful interviews open up a safe repository for participants' descriptions of their bodies and their journeys through illness.

When informants have discussions in a group setting, researchers can accumulate numerous accounts in a relatively short amount of time. It is possible to view how members of a sample interact with each other and serve as mutual springboards for ideas. Focus groups are also naturalistic occurrences of health communication. The group dynamic adds an important meta-communicative layer of information, as respondents talk to each other about the experiences they have had engaging with other people about their health. When working with cancer survivors (e.g., Donovan-Kicken et al., 2012), Erin (present chapter) has noticed that focus groups may spontaneously exhibit qualities of support group meetings, as participants swap experiences, validate each other's decisions, ask for advice, and even trade phone numbers so that they can stay in touch afterward.

Limitations

While it is true that some participants may prefer to be interviewed rather than complete a written or online questionnaire, certain drawbacks to interviews must be weighed. Interviewers are unlikely to hear from people who are not comfortable being interviewed, and this self-selection bias has implications for theory and practice. Individuals who volunteer for face-to-face interviews about sensitive health topics such as sexuality, for example, may be more knowledgeable about the topic and more self-confident in general (Catania, McDermott, & Pollack,

1986). People may be more likely to take part in interviews if they reject the stigma associated with their health condition, or if they are less physically debilitated than others with the same diagnosis.

Interviews are self-reports, and some scholars have argued that research has veered too much toward privileging what people say about what they do, in lieu of observing true behavioral practices. As Weiss (1994) noted, "The vagaries of respondent memory make for reports in which some observations are crystal clear while others are obscured or distorted or blocked. Respondents also may shade their responses to present a positive picture of themselves" (p. 149). Recall effects cannot be ruled out. A patient whose cancer battle has lasted four years may not be able to accurately recall the specifics of being diagnosed. Participants may reveal inconsistent information as the interview progresses. As Goldsmith, Miller, and Caughlin (2008) noted, "couples may say that 'we talk about everything (or we could)' but then describe reasons why they actively avoid some topics" (p. 93).

Whether some of those characteristics of interviews are strengths or limitations depends upon one's epistemology and research questions—sometimes, self-presentation and sense making are the object of inquiry, and, other times, participants' recall and interpretation of their experience are as influential as the "facts" of that experience. Researchers need to be clear that an interview is always an account given in a particular context, and this should condition claims made from interview data. The way a participant remembers experiencing a health event is meaningful, even if it is not a perfect rendering of what "actually" happened. Rather than viewing participants' contradictions as a fatal flaw of a study, it behooves researchers to see them as data in their own right, and subsequently attend to them, tease out their origins and meanings, and derive lessons from them (Barbour, 2001; Charmaz, 1995). Because it is possible to portray nuance while writing interview studies, findings can be precisely described within the context of each respondent's trajectory. This is valuable because some health experiences are extremely complex and may take years for people to fully grasp; yet the account that is offered during an interview does represent that person's knowledge at that time.

An additional limitation of interview methods is the way in which an interviewer's own contributions to the conversation may shape its course and content. For instance, interviewers should be aware that if they show approval, disapproval, surprise, or disinterest, this will likely influence what participants tell them (Weiss, 1994). It is also possible for interviewers to phrase questions in such a way that inadvertently prompts specific answers from participants (Ulin et al., 2005). Informal language may facilitate participants' understanding (e.g., "What do you and your spouse talk about?" rather than "What are the communication patterns between you and your spouse?"). Similarly, interviewer characteristics can influence participants' responses and participants may respond differently to different interviewers. For example, a female breast cancer patient may feel more at ease disclosing her fears and bodily changes with a female interviewer. In several of the interviews Daena conducted with recovering heart patients, she noticed it seemed awkward for men her father's age to talk with a woman their daughter's age about the impact of their heart condition on their sex lives. It is beyond the scope of this chapter to address the extent to which interviewers should strive for a neutral "unbiased" role, but reflexivity about the potential effects of one's own participation is critical.

Challenges and Lessons Learned

Some limitations of interviews about health communication cannot be overcome in a single study or even a series of interview studies. However, there are some considerations that are worth contemplating ahead of time so that the effects of these challenges can be minimized.

Face-to-face conversations with people about health and illness are challenging, enough so that some scholars eschew this type of research altogether. The subject matter is sensitive, and the conversation can be stressful. Participants who are thinking and talking about health, illness, and death may become distressed. They may get angry; they may cry. Researchers can strategize about appropriate ways of managing emotional conversations before, during, and after they occur: for instance, bringing tissues; asking participants whether they wish to stop the recording and take a break; and memoing about the episode while completing field notes after the interview. It may also be appropriate to provide a list of community referrals at the conclusion of the interview, so that, if distress prompted by the interview lingers, participants know whom they may contact for additional help.

There are practical and ethical challenges to recruiting interviewees. Like other research with people who are living with an illness, interviewers may need to consider exclusion criteria so that they can gather usable data. For example, it may be necessary to screen participants to make sure that they are not cognitively impaired from their condition (e.g., Step & Berlin Ray, 2011); alternatively, researchers may use cognitive impairment or physical debilitation as theoretical sampling criteria. When accessing and working with stigmatized or otherwise vulnerable populations (e.g., Kosenko, 2010), interviewers may need to take extra steps to ensure participant confidentiality and safety and to manage the power imbalance between researcher and participant (Leeman, 2011). When working with interviewees recruited via healthcare organizations, it may be necessary to explicitly say that their interview responses have no bearing on their medical treatment. Erin has found that, when she partners with hospitals and clinics to interview patients, participants sometimes need to be reminded that we are neither "doctors" in the medical sense, nor are we qualified to answer questions about individual health concerns.

Finally, one of the difficulties of conducting health communication research involves making the subject matter accessible to participants. Just as physicians ought to use layperson language in lieu of complex medical terms, researchers need to beware of their own tendencies toward jargon. Charmaz (2006) noted that the average person may not know what we mean if we ask what coping strategies he uses to manage his health stressors. One piece of advice Charmaz offered is to follow the lexicon of participants and use their words to rephrase questions in the terms that seem meaningful to members of that population. Hence, a fundamental advantage of interviews: the continuous back-and-forth between respondent and researcher, opening the door to reassure participants that we are interested in their experiences when they ask, as many do, "Is that what you mean? Am I answering the question you asked?"

Conclusion

Through in-depth interviews, health communication scholars have made important contributions to theory and practice. Interviews are ideally suited to drawing out the complexities of how people manage health, wellness, illness, and death—as individuals, in interpersonal relationships, and through their professional pursuits. In-depth interviews empower nuance, thus leading us down new investigative paths that may not have revealed themselves to us otherwise. They forge a connection between researcher and participant that permits the co-creation of knowledge. There is little doubt that a physician's capacity to heal is facilitated by constructive dialogue with a patient. Likewise, scholarship concerning health communication has been enriched by talking with patients, providers, and others who have a stake in individual and public health. As a complement to other methodologies and a rewarding enterprise in their own right, the value of in-depth interviews is apparent in the compelling words of the respondents who take the time to tell us their stories.

References

Al-Busaidi, Z. Q. (2008). Qualitative research and its uses in health care. *Sultan Qaboos University Medical Journal, 8*(1), 11–19.

Alvesson, M., & Sköldberg, K. (2009). *Reflexive methodology: New vistas for qualitative research.* Thousand Oaks, CA: Sage Publications.

Barbour, R. S. (2001). Checklists for improving rigour in qualitative research: A case of the tail wagging the dog? *BMJ, 322*(7294), 1115.

Baxter, L. A., & Babbie, E. R. (2004). *The basics of communication research.* Belmont, CA: Wadsworth/Thomson Learning.

Baxter, J., & Eyles, J. (1997). Evaluating qualitative research in social geography: Establishing 'rigor' in interview analysis. *Transactions of the Institute of British Geographers, 22*(4), 505–525.

Bowling, A. (2009). *Research methods in health: Investigating health and health services* (3rd ed.). New York, NY: McGraw Hill/Open University Press.

Brashers, D. E., Neidig, J. L., Cardillo, L. W., Dobbs, L. K., Russell, J. A., & Haas, S. M. (1999). "In an important way, I did die": Uncertainty and revival in persons living with HIV or AIDS. *AIDS Care, 11*(2), 201–219.

Bute, J. J. (2009). "Nobody thinks twice about asking": Women with a fertility problem and requests for information. *Health Communication, 24*(8), 752–763.

Bute, J. J., & Jensen, R. E. (2010). Low-income women describe fertility-related expectations: Descriptive norms, injunctive norms, and behavior. *Health Communication, 25*(8), 681–691.

Bute, J. J., Donovan-Kicken, E., & Martins, N. (2007). Effects of communication-debilitating illnesses and injuries on close relationships: A relational maintenance perspective. *Health Communication, 21*(3), 235–246.

Catania, J. A., McDermott, L. J., & Pollack, L. M. (1986). Questionnaire response bias and face-to-face interview sample bias in sexuality research. *The Journal of Sex Research, 22*(1), 52–72.

Charmaz, K. (1991). *Good days, bad days: The self in chronic illness and time.* New Brunswick, NJ: Rutgers University Press.

Charmaz, K. (1995). Grounded theory. In J. A. Smith, R. Harré, & L. van Langenhove (Eds.), *Rethinking methods in psychology* (pp. 27–49). London, England: Sage Publications.

Charmaz, K. (2006). *Constructing grounded theory: A practical guide through qualitative analysis.* Thousand Oaks, CA: Sage Publications.

Clark, M. S., & Reis, H. T. (1988). Interpersonal processes in close relationships. *Annual Review of Psychology, 39*(1), 609–672.

Corbin, J. M., & Strauss, A. (1990). Grounded theory research: Procedures, canons, and evaluative criteria. *Qualitative Sociology, 13*(1), 3–21.

Creswell, J. W., & Miller, D. L. (2000). Determining validity in qualitative inquiry. *Theory Into Practice, 39*(3), 124–130.

Denzin, N. K., & Lincoln, Y. S. (Eds.) (2008). *Strategies of qualitative inquiry* (3rd ed.). Thousand Oaks, CA: Sage Publications.

Donovan-Kicken, E., Tollison, A. C., & Goins, E. S. (2011). A grounded theory of control over communication among individuals with cancer. *Journal of Applied Communication Research, 39*(3), 310–330.

Donovan-Kicken, E., Tollison, A. C., & Goins, E. S. (2012). The nature of communication work during cancer: Advancing the theory of illness trajectories. *Health Communication, 27*(7), 641–652.

du Pré, A., & Crandall, S. J. (2011). Qualitative methods: Bridging the gap between research and daily practice. In T. L. Thompson, R. Parrott, & J. F. Nussbaum (Eds.), *The Routledge handbook of health communication* (2nd ed.), (pp. 532–545). New York, NY: Routledge.

Eggly, S. (2002). Physician–patient co-construction of illness narratives in the medical interview. *Health Communication, 14*(3), 339–360.

Frank, A. W. (1995). *The wounded storyteller: Body, illness, and ethics.* Chicago, IL: University of Chicago Press.

Geertz, C. (1973). Thick description: Toward an interpretive theory of culture. *Culture: Critical Concepts in Sociology, 1*, 173–196.

Glaser, B. G., & Strauss, A. L. (1967). *The discovery of grounded theory: Strategies for qualitative research*. New York, NY: Aldine Publishing Company.

Goldsmith, D. J., & Domann-Scholz, K. (2013). The meanings of "open communication" among couples coping with a cardiac event. *Journal of Communication, 63*(2), 266–286.

Goldsmith, D. J., Lindholm, K. A., & Bute, J. J. (2006). Dilemmas of talking about lifestyle changes among couples coping with a cardiac event. *Social Science & Medicine, 63*(8), 2079–2090.

Goldsmith, D. J., Miller, L. E., & Caughlin, J. P. (2008). Openness and avoidance in couples communicating about cancer. In C. Beck (Ed.), *Communication Yearbook 31* (pp. 62–117). New York, NY: Lawrence Erlbaum Associates.

Graneheim, U. H., & Lundman, B. (2004). Qualitative content analysis in nursing research: Concepts, procedures and measures to achieve trustworthiness. *Nurse Education Today, 24*(2), 105–112.

Gubrium, J. F., & Holstein, J. A. (Eds.) (2002). *Handbook of interview research: Context & method.* Thousand Oaks, CA: Sage Publications.

Hsieh, E., & Kramer, E. M. (2012). Medical interpreters as tools: Dangers and challenges in the utilitarian approach to interpreters' roles and functions. *Patient Education and Counseling, 89*(1), 158–162.

Janesick, V. J. (2000). The choreography of qualitative research design: Minuets, improvisations, and crystallization. In N. K. Denzin & Y. S. Lincoln (Eds.), *Handbook of qualitative research* (pp. 379–399). Thousand Oaks, CA: Sage Publications.

Karp, D. A. (1996). *Speaking of sadness: Depression, disconnection and the meanings of illness.* New York, NY: Oxford University Press.

Kitzinger, J. (1994). The methodology of focus groups: The importance of interaction between research participants. *Sociology of Health & Illness, 16*(1), 103–121.

Kleinman, A. (1988). *The illness narratives.* New York, NY: Basic Books.

Kosenko, K. A. (2010). Meanings and dilemmas of sexual safety and communication for transgender individuals. *Health Communication, 25*(2), 131–141.

Leeman, M. A. (2011). Balancing the benefits and burdens of storytelling among vulnerable people. *Health Communication, 26*(1), 107–109.

Liamputtong, P., & Ezzy, D. (2005). *Qualitative research methods* (2nd ed.). New York, NY: Oxford University Press.

Lichstein, P. R. (1990). The medical interview. In H. K. Walker, W. D. Hall, & J. W. Hurst (Eds.), *Clinical methods: The history, physical, and laboratory examinations* (3rd ed.) (Chapter 3). Boston, MA: Butterworths. Available from: http://www.ncbi.nlm.nih.gov/books/NBK349/

Lincoln, Y. S., & Guba, E. G. (1985). *Naturalistic inquiry.* Beverly Hills, CA: Sage Publications.

Lindlof, T. R., & Taylor, B. C. (2002). *Qualitative communication research methods* (2nd ed.). Thousand Oaks, CA: Sage Publications.

Lofland, J., & Lofland, L. H. (1995). *Analyzing social settings: A guide to qualitative observation and analysis.* (3rd ed.). Belmont, CA: Wadsworth.

MacCracken, G. D. (1988). *The long interview.* Newbury Park, CA: Sage Publications.

Marshall, A. A., Smith, S. W., & McKeon, J. K. (1995). Persuading low-income women to engage in mammography screening: Source, message, and channel preferences. *Health Communication,* 7(4), 283–299.

Mays, N., & Pope, C. (1995). Rigour and qualitative research. *BMJ, 311*(6997), 109–112.

Miller, L. E. (2012). Sources of uncertainty in cancer survivorship. *Journal of Cancer Survivorship: Research and Practice, 6*(4), 431–440.

Miller, L. E. (2014). Uncertainty management and information seeking in cancer survivorship. *Health Communication, 29,* 233–243.

Miller, L. E., & Caughlin, J. P. (2013). "We're going to be survivors": Couples' identity challenges during and after cancer treatment. *Communication Monographs, 80*(1), 63–82.
Mishler, E. G. (1984). *The discourse of medicine: Dialectics of medical interviews.* Norwood, NJ: Ablex Publishing.
Noller, P., & Feeney, J. A. (2004). Studying family communication: Multiple methods and multiple sources. In A. L. Vangelisti (Ed.), *Handbook of family communication* (pp. 31–50). Mahwah, NJ: Lawrence Erlbaum Associates.
Oskouie, F., Zeighami, R., & Joolaee, S. (2011). Outcomes of parental mental illness on children: A qualitative study from Iran. *Journal of Psychosocial Nursing and Mental Health Services, 49*(9), 32–40.
Patton, M. Q. (1999). Enhancing the quality and credibility of qualitative analysis. *Health Services Research, 34*(5) (Pt 2), 1189–1208.
Rich, E. C., Crowson, T. W., & Harris, I. B. (1987). The diagnostic value of the medical history: Perceptions of internal medicine physicians. *Archives of Internal Medicine, 147*(11), 1957–1960.
Riessman, C. K. (2007). *Narrative methods for the human sciences.* Los Angeles, CA: Sage Publications.
Romo, L. K. (2012). "Above the influence": How college students communicate about the healthy deviance of alcohol abstinence. *Health Communication, 27*(7), 672–681.
Scott, A. M., Martin, S. C., Stone, A. M., & Brashers, D. E. (2011). Managing multiple goals in supportive interactions: Using a normative theoretical approach to explain social support as uncertainty management for organ transplant patients. *Health Communication, 26*(5), 393–403.
Sharf, B. F., Harter, L. M., Yamasaki, J., & Haidet, P. (2011). Narrative turns epic: Continuing developments in health narrative scholarship. In T. L. Thompson, R. Parrott, & J. F. Nussbaum (Eds.), *The Routledge handbook of health communication* (2nd ed.), (pp. 36–51). New York, NY: Routledge.
Silverman, D. (1997). *Qualitative research: Theory, method, and practice.* London, England: Sage Publications.
Step, M. M., & Berlin Ray, E. (2011). Patient perceptions of oncologist–patient communication about prognosis: Changes from initial diagnosis to cancer recurrence. *Health Communication, 26*(1), 48–58.
Strauss, A. L., & Corbin, J. M. (1990). *Basics of qualitative research: Grounded theory procedures and techniques.* Newbury Park, CA: Sage Publications.
Suddaby, R. (2006). From the editors: What grounded theory is not. *Academy of Management Journal, 49*(4), 633–642.
Taylor, S. J., & Bogdan, R. (1998). *Introduction to qualitative research methods* (3rd ed.). New York, NY: John Wiley.
Ulin, P. R., Robinson, E. T., & Tolley, E. E. (2005). *Qualitative methods in public health: A field guide for applied research.* San Francisco, CA: Jossey-Bass.
Vanderford, M. L., Jenks, E. B., & Sharf, B. F. (1997). Exploring patients' experiences as a primary source of meaning. *Health Communication, 9*(1), 13–26.
Weiss, R. S. (1994). *Learning from strangers: The art and method of qualitative interview studies.* New York, NY: Free Press.
White, J., Levinson, W., & Roter, D. (1994). "Oh, by the way . . .": The closing moments of the medical visit. *Journal of General Internal Medicine, 9*(1), 24–28.
Wittenberg-Lyles, E.M., Goldsmith, J., Ragan, S. L., & Sanchez-Reilly, S. (2010). *Dying with comfort: Family illness narratives and early palliative care.* Cresskill, NJ: Hampton Press.

THE CASE STUDY IN HEALTH COMMUNICATION RESEARCH

Leigh Arden Ford, Mindi Ann Golden, and Eileen Berlin Ray

Imagine a group of ten women, all in their 30s and 40s, receiving weekly chemotherapy treatment for breast cancer at the same oncology center. They introduce themselves and, over the course of several weeks, talk about their diagnosis, treatment experiences, and emotional responses to the disease. The women decide to form a support group and start meeting once a month, away from the oncology center. They continue to meet throughout the first year of their illness. Researchers using a case study approach to health communication would argue that there is much to be learned from this single breast cancer support group. How, for example, is a sense of community and shared identity constructed within the group's communication, given varied diagnoses, treatment plans, and prognoses? How is social support communicated within the group, and what are the impacts of social support for coping? How is uncertainty communicated and managed within the group?

The case study as a research method is found in disciplines as diverse as sociology, education, management, nursing, and law. Although sometimes controversial when first introduced, case study research, when conducted with care, is now viewed as a valuable methodological option (Simons, 2009; Yin, 1994). The central purpose of this chapter, then, is to present the case study as a health communication research method. First, the nature of the case study method is examined, including its description; assumptions; and procedures for data gathering, data analysis, and presentation of results. Second, we provide a framework for evaluating the method and describe various challenges in creating sound case study research. Third, the chapter concludes with a discussion of the promises and potentials of case study research.

Note: The authors, listed alphabetically, contributed equally to this chapter.

The Case Study in Health Communication Research: Method or Approach

The case study has different meanings for researchers in different disciplines (see Simons, 2009, for a review of these definitions). For example, Stake (1995) focuses his definition on the complexities and details of a specific context. Yin (1994) suggests that a case study "investigates a contemporary phenomenon in its real life context, especially when the boundaries between phenomenon and context are not clearly evident" (p. 13). Other definitions include the importance of historical data to a case, or emphasize the in-depth, holistic, descriptive nature of the case study method (Merriam, 1988). Despite these differences, definitions of the case study as a research method share important common characteristics.

The first, and perhaps most critical, shared definitional characteristic of the case study method is "boundedness" (Yin, 2003), meaning the phenomenon under examination is contextualized. A researcher chooses to use the case study as a research method because the phenomenon can only be well understood within its context and with respect to multiple perspectives within that context.

Second, definitions of the case study method share a commitment to addressing "how" and "why" questions (Yin, 2003). In contrast, many methods used to study health communication focus on *what* questions. Survey or experimental research regarding provider–patient interaction, for example, can link independent variables to the dependent variable of patient satisfaction. As a result, we have knowledge of *what* factors influence patient satisfaction (Duggan & Thompson, 2011). Case study research, on the other hand, would maintain the holistic character of human communication in a specific context (Yin, 2003), allowing for a complex and detailed sense of how patient satisfaction is interactively achieved. Smith-Dupre and Beck (1996), for example, explore naturally occurring interactions between a physician and his or her patients, demonstrating *how* they enable attention to both parties' goals, resulting in interpersonal satisfaction.

Third, definitions of the case study method share a focus on a particular and singular phenomenon, whether it is an individual, relationship, group, or organization, and the emphasis is on understanding the complexity and uniqueness of that phenomenon (Simons, 2009). In pursuit of the phenomenon of central interest, a researcher may examine historical documents and data, but more typically is focused on contemporaneous actions and the consequences and meaning of those actions for the participants.

A fourth shared characteristic is that a case study is not defined by its methods (i.e., methods of data gathering and analysis vary and may include quantitative or qualitative methods, or both). Further, the use of multiple forms of data to understand the phenomenon studied is an expectation of case study research (Stake, 1995;Yin, 1993) and is a signal difference between the case study method and other qualitative research methods (with the exception of rare cases where triangulation of methods is utilized). That the case study is not defined by its methods leads Simons (2009) to argue that the term "case study method" creates confusion. Because researchers use a variety of techniques (i.e., methods) to gather and analyze data, she posits that "case study approach," a broader term, reflects the actual nature of the case study as research and is more appropriate. Henceforth in this chapter, we will use "approach" when we refer to the totality of the case study research enterprise, and will use "method" to refer to specific data-gathering techniques.

In sum, the case study approach captures the reality of a given phenomenon for participants from multiple points of view (Simons, 2009) within a larger social context that is bounded by space and time. Based on these key characteristics, it is clear that many phenomena of interest to health communication researchers would be well served by the case study approach. Consider the hypothetical support group described at the start of this chapter. Over the course of the year, a researcher might attend the support group's meetings, interview individual members, and review materials and documents shared by group members. The researcher could use all of these data to understand and describe the content and experience of social support for this particular group of women, as well as perceived impacts of support on personal identity, coping, and uncertainty.

In another example, a health communication researcher might be interested in the introduction of a new hand-off procedure as patients are moved from the emergency department to wards at a metropolitan hospital, and the effects of that procedure on nurse–nurse communication practices. The researcher might examine past hand-off practices and the data reports regarding patient outcomes, hold a focus group with the nurses involved in the new procedure, and interview hospital administrators, all with the goal of describing how the new procedure impacts communication and outcomes. In both the case focusing on our breast cancer support group and the case focusing on the new hand-off procedure, the researcher is (a) interested in "how" or "why" questions, (b) examining a singular phenomenon in its real-life context, (c) using multiple data-gathering methods, and (d) analyzing and reporting the data in an integrated way to inform our understanding of the phenomenon. This is the case study approach in practice.

Using the Case Study Approach in Health Communication Research

Assumptions

The case study approach we explicate in this chapter is grounded in the assumptions of the interpretive paradigm and the methods associated with naturalistic inquiry (Baxter & Jack, 2008; Payne, Field, Rolls, Hawker, & Kerr, 2007; Simons, 2009). Specifically, health communication theory and research within the interpretive paradigm assumes that (a) the nature of truth is subjective, (b) participants may hold multiple and varied meanings and must communicate to co-construct a shared social reality, (c) meaning is situated or contextualized, and (d) the goal of research is to reveal and make understandable lived experiences and participant understandings of their own lives (Lindlof & Taylor, 2011; Tracy, 2013).

In naturalistic inquiry, the boundary between researcher and participants is permeable and that permeability varies in degree. The boundary permeability of naturalistic inquiry coupled with the centrality of boundedness in the case study approach suggests that a variety of qualitative methods might be used to gather data, including but not limited to semi-structured interviews, focus groups, participant observation, and document analysis. Quantitative research methods may be included in a case study or form the data base for some case studies (see Yin, 2003); however, quantitative data more frequently appear as adjunct to qualitative data in the case study approach, functioning as additional or alternative evidence that illuminates understandings gleaned from participants via other methods (Simons, 2009).

Research Design

Research design in the case study approach follows the general steps found across paradigms and across research goals and methods. To facilitate understanding of the research design stages, we will use our example of a case study regarding breast cancer patients forming a support group through the first year of their illness.

In the first design step, the researcher must determine the question or problem to be addressed by the research. In health communication case studies, research questions arise from observation, previous research findings, and theoretical concerns. The research questions at the heart of health communication case studies may emphasize interpersonal relationships (e.g., spouses, parent–child, provider–patient, family), group dynamics (e.g., healthcare teams, support groups), organizational structures and processes (e.g., urban medical centers, free clinics, physician-owned medical service centers), or public health campaigns (e.g., organ donation, HIV prevention, diabetes testing).

Within any health communication context, the potential questions that present themselves are nearly limitless; hence, case study methodologists recommend two interrelated means for limiting the scope of the potential case study. The researcher must identify the unit of analysis by engaging in the iterative process of answering the questions: "What is the case?" and "What is not the case?"; this is termed "binding the case" (Baxter & Jack, 2008). The iterative process may seem simplistic, but in fact requires the researcher to be conscious of the unit of analysis as the case must have the characteristics noted in the opening definition section of this chapter. Specifically, the case must be focused on a single "phenomenon … occurring in a bounded context"

(Miles & Huberman, 1994, p. 25). Thus, in our support group example, the researcher has question options. She might be interested in how the group defines "illness" and "health" over the course of the year. Alternatively, she might be interested in the way communication creates the structures and norms of the group. The researcher would refine these questions as she excludes some forms of data while including others—"binding" the case to the key question of concern within the context of this group's meetings and discussions over the course of a single year. In short, in the case study approach, defining the boundaries of the case is equally important to developing the research questions/problem identification.

In the second step of study design, the researcher is charged with identifying the overarching purpose of the case study. Based on the assumptions of naturalistic inquiry, and the characteristics of the case study approach described previously in this chapter, the research purposes of a case study typically are to explore, explain, describe, illustrate, or evaluate a contemporary phenomenon in depth and in context (Baxter & Jack, 2008; Simons, 2009; Stake, 1995; Yin, 2003). Simons (2009) suggests two further categories for distinguishing the purpose or type of case study: the theory-led case and the theory-generating case. In the theory-led case study, a theory may be a sensitizing tool used to explore a contemporary phenomenon or the case may be an exemplification of a theory. Such a case study supports and extends our understanding of the phenomenon of interest while also supporting the concepts, principles, and purpose of the theory. In the theory-generating case study, the research purpose might be to develop theory using a grounded theory approach (Glaser & Strauss, 1967) or a constructivist grounded theory (Charmaz, 2006). A theory-generating case leads to the development of theoretical constructs and perhaps their relationship to one another.

Theory-led "case studies"[1] have been more common in health communication research as researchers explore, explain, and/or describe a health communication phenomenon framed by a specific theory (see, e.g., Golden, 2010; Harrison et al., 2010; Nicotera & Clinkscales, 2010); however, there is rich potential for theory-emergent health communication research.[2] In an example of theory-led research, Golden (2010) draws upon Relational Dialectics Theory to detail one spouse-caregiver's experience moving her husband with dementia to an assisted-living facility. Focusing on the caregiver's communication as she wrestles with her decision to place her husband, the communication between them on the day of placement, and communication between them in the weeks following placement, Golden is able to highlight the interplay of autonomy and connection underlying the emotional difficulty of the transition for both parties. This study uses Relational Dialectics Theory to contextually specify the general experience of dementia caregiving (Baxter, Braithwaite, Golish, & Olson, 2002), and details how dialectical tensions are communicatively created in the moment.

As the initial research focus and purpose become more clear, some researchers develop a set of propositions as a third stage of the case study design. A proposition bears some resemblance to a hypothesis in that it identifies the potential relationships between two concepts or ideas. This relationship typically arises from previous research and theorizing found in the literature, or, alternatively, is derived from observation and logic (Baxter & Jack, 2008). In our case study example of the breast cancer support group, a possible proposition might be as follows: Women in a breast cancer support group mutually manage uncertainty as they co-construct their illness identities. Such a proposition would draw on previous research literature and communication theories used in efforts to understand illness and uncertainty (see, e.g., Babrow, Kasch, & Ford, 1998; Ford, Babrow, & Stohl, 1996). While hypothesis-like, a case study proposition is not designed to be empirically tested; instead, propositions guide our data gathering and analysis. This guidance may be problematic, as it limits the researcher's capacity for openness to alternative understandings of the data; hence, propositions should be used with caution in case study research (Baxter & Jack, 2008).

In sum, case study researchers begin by specifying their focus and purpose, and may articulate propositions. In the next section of this chapter, a description of the diversity of data-gathering and analysis methods in case study research as well as a discussion of the presentation of research results are offered. Because the case study approach arises from the interpretive paradigm, Simons (2009) and other scholars remind us that data gathering and analysis occur simultaneously; hence, as we engage research questions via our selected methods, our questions may change and the research design itself is emergent and subject to revision (Baxter & Jack, 2008; Hancock & Algozzine, 2006; Simons, 2009).

Data Gathering, Analysis, and Presentation of Results

As case study researchers move the study design from what is essentially argument to action and process, they have several choices for gathering data, analyzing data, and, ultimately, presenting the results of the case study. At each decision point, the case study's purpose and questions should guide researchers' choices while acknowledging emergent understandings as the research process unfolds.

Data-Gathering Methods in the Case Study Approach

As previously noted, the case study approach provides several options for data gathering: participant observation, in-depth interviews, focus groups, historical/document research, as well as other qualitative methods. A central characteristic of the case study approach is its reliance on more than one method for data gathering. Further, individual methods for the case study are selected for their capacity to illuminate various aspects of the study question(s) and for their capacity to provide complementary, contrastive, and integrated insights (Baxter & Jack, 2008; Payne et al., 2007; Simons, 2009).

Current health communication research provides a variety of exemplars where a particular study uses a specific data-gathering method and also meets one or more of the key definitional characteristics of the case study approach. For example, Vande Berg and Trujillo (2008) employ narrative methodology (see Yamasaki, Sharf, & Harter, this volume), each telling their own story, then interweaving their shared story of Vande Berg's diagnosis of and treatment for ovarian cancer, and, ultimately, her death. In this narrative, we are privy to their individual perceptions of the situation and of each other, and are given honest insight into love, life, and death in the context of terminal cancer.

In another case study, Pitts (2011) relies primarily on in-depth interviews (see Donovan-Kicken, Miller, & Goldsmith, this volume) with members of one family to describe how they create shared meanings of death and dying. Pitts describes how Gigi Balin, the matriarch, and her family openly communicate about death and dying, share spiritual insights and experiences, and create shared family metaphors (e.g., death is making it home) to facilitate positive perceptions of life and death. In a culture where talk of death and dying is often avoided, uncomfortable, or cloaked in metaphor (Sexton, 1997), Pitts' study of one family's belief system and communication practices enables detailed understanding of an alternative meaning framework, constructed in contrast to the dominant cultural frame.

Using critical discourse analysis as method, Dixon (2004) addresses issues of provider–patient interaction (see Bell & Kravitz, this volume). Focusing on an interaction between a White, middle-class, male physician and an African American, female patient, Dixon walks through the patient's medical visit step by step. In her analysis, Dixon argues that age, gender, race, and socio-economic differences all contribute to the unraveling of this provider–patient interaction. As a case study, Dixon richly illustrates how, despite the best of intentions, an unsatisfactory healthcare visit, with potentially profound health consequences for the patient, is created and situated in the larger social, cultural, and political context.

In an exemplar organizational health communication case study, Chapkis and Webb (2008) use ethnographic research (see Ellingson & Rawlins, this volume) to examine the Wo/men's Alliance for Medical Marijuana [WAMM], a cooperative in Santa Cruz, California, where chronically and terminally ill members and their caregivers cultivate medicine and provide one another emotional and physical care. Medical research, legal history, social debates, and tensions between state and federal law enforcement are a backdrop as WAMM members work in the garden, if their health allows, and meet to build community as they receive their medicine at no charge. Chapkis and Webb help us experience and understand communication practices and perspectives within this caregiving collective as members support one another and a larger cause.

Each of these exemplars using different data-gathering methods supports the notion that the case study approach has utility and relevance for health communication research. In these examples, contextualization is key to building the bounded case and to understanding the data interpretively. In some of these exemplars, the inclusion of data from multiple sources and of multiple types is present, while, in other exemplars, the addition of data gathered through other methods could potentially increase our understanding of these compelling and challenging health communication contexts. In sum, health communication case study researchers can use multiple data-gathering techniques that yield a rich and complex data set. The methods should both complement and complicate our understanding of the questions posed.

Data Analysis in the Case Study Approach

The case study approach with its multiple data-gathering possibilities moves a study beyond triangulation of methods to a more fully integrated analytical strategy that potentially provides more complex understandings of a phenomenon. The complexity (and, in many instances, the sheer amount of data collected) requires an analytic strategy that integrates the data rather than addressing each source individually. This goal of data convergence distinguishes the case study approach from other study designs where more than one data-gathering technique is employed, but the results of each method are reported separately or layered as a value-added element to the study.

Convergence in data analysis emerges from the researcher's efforts to, first, examine an individual data source within and against the multiple data sources and, second, integrate these individual strands in light of the larger context of the case. Various experts have described analytic techniques that fit specific case study purposes and types (see Simons, 2009; Yin, 2003). The specific steps of each technique are beyond the scope of this chapter, but Hancock and Algozzine (2006) provide a useful set of questions that may facilitate the researcher's efforts toward integration and synthesis of information. Whatever the specific data analysis technique(s) employed, case study researchers are cautioned that integration and management of various data sources and perspectives is complicated and can overwhelm even an experienced researcher. Therefore, an essential part of the research design includes a data management plan that has been established during the initial stages of research design.

Presentation of Results in the Case Study Approach

The final stage of the case study approach in practice is the presentation of the research findings. Strategies for communicating case study findings take several forms, including but not limited to the formal report, the conclusion-led case, the descriptive portrayal, and storytelling (Hancock & Algozzine, 2006; Simons, 2009; Yin, 1993).

The formal report most closely resembles the traditional structure of research reporting found in most academic journals (i.e., the post-positivist frame). In the formal report, an in-depth description of the nature of the problem, the research literature informing the problem, and the research questions drawn from this examination are presented, followed by the methods of data collection and analysis. The report of the research results then provides an extensive description of the case elements: (a) the individual, group, or organization as the focus of the case; (b) the context, including the immediate environment and the larger historical, cultural, sociopolitical context; (c) the issues (e.g., factors facilitating or impeding the resolution of the problem); and (d) conclusions and implications (i.e., present and potential consequences in the case; Hancock & Algozzine, 2006; Simons, 2009; Yin, 1993).

The conclusion-led case report has similarities to the formal report in that it emphasizes description and explanation. However, the explanation is typically driven by a theoretically-based analysis. For example, if our case study example of the breast cancer support group was examined using Problematic Integration Theory (Babrow, 2007) as a lens for understanding, we might in our analysis identify several theory-based themes represented in our data. In our report, we would organize the telling of the case around those themes and we would present supporting evidence in the form of excerpts from group interactions that illustrate the theoretical themes. In this form, the use of representative quotations and excerpts engage the reader and enliven the experiences of the participants.

The descriptive portrayal features elements of both the formal report and the conclusion-led report. It resembles the formal report in that minimal researcher interpretation is placed on the data; the goal is to display the data itself. It resembles the conclusion-led report in that the words and lived experiences of the participants are primary; in effect, the participants reveal the elements of their own case/story. In a descriptive portrayal, the researcher may present a series of vignettes, juxtapose different participants' perspectives, provide descriptions of places and people, or may include all of these forms displayed in collected and contrasting ways. The reader engages the case and the underlying themes and conclusions emerge from the data itself (Simons, 2009). In our example, we might juxtapose two women's stories of diagnosis against each other and against a report of the general characteristics of the communication of a breast cancer diagnosis as experienced by all of the women in the support group as one element of our explanation of the first year of living with breast cancer.

Finally, narrative (i.e., storytelling) is also a typical presentation form for a case study as research method. In this form, the research findings and data are presented within narrative structure. The researcher is held to the standards of narrative coherence and fidelity (Fisher, 1987). In this format, the goal is to engage the reader intellectually and emotionally in lived experience. As a qualitative research method, the case study values narrative form and interpretation, but also grounds the story in the actual data collected for the research study. While anonymity for the participants, organization, and/or community may be assured by disguising names and identifying details, the narrative should present the research findings in a manner that reflects participants' perspectives and voices and is recognized as such by those participants.

A range of options exists for reporting case study results. Case study methodologists agree that two factors help guide the choice of reporting style: (a) the nature of the audience for whom the report is being prepared and (b) the original purpose of the study (Hancock & Algozzine, 2006; Simons, 2009; Yin, 1993). The researcher should determine these factors a priori and then reflect on them throughout the various stages of the research project.

Evaluating the Case Study Approach: Criteria and Challenges

In this section of the chapter, criteria typically applied to evaluate the quality and findings of case study research are reviewed, then the challenges of producing "trustworthy" research throughout the case study's planning, enactment, and presentation are outlined.

Criteria for Evaluation: What Constitutes "Good" Case Study Research

The most common critique of case study research is lack of generalizability, a post-positivist evaluation criterion. In other words, what is captured in one case cannot be claimed as true of all cases. Yin (2003) argues that this criticism is overstated, pointing out that, although experimental research is associated with establishing generalization, scientific facts are rarely based on the findings of a single experiment. Regardless of this debate, as we have demonstrated in this chapter, case studies are rich, specific descriptions of communication processes and experiences in a particular context; they are "not intended to be . . . used as a 'sample' of something else" (Chen & Pearce, 1995, p. 141). Hence, evaluation of case study research should be determined by criteria commonly associated with the naturalistic paradigm and the use of qualitative methods.

For qualitative research, generally, and case study research, specifically, validity appears to be the prime criterion for evaluation of research quality. In case study research, this criterion frequently is defined as: Does the case reveal a trustworthy understanding of the phenomenon of interest and the social, political, cultural context within which it occurs (Baxter & Jack, 2008; Simons, 2009)? "Trustworthiness," according to Lincoln and Guba (1985), includes dimensions of credibility, transferability, dependability, and confirmability.[3] In a revision of their criterion in 1989, Guba and Lincoln suggest that "authenticity" moves evaluation away from a set of dimensions somewhat parallel to criteria used to judge quantitative research.

Authenticity includes fairness, respect for participants' perspectives, and empowering participants to act (Simons, 2009). All of these dimensions have potential value for assessing the quality of a case study. The key is to establish at the beginning of the research project which of the dimensions of validity will be applied.

Challenges in Case Study Research: Achieving Trustworthiness

Given the primary focus on validity when determining "good" case study research, a review of the likely threats to validity and/or possible strategies to prevent those threats is warranted. These threats are addressed within three phases of the research process: planning, enactment, and presentation.

Planning Stage

Establishing validity begins with a careful study design and clearly defining the research question (Baxter & Jack, 2008; Simons, 2009). Central to an appropriate study design is the notion of boundedness, as defined early in this chapter. Boundedness establishes both the limits of the case (i.e., the boundaries) and the context of the case (i.e., the environmental, cultural, sociopolitical context). This "case/not case" definition should be revisited across all phases of the research to increase claims of validity.

Enactment Stage

When gathering and analyzing data, possible threats to trustworthiness and authenticity arise from several sources. First, the researcher must have the capacity to spend sufficient time in the field with the case. Limited time in the field leads to a narrower understanding of the context and the phenomenon of interest. Second, in some respects, the key to increasing validity rests on the capacity of the researcher to organize and manage effectively the large amount of data typically collected to understand the case (see Hancock & Algozzine, 2006, and Simons, 2009, for suggestions, including computer-mediated management systems). Even experienced researchers can be overwhelmed by the amount and complexity of multiple sources of data and its analysis.

Third, the case study approach requires the researcher to demonstrate expertise in varied data-gathering methods and data analysis, a skill demand that is atypical for most research studies. Failures in execution of one method could potentially infect other data gathered in the analysis phase. Fourth, throughout the entire research process, the researcher must practice reflexivity and be open to emergent findings that may affect the study design and analysis going forward as well as the ultimate interpretation of the study results. The researcher must always acknowledge his or her role and subjectivity while simultaneously using the self effectively to foreground the voices and experiences of the participants.

In order to support and enable openness and acknowledge subjectivity, case study researchers suggest using a peer to check field notes and preliminary analyses, as well as, under some circumstances, asking peers to serve as independent coders (Baxter & Jack, 2008; Hancock & Algozzine, 2006). Alternatively, the researcher might use a double coding technique. In this effort to increase validity, the researcher codes/categorizes/thematizes data, then leaves the findings and data alone for several weeks. After this time away, the researcher then codes the same data again and compares these findings to the previous analysis (Baxter & Jack, 2008). With each technique briefly described here, the goal is to check/re-check, review, and reflect.

Presentation Stage

In this chapter, we have suggested several options for presenting case study research results. While these formats are varied in structure, and in presentation of data and evidence within the structure, they share one technique for validating the research and its reporting: member checks. This method of assessing validity is common to several qualitative research methods, so it is not surprising that it is offered as a validity check in case study research. That said, because the case study focuses on a singular phenomenon bounded by space and time, the centrality of the participants' perspectives in gathering the data, analyzing the data, and presenting the data are intensified within the case study approach. It follows that the researcher is obliged to conduct member checks throughout the research process, but especially during the presentation stage. Participants should recognize their lived experiences, presented in a credible, authentic way, regardless of the case study's purpose.

In sum, while threats to validity are significant in the case study approach, the enactment of multiple counterstrategies noted in this section should create important safeguards and provide confidence in the case study as a qualitative health communication research method.

The Promise and Potential of Case Study Research in Health Communication

The potential contributions of the case study approach to health communication research are several. The case study, because of its use of multiple methods, matches the complexity of the situations experienced within the realm of health and illness. Further, the case study approach uncovers localized understandings that may have macro implications for participants and for the larger context within which these experiences occur. The case study also provides a rich environment for theory development and theory application. Careful attention to everyday experiences through case study research can lead to insights for researchers and participants alike. Cases offer participants the opportunity to communicate and understand their own lives more clearly, and, perhaps, to change their meanings, experiences, and understandings where needed. Finally, there are human experiences that defy the ordinary and routine, requiring a research approach that values unique and extraordinary experiences, where the single case can illuminate communication and human connection to the social context.

Another powerful potential contribution of case study research is the ability to translate research findings to pedagogy (see Berlin Ray 1993, 1996, 2005; Brann 2011). Pedagogical case studies are meant for classroom use (i.e., students read a case and discuss it in terms of relevant health communication issues, concepts, and theoretical frameworks), emphasizing the dynamics and complexities of communication issues related to health-related concerns. Unlike the case study method and approach, the pedagogical case study must meet pragmatic goals. Good pedagogical case studies raise questions that lead to discussion and expose students to new topics and situations (Boehrer & Linsky, 1990; Sypher, 1997). By focusing on complex, real-world health communication problems, pedagogical case studies enable students to apply their knowledge beyond the classroom walls.

The case study approach to research enables exploration of the complexity and consequentiality of communication in health contexts. It can further the application of theory, potentially develop theory, and result in concrete application. Case study research can capture the interplay of individual, group, organizational, and/or social contexts. Because of its boundedness, the case study approach can also be the basis for creating pedagogical health communication case studies, linking health contexts and the health communication classroom in meaningful ways.

Conclusion

In this chapter, the case study approach to health communication research—including assumptions, procedures, challenges, and potentials—have been overviewed. The case study approach to research emphasizes boundedness (i.e., examining a contextualized, single phenomenon) and enables focus on "how" and "why" questions. Grounded in the interpretive paradigm and naturalistic inquiry, case study research relies on data collection and analysis procedures associated with qualitative research. In fact, use of multiple data-gathering methods can yield rich, integrated pictures of health communication phenomena. Validity is the key criterion for evaluating case study research. And, although case study research in health communication has been largely theory led, poignant "defining moments" described by researchers may serve as cornerstones for future theory-generating case studies. The case study research approach illu-minates the complexity and detail of communication in a health context, producing unique research findings and creating enormous potential for translation to pedagogy.

There is a great deal to be learned from a single case. Our hypothetical support group has much to teach us about support, identity, and uncertainty in the first year of breast cancer diagnosis and treatment. How does communication with similar others shape what it means to have breast cancer or be a breast cancer "patient"? How does communication within the support group influence how members think about their own identities and their sense of self in the larger contexts of their families and Western society? How does the social support communicated within the group relate to coping, decision making, and uncertainty management? What new theories regarding humor, group dynamics, and individual health management might emerge from the study of this single group? The "how" and "why" questions are many, and the case study approach to research provides a means of addressing them.

Notes

1. The term "case study" is frequently used in health communication research, but may or may not meet all of the definitional characteristics of the case study approach.
2. Although we are unaware of health communication case studies that have generated theory, we believe the "Defining Moments" published in the journal *Health Communication* may provide an exciting first step in this direction. Defining moments are narrative essays describing poignant experiences in health contexts. These defining moments may contain unique experiences and novel ideas, laying the cornerstone for generating further examples and, ultimately, new theory (Bavelas, 1987).
3. These dimensions are applicable to all forms of qualitative research methods.

References

Babrow, A. S. (2007). Problematic integration theory. In B. B. Whaley (Ed.), *Explaining communication: Contemporary theories and exemplars* (pp. 181–200). Mahwah, NJ: Lawrence Erlbaum Associates.

Babrow, A. S., Kasch, C. R., & Ford, L. A. (1998). The many meanings of uncertainty in illness: Toward a systematic accounting. *Health Communication, 10*(1), 1–23.

Bavelas, J. B. (1987). Permitting creativity in science. In D. N. Jackson & J Philippe Rushton (Eds.), *Scientific excellence: Origins & Assessment* (pp. 307–327). Newbury Park, CA: Sage Publications.

Baxter, L. A., Braithwaite, D. O., Golish, T. D., & Olson, L. N. (2002). Contradictions of interactions for wives of elderly husbands with adult dementia. *Journal of Applied Communication Research, 30*(1), 1–26.

Baxter, P. & Jack, S. (2008). Qualitative case study methodology: Study design and implementation for novice researchers. *The Qualitative Report, 13*(4), 544–559.

Berlin Ray, E. (1993). *Case studies in health communication.* Hillsdale, NJ: Lawrence Erlbaum Associates.

Berlin Ray, E. (1996). *Case studies in communication and disenfranchisement: Applications to social health issues.* Mahwah, NJ: Lawrence Erlbaum Associates.

Berlin Ray, E. (2005). *Health communication in practice: A case study approach.* Mahwah, NJ: Lawrence Erlbaum Associates.

Boehrer, J., & Linsky, M. (1990). Teaching with cases: Learning to question. *New Directions for Teaching and Learning, 42*, 41–57.

Brann, M. (Ed.). (2011). *Contemporary case studies in health communication: Theoretical and applied approaches*. Dubuque, IA: Kendall Hunt.

Chapkis, W., & Webb, R. J. (2008). *Dying to get high: Marijuana as medicine*. New York, NY: New York University Press.

Charmaz, K. (2006). *Constructing grounded theory: A practical guide through qualitative analysis*. London, England: Sage Publications.

Chen, V., & Pearce, W. B. (1995). Even if a thing of beauty, can a case study be a joy forever? A social constructionist approach to theory and research. In W. Leeds-Hurwitz (Ed.), *Social approaches to communication* (pp. 135–154). New York, NY: Guilford Press.

Dixon, L. D. (2004). A case study of an intercultural health care visit: An African American woman and her white male physician. *Women and Language, 27*(Pt 1), 45–52.

Duggan, A. P., & Thompson, T. L. (2011). Provider–patient interaction and related outcomes. In T. L. Thompson, R. Parrott, & J. F. Nussbaum (Eds.), *The Routledge handbook of health communication* (2nd ed.) (pp. 414–427). New York, NY: Routledge.

Fisher, W. R. (1987). *Human communication as narration: Toward a philosophy of reason, value, and action*. Columbia, SC: University of South Carolina Press.

Ford, L. A., Babrow, A. S., & Stohl, C. (1996). Social support messages and the management of uncertainty in the experience of breast cancer: An application of problematic integration theory. *Communication Monographs, 63*(3), 189–207.

Glaser, B. G., & Strauss, A. L. (1967). *The discovery of grounded theory: Strategies for qualitative research*. Chicago, IL: Aldine Publishing Company.

Golden. M. A. (2010). Dialectical contradictions experienced when placing a spouse with dementia in a residential care facility. *Qualitative Research Reports in Communication, 11*(1), 14–20.

Guba, E. G., & Lincoln, Y. S. (1989). *Fourth generation evaluation*. Newbury Park, CA: Sage Publications.

Hancock, D. R., & Algozzine, B. (2006). *Doing case study research: A practical guide for beginning researchers*. New York, NY: Teachers College Press.

Harrison, T. R., Morgan, S. E., King, A. J., Di Corcia, M. J., Williams, E. A., Ivic, R. K., & Hopeck, P. (2010). Promoting the Michigan organ donor registry: Evaluating the impact of a multifaceted intervention utilizing media priming and communication design. *Health Communication, 25*(8), 700–708.

Lincoln, Y. S., & Guba, E. G. (1985). *Naturalistic inquiry*. Beverly Hills, CA: Sage Publications.

Lindlof, T. R., & Taylor, B. C. (2011). *Qualitative communication research methods* (3rd ed.). Thousand Oaks, CA: Sage Publications.

Merriam, S. B. (1988). *Case study research in education: A qualitative approach*. San Francisco, CA: Jossey-Bass.

Miles, M. B., & Huberman, A. M. (1994). *Qualitative data analysis: An expanded sourcebook* (2nd ed.). Thousand Oaks, CA: Sage Publications.

Nicotera, A. M., & Clinkscales, M. J. (2010). Nurses at the nexus: A case study in structurational divergence. *Health Communication, 25*(1), 32–49.

Payne, S., Field, D., Rolls, L., Hawker, S., & Kerr, C. (2007). Case study research methods in end of life care: Reflections on three studies. *Journal of Advanced Nursing, 58*(3), 236–245.

Pitts, M. J. (2011). Dancing with the spirit: Communicating family norms for positive end-of-life transitions. In M. A. Miller-Day (Ed.), *Family communication, connections, and health transitions* (pp. 377–404). New York, NY: Peter Lang.

Sexton, J. (1997). The semantics of death and dying: Metaphor and mortality. *ETC: A Review of General Semantics*, *54*(3), 333–346.

Simons, H. (2009). *Case study research in practice.* Los Angeles, CA: Sage Publications.

Smith-Dupre, A., & Beck, C. S. (1996). Enabling patients and physicians to pursue multiple goals in health care encounters: A case study. *Health Communication*, *8*(1), 73–90.

Stake, R. E. (1995). *The art of case study research.* Thousand Oaks, CA: Sage Publications.

Sypher, B. D. (Ed.) (1997). *Case studies in organizational communication 2: Perspectives on contemporary work life.* New York, NY: Guilford Press.

Tracy, S. I. (2013). *Qualitative research methods: Collecting evidence, crafting analysis, communicating impact.* Malden, MA: Wiley-Blackwell.

Vande Berg, L., & Trujillo, N. (2008). *Cancer and death: A love story in two voices.* Cresskill, NJ: Hampton Press.

Yin, R. K. (1993). *Applications of case study research.* Thousand Oaks, CA: Sage Publications.

Yin, R. K. (1994). *Case study research: Design and methods* (2nd ed.). Thousand Oaks, CA: Sage Publications.

Yin, R. K. (2003). *Case study research: Design and methods* (3rd ed.). Thousand Oaks, CA: Sage Publications.

ETHNOGRAPHY IN HEALTH COMMUNICATION RESEARCH

Laura L. Ellingson and William K. Rawlins

Nature of Method

Ethnography is a naturalistic method of inquiry that involves close observation and interaction in a setting in order to learn about participants' social construction of meaning as it relates to (some aspect of) health. Denzin's (1997) definition of "ethnography" emphasizes the dual nature of ethnography as both process and product: "that form of inquiry and writing that produces descriptions and accounts about the ways of life of the writer and those written about" (p. xi). Health communication researchers can utilize ethnography for the purposes of learning about and assisting in the development or enhancement of communication processes in provision of health care, the construction and targeting of health messages, and the many mundane sites in which people experience culturally specific meanings of (and threats to) health and illness. Thus, this chapter explores how and for what purposes health communication researchers conduct ethnography in hospitals, clinics, and other health-related settings, including homes, workplaces, and schools.

Theoretical Assumptions

Ethnography assumes a naturalistic paradigm (see Lincoln & Guba, 1985), meaning that it involves studying groups of people in their natural contexts (Atkinson, Coffey, Delamont, Lofland, & Lofland, 2001). Ethnography requires being present in the space(s) being studied, for the ability to make knowledge claims is grounded in researchers' direct observation of that space and the interactions within (e.g., Lindlof & Taylor, 2011). Early ethnographers made positivist claims of discovering "the truth" about their subjects' culture, but contemporary ethnographers acknowledge (to varying degrees) the role of the ethnographer in co-constructing meaning in research (Denzin & Lincoln, 2011).

Ethnographers may construct a nuanced range of methodological possibilities to describe what traditionally have been socially constructed as dichotomies, such as art/science, hard/soft, truth/fiction, and qualitative/quantitative (Potter, 1996). Building upon Ellis's (2004) representation of the two ends of the qualitative continuum (i.e., art and science) and the analytic mapping of the continuum developed in Ellis and Ellingson (2000), we posit the continuum as having three primary areas, with infinite possibilities for blending and moving among them (Ellingson, 2009). Such a methodological continuum of approaches to ethnography is made up of a vast and varied middle ground, with art and science representing only the extreme ends of the methodological and representational range, rather than each constituting half of the ground with a sharp delineation between the halves. The goals, questions posed, methods, writing styles, vocabularies, role(s) of researchers, and criteria for evaluation vary across the continuum as we move from a (post-)positivist social science stance toward ethnography on the far right (functional/realist ethnography), through a social constructionist middle ground (interpretive ethnography), to an artistic paradigm on the left (narrative ethnography, autoethnography). Middle-ground approaches that incorporate both artistic and scientific sensibilities need not represent compromise or a lowering of standards. Rather, they can signal innovative approaches to sense making and representation.

Ethnographies cannot be separated into ideal types or located at precise spots along an epistemological and methodological continuum. Rather, ethnography can be thought of as a toolbox that allows for significant choice in how data is gathered, analyzed, and represented, while also responding to cultural, organizational, interpersonal, and intrapersonal forces on the ethnographer and on the process of ethnography.

Applications

When to Use Ethnography

Ethnography tends to be employed when researchers face questions about complex communicative processes in real-world settings that do not lend themselves to precise definition of variables or measurements. Through participant observation in the chosen setting (e.g., a clinic, a school) or with people of a particular type (e.g., people living with diabetes), ethnographers can observe and develop rich descriptions of behavior and language as they occur. The benefit of this approach over researcher-controlled data generation (e.g., surveys, experiments) is the opportunity to participate in joint sense making with participants in the actual settings and circumstances in which they normally engage in the types of communication that constitute the focus of the research. Ethnography can shed light on taken-for-granted patterns of verbal and nonverbal communication by participants and often yields vital insights into health behaviors and healthcare delivery.

In health communication research, ethnography has been utilized for the purpose of studying interactions within groups, including interdisciplinary teams (Gardezi, Lingard, Espin, Whyte, Orser, & Baker, 2009; Opie, 2000), nursing care teams (Propp, Apker, Zabava Ford, Wallace, Serbenski, & Hofmeister, 2010), and social support groups for patients and caregivers (Arrington, Grant, Vanderford, 2005; Golden, 2010). Ethnography also offers access to informal or "backstage" communication (outside of formal meetings) among healthcare providers in healthcare organizations (Ellingson, 2005; Morgan-Witte, 2005; Wittenberg-Lyles, Cie' Gee, Oliver, & Demiris, 2009). Health communication ethnographers also study patient–healthcare provider interactions (The, Hak, Koëter, & van der Wal, 2001), including uses of humor (du Pré, 1998) and the impact of electronic medical records on interaction (Ventres, Kooienga, Vuckovic, Marlin, Nygren, & Stewart, 2006). A particularly intimate health communication topic explored through ethnography is death and dying (Foster, 2007). Autoethnography, a subgenre of ethnography that uses ethnographic techniques to study one's own health experiences, yields insightful, often painful stories of death and dying (Golden, 2009; Vande Berg & Trujillo, 2008), as well as intimate portraits of suffering due to trauma, such as rape and sexual abuse (Minge, 2007; Rambo Ronai, 1995). Finally, ethnography may be used in multi-method health communication studies as a way to gather data and findings to guide development of questionnaires and measures and to enhance understanding of survey or epidemiological data (e.g., Hesse-Biber, 2010).

Ethnographic Exemplars

Social Constructivist/Post-Positivist Ethnography

Considine and Miller (2010) conducted an ethnographic study of hospice workers and volunteers, and posed the research question: "How do caregivers communicate in providing comfort to patients and families at the end of life?" (p. 167). They enriched their data further with interviews and a review of documents produced by the hospice organization. As is typical in ethnography, however, the researchers found themselves accumulating such a wealth of data about communication in end-of-life care, with all its contradictions and complexities, that further decisions about the focus and goals of the inquiry became necessary. Choosing dialectical theory (e.g., Baxter & Montgomery, 1996) to help frame their analysis, they revised their research question to more specifically guide their inquiry: "How do hospice workers and volunteers manage the dialectics of interaction in discussing issues of spirituality with patients and families at the end of life?" (p. 167). Their findings richly illuminated the active and ongoing negotiation of a dialectical tension between "leading" and "following" patients and their loved ones as caregivers participated in end-of-life conversations and sought to give comfort. Considine and Miller then situated their findings by linking them to research on other aspects of end-of-life care in which researchers have found the lead/follow dialectic to be present, such as decision making with physicians.

Narrative Ethnography/Autoethnography

Taking a step toward the artistic pole of the methodological continuum, some ethnographers use more personal and artistic techniques to illuminate health communication issues from a more personal lens. As the son of a family physician, Rawlins (2005) combined narrative ethnography and autoethnography to examine the patient-centered care he perceived his father performed and described while he was growing up. His investigation found Rawlins returning to his childhood home to interview his father and listen to his stories about his medical practice in the very setting where this doctor's son (the study's author) heard him give advice to patients on the phone and leave for and return from house calls. Using a narrative ethnography approach, Rawlins juggled the multiple forms of temporality, as well as personal and scholarly decisions patterning his experiences conducting, living, and rendering this study. For example, while developing the interview protocol, Rawlins experienced physical discomfort that warranted calling his dad for medical advice. During this phone conversation, he remembered several health-related episodes involving calling his dad or receiving his care, which became important for conceptual reflection. During their face-to-face interview, his father told stories that colorfully dramatized his practices, concerns, and convictions as a family physician, which also became grist for analysis. Throughout this investigation, Rawlins' reflections articulated the significance of what he was hearing simultaneously as a son, patient, and interviewer. These various perspectives ground the study in his own lived experience in ways that complemented the accounts of his father's storytelling. Meanwhile, Rawlins placed concrete understandings he gleaned as a vulnerable middle-aged man conversing with his father in dialogue with diverse theoretical discourses pertaining to healthcare and communication.

Employing the Method

Ethnographers embrace a continuum of approaches at every stage of the ethnographic process, and, hence, methodological practices vary tremendously. That said, certain common elements figure centrally in all health ethnography (see Bloor, 2001). We provide here a middle-ground (i.e., social constructionist) perspective that highlights techniques commonly used in health communication ethnography while acknowledging differences and commonalties of approaches closer to art and science ends of the methodological continuum.

Question/Purpose

Health communication ethnographies begin with a general research question that often gets refined or developed into a set of related questions after ethnographers undertake preliminary fieldwork and focus on concrete aspects of communication. However, in our experience health communication ethnographies are just as likely to begin through synchronicity—a chance meeting of a person, a loved one developing a disease about which little is known, stumbling onto an organization's website, noticing a flyer for an upcoming event, or reading a news article. Ethnographers often encourage their students to "start where you are," or to consider the mundane aspects of daily communication (Warren & Karner, 2009), a strategy well suited to health communication research. And, of course, myriad questions about people's daily health behaviors and healthcare delivery yield rich traditions of research investigating patient–healthcare provider communication, professional collaboration, social support, and organizational aspects of healthcare. We recommend beginning with a broad question about an aspect of health communication, but being open to adapting that question as fieldwork progresses and opportunities arise (and disappear). For example, the first author of the present chapter began her study of communication on a geriatric oncology team intending to explore team communication with patients, but shifted to look at the "backstage" communication among team members and how that related to patient–team member communication (Ellingson, 2005). While realist/scientific ethnographies likely pursue a more specific set of research questions grounded directly in current health communication research and theory, more artistic or narrative ethnographies tend to emerge based on personal experience or serendipitous opportunity.

Access

Ethnographers must obtain access, traditionally known as *gaining entre* to the setting or group they wish to study (Agar, 1980). This access typically is done via a *gatekeeper*, a person with formal or informal power to grant the ethnographer permission to conduct research. For example, a hospital administrator may be gatekeeper to an outpatient clinic, or a counselor may be a gatekeeper for a support group. The gatekeeper will likely provide parameters, such as the areas in which researchers are allowed, the patients they may approach, and the times/days that are best for fieldwork. Such access may be serendipitous, but it may also be difficult to come by. "Cold calling" to request access does not boast a high degree of success, particularly given the sensitive nature and privacy concerns involved within healthcare. You would do well to access your networks within academia and beyond to find someone with connections who can introduce you to a likely gatekeeper. Also consider contacting other ethnographers who conduct similar research to learn how they secured access.

Data Gathering

Once access is obtained, the ethnographer begins observing and participating in the setting. Actually being in the space or with the group you are studying is referred to as "conducting ethnography," participant observation, or fieldwork. Unlike in survey or experimental research, there is little formal design; instead, the ethnographer hangs out in a space (Coffey, 1999). You will likely find that certain participants are designated as, agree to become, or over time emerge as "key informants" (Lindlof & Taylor, 2011). These people allow you to hang around or shadow them while observing their interactions with others, engaging them in conversation, and asking lots of questions. You should keep in mind that the person(s) you spend the most time with occupy specific positions within the group or space, and that no single perspective offers "the truth" of what happens there. We recommend that you try to observe and converse in *informal interviews* with participants in as many different positions as possible within the group to facilitate a richer understanding. You may also want to invite participants during or after your fieldwork to participate in formal, recorded interviews to complement your ethnographic data.

As the ethnographer, you may have a designated *role* as a volunteer or informal helper, or you may need to work to position yourself as a student of the group's practices or just a friendly and respectful companion. Keep in mind that your participants will make sense of you every bit as much as you will make sense of them, and that you will not always like the role to which you are assigned. You will likely encounter impressions that you will need to counter, such as entry-level employees who think you are a spy from management or factions that wish to have you report their side of conflicts and to discount others' perspectives. Still others may be intimidated by your expertise and respond defensively or antagonistically to your presence. The first author of this chapter found it beneficial to have a simple explanation for why she was observing in a clinic and what she intended to do. For example, she explained to dialysis staff (whose shifts changed weekly), visitors, patients, and visiting physicians that she was interested in the mundane or everyday aspects of communication, or what she called "the little things that you do all day without thinking about it in order to get your job done" (Ellingson, 2011).

Remember that the ethnographer is an embodied presence in the field (Bresler, 2006; Ellingson, 2006; Sharma, Reimer-Kirkham, & Cochrane, 2009). We tend to talk about knowledge as though it were obtained through some sort of disembodied, immaculate process, instead of the complex, human processes that it involves. In a very real sense, the ethnographer is the research instrument; her body, mind, and cultural signifiers become the tools through which perceptions and information are taken in, made sense of, and rendered meaningful. Gender, race, and bodily comportment matter. Moreover, open up all your senses to take in knowledge beyond what you see and hear—what do textures of the furniture feel like? How comfortable is the seating, how crowded is the room? What smells can you detect? What is the temperature? What sounds besides voices permeate the space? How would you describe the quality of the light—harsh, yellow, natural, bright? Get as many of these details down as you can and remember that *all* senses are part of sense making.

Advice on how long to make fieldwork sessions varies, but we recommend that you not spend more than a couple of hours at a time without a break. Scratch notes, or jottings, are the abbreviated ideas, key phrases, and descriptions that you jot down surreptitiously while in the field—or sometimes hiding in the restroom, back room, or some other (sort of) private space during observations (Emerson, Fretz, & Shaw, 2011). The longer you stay, the more you need to jot in order to prime your memory for writing field notes. Most ethnographers are surprised at how much they can recall when they focus on reconstructing their memories. With practice, you will be able to attend to many details and to notice many aspects of verbal and nonverbal communication within your ethnographic setting. As fieldwork continues, you eventually will focus on a few key aspects of communication, and your subsequent observations and conversations will concentrate on those in developing your findings. Also, as you become more familiar with your setting and participants, you will find that you quickly are able to recognize routine types of interactions, processes, and events, and thus your mind is freed to notice the ways in which a typical incident is both unique and similar to previously observed incidents.

Data Construction: Logbook, Field Notes, Reflections

Logbook

Before the ethnography begins, set up a logbook for the project, which will serve as a designated space for information on the human subject review board, grant applications, schedules for observation and/or interviews, designated pseudonyms for participants, details you need to follow up on, questions or information you need to find. Other things you may include: organizational/group documents, artifacts, participatory artwork, interview transcripts. Traditionally, logbooks have been three-ring binders or hard-copy files, but increasingly ethnographers save all information electronically, retaining computer files and scanning hard-copy materials to store as PDF files.

Field Notes

While in the field, take scratch notes whenever possible—jotted words or phrases to jump-start your memory later. Field notes are not neutral but motivated written accounts of your observation and participation within the setting (Emerson et al., 2011). Indeed, in many ways, field notes say as much or more about the ethnographer as they do about the observed participants, as the choices of details to note and the words used to describe those details are grounded in the researcher's standpoint (Behar, 1996). Immediately upon exiting your setting/group, write your field notes. Do not wait, as your ability to recall, especially the order of events, declines rapidly over time (Warren & Karner, 2009). Field notes should be labeled with the date and time of observation. Begin writing all you can recall, using your scratch notes as a guide and then adding in details. Develop shorthand for commonly used terms and for key participants' names to speed up your writing. Resist the urge to edit yourself, and, instead, write down everything, reserving judgment on what is important until later. Some ethnographers prefer to segment their notes by type, while others (including us) prefer to write narratively as thoughts come to us, freely mixing personal reactions—fear, disgust, frustration, embarrassment—with theoretical linkages, analytical insights, and specific details from that day's time in the field.

Research Journal

You should also begin a research journal. In a separate notebook or computer file, give yourself a space for free-ranging reflexivity, recording any and all ongoing thoughts and ideas, emotions, preliminary themes, or key ideas as they emerge for you. Such reflections may address the ongoing progress of the study, decisions about organizing and analyzing site visits and data, evolving perceptions about oneself and the participants. Any ideas—no matter how big or seemingly small—should be recorded. There is a reason they gave you pause. You may think you will always remember the great idea or keen perception you just had, but there are so many things happening that it will likely vanish if not recorded. We have found our journals to be invaluable in our studies. They often serve as the basis for recounting many methodological decisions and practices. And some of the analytical notes made here assume notable significance later on as related events occur.

A final note on procedure: We have learned from painful experience to be sure to maintain a back-up of all information, forms, field notes, and other data to protect your project. In addition, be sure to maintain a master copy that you do not alter in any way as you engage in analysis. Use separate copies of electronic or paper files on which to make notes, cut and paste quotes from, etc., so as not to risk accidentally destroying part of your data.

Analysis and Sense Making

Analysis of field notes, interview transcripts, organizational documents, and other data can be accomplished using one or a combination of data analysis methods, depending upon the questions addressed and the ideological and methodological commitments of the researcher. As with all interpretative methods, ethnography involves a nonlinear, inductive process. Importantly, analysis does not begin after data collection, but is concurrent with it in the form of notes, reflections, and analytic memos. We concur with Richardson (2000) that writing is not merely a "mopping up" phase, but begins with the writing of notes and reflections.

In his classic treatise on social science methodology, Kaplan (1964) distinguishes between "logic-in-use," the "more or less logical" way of thinking people employ to solve problems, and "reconstructed logic," which attempts to "formulate it explicitly" after the fact. He notes that "comparative ethnology made us painfully aware" that there is no such thing as "a universal rationality" (p. 8). Instead, numerous logics-in-use inform health communication practices as well as our research about them. Reconstructed logics developed after our studies guide future activities for healthcare participants and scholars. In describing ethnography as a method for understanding health communication in its lived contexts, we find it vital to recognize the mutually conditioning relationships between logics-in-use and reconstructed logics. Our accounts and those of our participants in describing their activities (as well as our own) are always reconstructions of practices addressing with diverse mixtures of reason and emotion the moment at hand.

Ethnographers used to refer to such work simply as "ethnographic analysis," and some still do, but it is far more common now to designate a specific tradition, such as grounded theory or constant comparative analysis (Charmaz, 2000), narrative analysis (see Yamasaki, Sharf, Harter, this volume), or critical analysis (e.g., Madison, 2005). Traditionally, it was common practice for ethnographers to produce "confessional tales" published separately from their findings (Van Maanen, 1989). Of course, researchers can and do produce separate reflection pieces, sometimes as autoethnography, but others now blend reflections on their own sense making and personal experiences with their ethnographic findings (Lindlof & Taylor, 2011). Although many options exist for analysis of ethnographic data, we will explain two that occupy different ranges of the epistemological/methodological continuum: grounded theory (i.e., constant comparative) analysis, and narrative ethnography.

Grounded Theory

Grounded theory (GT) can be thought of as middle, with nods to both the interpretive and the more scientific post-positivist perspectives. GT has a rich history and trajectory in ethnographic research (Charmaz & Mitchell, 2001). While there are important variations in GT, all have certain commonalties in process. Charmaz (2006) revised Glaser and Strauss' (1967) initial framing of GT methodology, placing it within a social constructivist framework and forming a more flexible, reflexive practice of GT. The steps of traditional GT analysis outlined by Corbin and Strauss (2008) and Charmaz (2006) resemble each other and other conceptualizations of GT. Analysis should occur throughout the data-gathering period, rather than beginning afterward.

First, engage in open coding of data, including field notes, transcripts, and any other documents. This coding can be done using a specially designed qualitative analysis software package, such as ATLAS.ti or HyperRESEARCH, and you can do it the traditional way of writing descriptive words and phrases in the margins of printed copies of data. The goal is to radically reduce your data so that you can detect themes and patterns. We urge our students to make codes of no more than three words each, thus requiring them to be thoughtful and precise. Ideally, ethnographers do "line by line" coding, meaning that they code each printed line of data. However, most of us are somewhat looser in actual practice, often summarizing two or three lines with a single code.

Next, develop preliminary inductive categories or themes and write memos in which you explicate each theme and examine several pieces of data (quotations from participants, field note descriptions, etc.) as they exemplify the category. As you notice what data does and does not fit in each of your categories, you will then engage in the third step. This step involves continually revising the definitions and parameters of categories; at times, combining one or more into a single category, breaking a single category into distinct subcategories, and/or shifting the scope and angle of a category to accommodate additional data pieces and remove others. As you collect data and analyze, you should engage in ongoing comparison of data within the data set and to existing research, concepts, and theory in order to inductively construct meaningful findings (Corbin & Strauss, 2008). No substitute exists for this messy, frustrating, and often highly engaging experience of building and rebuilding patterns until you arrive at a conceptual typology that describes (much of) your data. As you continue collecting data and discerning a focus for your inquiry, continue writing memos and revising categories until you reach "saturation," meaning that further data collected fit well with existing findings (Kerr, Nixon, & Wild, 2010). Axial coding entails thoughtful consideration of how your codes interrelate and come together to form a meaningful typology and collectively constitute a theory (Charmaz, 2006).

Further, it is impossible simply to "discover" patterns in data; you must co-construct them. We encourage ethnographers to engage in reflexive consideration of their own roles in data gathering and analysis to enhance attention to the subtleties of meaning in data (Corbin & Strauss, 2008). For example, in a study of a dialysis clinic, Ellingson (2011) reflected upon issues that influenced her sense making—such as differences between her formal educational attainment and that of the paraprofessionals, her freedom to come and go freely from the clinic, her White privilege in a markedly diverse group of patients and staff that often included people of eight or more ethnicities at any one time in the clinic, and her own limping, scarred, cancer-survivor body—as a part of her interactions with patients and staff. Most grounded theory analyses are written in conventional research reporting genres, but, increasingly, some are engaging with artistic genres and multimedia representations. Such investigations blend traditional report writing with photography in a study of the quality of life among African American breast cancer survivors (López, Eng, Randall-David, & Robinson, 2005) or perform poetic transcription in a study of professionalism among dialysis care technicians (Ellingson, 2011). We return to such efforts in our concluding section on current trends.

Narrative Ethnography

Narrative ethnography emphasizes that all human beings are storytellers, which importantly shapes its analytical materials and practices. Narrative ethnographers believe the persons and settings they investigate are best understood through examining the stories participants tell about themselves and their lived experiences. Viewed as products of their storytelling in the field or in formal interviews, and as objects for analysis, stories can provide extensive information about participants' recalled experiences communicating about illness, and delivering or receiving health care in actual settings. Such stories offer distinctive attributes for analysis: (a) they uniquely portray the meanings and significance that persons assign to events in their lives, (b) they embody specific points of view of the teller and emphasize particular features of the cultural context being described, (c) they reveal choices that were made and how events unfolded over time according the storyteller, and (d) they display versions of the storyteller's identity as a character in the story and in the role of storyteller (Rawlins, 2009).

When viewed as finished *products*, individual stories collected from research participants can be analyzed in various ways. Stories may be coded as representing certain themes or subthemes; for example, a story about a caring and sensitive healthcare provider, or a story depicting the inaccessibility of certain kinds of treatment for specific persons. Alternatively, investigators may identify standard literary devices appearing in the stories: Who are the main characters—protagonists and antagonists, heroes, and villains? How does the story's setting shape the characters' possibilities for action? What is the basic plot, conflict, quest, or climax of the story? Charon (2006) advocates "close reading" of narratives to discover how the teller frames narrated events, assigns motives to characters, and conveys the coda, point, or moral of the story. The unique attributes of stories allow for multiple readings based on different research questions and participants' and investigators' points of view. Confronting the richness of information offered by narratives, researchers have to make choices.

When narrative ethnographers emphasize the communicative *process* of storytelling over stories as finished products, they explore the ongoing dialogical potentials of storytelling relationships for co-constructing meanings and knowledge (Frank, 2000). While owning their role in the process, researchers seek to understand what matters to *this* storyteller at *this* place and time in voicing *this* narrative. Listening respectfully to others' renderings of their own lives is a primary responsibility in this form of narrative analysis (Thomas, 2010), yielding distinctive questions. How is the listener implicated in this moment of telling? To what extent does the storyteller seem to invite the listener to reaffirm a world they share, or to recognize and feel the depth and complexities of their differences (Frank, 2000)? Should this story be understood as a call for witnesses to this person's or group's struggles and triumphs? How are the identities and convictions of all the participants affected by engaging in the meaning-making activities of storytelling?

Narrative-as-process ethnographers perform their analyses by involving narrative activity throughout their work. Writing is a way of knowing and a significant part of one's method. As one jots down field notes, transcribes interviews, and examines documents, an investigator is always already co-telling, analyzing, making sense of and appraising events, noting converging and diverging accounts. Engaging with multiple materials, types of discourse, details, feelings, events, and timelines, writing as analysis is neither linear nor pre-determined, which can drastically limit what may be learned; "The form will evolve during the research process" (Ellis & Bochner, 2000, p. 757). Narrative ethnographers render a story about what they have learned through co-constructing, attending to, and analyzing their participants' stories, as well as their own role in the process. Their meta-stories about their research impose the closure of writing on human activities that always remain open to other interpretations (Clifford & Marcus, 1986).

Observation, writing field notes, and conducting analysis all involve thoughtful processes that necessitate extensive practice before ethnographers become proficient. With patience and experience, ethnographers generate rich findings that make significant contributions to health communication research and practical applications to healthcare delivery, health campaigns, and everyday experiences of health and illness.

Ethnographic Validities

Reliability and validity are traditional standards for assessing the trustworthiness of data analysis procedures. The validity of ethnography is grounded in the claim that a researcher has *been there*—wherever "there" might be (Lindlof & Taylor, 2011). Being there and writing about what one sees, hears, feels, smells, and tastes there constitute the essence of ethnography. Reliability—the degree to which a scale obtains a similar result when participants are retested or a coding scheme is applied consistently by multiple researchers—is not applicable to ethnography. As an interactive study of naturally occurring groups, ethnography cannot be repeated. Moreover, the fact that multiple ethnographers would generate somewhat (or very) different results is not considered a weakness but an inherent aspect of the naturalistic paradigm (Lincoln & Guba, 1985). Here, we briefly review three approaches to ethnographic validity.

Post-Positivist/Constructivist Validities

Fitch (1994) established the following standards for qualitative data analysis: (a) researchers should have been deeply involved with the group or topic; (b) at the same time, researchers also must achieve sufficient distance from participants to gain a broader perspective; (c) claims should be saturated in data; (d) data should be preserved as accessible records; and (e) data and analysis should include consideration of inferences and interpretations, as well as concrete phenomena (p. 36). Charmaz (2005) offers four criteria for evaluation that reflect a somewhat broader and more applied focus on what is valuable: credibility of the data collection, analysis, and representation processes; originality of the analysis and of its significance; resonance of the analysis with participants and larger social trends; and usefulness of findings for both everyday life and further research (p. 528). Each set of standards emphasizes careful attention to researcher processes; these guidelines are structured yet flexible, grounded in intersubjectivity and accountability.

Narrative Validity

Narrative validity in ethnography involves distinctive assumptions about narrative truth and doing justice to lived experiences. First, all storytelling, including ethnography, transpires in a narrative present—a here and now that occasions the narration. We tell stories at given moments to reconcile past, present, and future actions. Whereas historical truth seeks to accurately reflect past events, narrative truth articulates their significance for the storyteller's present situation and emerging choices—how they might inform future actions with others (Spence, 1982). Next, instead of viewing life as lived first and then narrated, narrative truth assumes the interdependence of living and telling. Persons narrate current events in their lives, clarifying thoughts and feelings while they occur. Previous actions also may take on different meanings due to their emerging consequences and present accounting, which may, in turn, alter future possibilities. This inter-animation of living and narrating blurs distinctions between fact and fiction. What matters are the meanings continuously made and shared. Third, avoiding abstraction through concrete and evocative writing, compelling narratives invite dialogue. A key feature of narrative validity is the capacity of the story to involve others and enable them to think, feel, and converse with the story

(Frank, 1995, 2000). Given narrative ethnography's respect for diverse lived experiences, valued narratives demonstrate a dialogic capacity for displaying and engaging with multiple meanings and worldviews among participants, authors and readers (Ellis & Bochner, 2000; Frank, 2000). Finally, narrative ethnographies gain validity through authors reflexively owning and interrogating their positionality, communicative practices with research participants, and the contingencies of producing their accounts.

Artistic/Interpretive Validity

Richardson (2000) offers a useful set of criteria for evaluating the quality of what she calls "creative analytic practices," or forms of representation that accompany or replace traditional report writing with narratives, performance, poetry, photography, and other artwork. First, "substantive contribution" concerns the degree to which the reader/audience is offered meaningful knowledge about the topic under investigation, such as communication among healthcare providers working together in a clinic. Second, "aesthetic merit" assesses the value of the representation using literary and artistic standards of quality, much as one would evaluate a novel or painting. This criterion embodies an axiom that, in order to be a valid creative representation of findings, the representation must succeed as art. "Reflexivity" is the third standard of validity, and this refers to the capacity of the work to demonstrate to the audience that the researchers critically reflected upon their own role in the construction of findings.

Next, "impact" on the audience is vital; this standard asserts that validity comes, in part, from the work's ability to engender an emotional, cognitive, physical, or spiritual response from those who view, listen, or read it. Finally, Richardson offers the criterion of "expression of reality," meaning that representations should be judged on how they present, or fail to present, a rich, embodied, realistic portrayal of participants' lived experiences. Another concept we find useful in assessing validity of artful health communication ethnography is "catalytic validity," which "refers to the degree to which the research process re-orients, focuses, and energizes participants in what Freire (1973) terms 'conscientization,' knowing reality in order to better transform it" (Lather, 1986, p. 67). That is, empowering participants to act on behalf of themselves and their communities is a valuable outcome of research and constitutes evidence of an ethical and pragmatic research validity.

Strengths and Limitations of Ethnography

Strengths

Ethnography has much to offer the field of health communication as a complement to the positivist and post-positivist methodological perspectives that underlie the vast majority of extant research. We find it most productive not to think about (or represent) ethnographic work as being in competition with or critical of research that falls closer to the science pole of the continuum. Instead, we promote dialogue with more traditional researchers in health communication, medicine, nursing, and allied health by explaining some of the unique contributions made by ethnographic work. Leading the list is "thick description" (Geertz, 1973), the rich, vivid accounts of communication that provide necessary details for understanding complex phenomena, such as suffering, dignity, or collaboration, that do not reduce readily to discrete variables. Moreover, these thick descriptions are of *actual interactions*; they are not artificial conditions created by researchers for the purpose of testing responses, but, instead, involve people behaving in the very settings that researchers seek to help understand and improve. Further, these descriptions often are *embodied*, highlighting the ways in which our corporeal selves are inescapably part of every interaction. Next, ethnographic descriptions allow for *multiple perspectives* to be shared in an account. Ethnographers can describe varied versions of an interaction, illustrating it from, for example, the perspectives of a physician, patient, patient's loved one, nurse, and researcher in order to demonstrate how differently meaning can be constructed from diverse standpoints. Ethnographers also offer *depth of understanding* of a specific space; what we may sacrifice in breadth and generalizability we more than make up for with clarity, complexity, and *depth*. Finally, ethnography is tremendously *pragmatic* in its implications. Ethnographic accounts reveal patterns that suggest concrete organizational policies, practice guidelines, opportunities for training and development, and process remedies that may improve communication within a range of comparable settings.

Limitations

Two primary limitations of ethnography persist. First is the credence of method. Because it is interpretative and hence generates neither generalizable findings nor evidence of causal relationships among variables, ethnographic methods are not accepted in some professional journals and are looked at with disfavor by some universities, foundations, institutes, and funding agencies, or seen as merely preliminary to more stringent tools of research. Second, ethnography is painstaking, time intensive, and requires both a high tolerance for ambiguity on the part of the researcher and openness to continual scrutiny by participants. These factors make it a challenging method to utilize, particularly for busy academics with competing time commitments, but, for us, the rewards of ethnography outweigh the costs.

Recent Developments and Controversies

In concluding, we discuss two recent trends in ethnography of health communication: first, disseminating ethnographic research in multiple genres to multiple stakeholder communities within a framework that considers all forms of representation and puts them "in conversation" with each other; and, second, utilizing social justice and participatory methods that empower participants and highlight their voices.

Cultivating Representational Possibilities Through Multi-Genre Crystallization

Ethnographic work may be enhanced through a postmodern-influenced approach to triangulation that Ellingson (2009) terms "crystallization." This approach urges researchers to complement research reports of findings with community performances and presentations, articles in newsletters, narratives, websites, organizational reports, professional trainings, videos, and other forms of representation for a wide variety of stakeholders (Ellingson & Quinlan, 2012). At the same time, the approach claims all of these varied representations not merely as public dissemination required by funding agencies or civic duty, but also as collectively constituting a postmodern validity to interpretative research. Richardson (2000) invoked the crystal as alternative metaphor to the two-dimensional, positivist image of a triangle as the basis for methodological rigor and validity. Ellingson (2009) further articulated this alternative to triangulation:

> Crystallization combines multiple forms of analysis and multiple genres of representation into a coherent text or series of related texts, building a rich and openly partial account of a phenomenon that problematizes its own construction, highlights researchers' vulnerabilities and positionality, makes claims about socially constructed meanings, and reveals the indeterminacy of knowledge claims even as it makes them.
>
> *(p. 4)*

Crystallization thus promotes diverse perspectives on topics that represent multiple points on the methodological continuum, while destabilizing those same claims. The framework enhances research validity through pragmatic, ethical, and representational rigor (see also Janesick, 2000; Saukko, 2004).

Crystallization features two primary types. *Integrated crystallization* refers to multi-genre texts that incorporate the above principles in a single, coherent representation (e.g., a book, a performance). It may take one of two basic forms: woven, in which small pieces of two or more genres are layered together in a complex blend; or patched, in which larger pieces of two or more genres are juxtaposed to one another in a clearly demarcated sequence. In an ethnography of backstage teamwork on an interdisciplinary geriatric oncology team, Ellingson (2005) highlighted the constructed nature of accounts via patched crystallization, juxtaposing genres in a series of chapters—ethnographic narrative, grounded theory analysis, autoethnography, and feminist critique. This structure demonstrated how all the accounts inevitably invoked authorial power (Ellingson, 2005; see also Bach, 1998; Lather & Smithies, 1997). *Dendritic crystallization* refers to the dispersed process of making meaning through multiple forms of analysis and multiple genres of representation without (or in addition to) combining genres into a single text. A particular benefit of conceptualizing the production of a series of separate representations as collectively constituting postmodern methodological triangulation is scholarly legitimacy and support for academics to reach multiple audiences within and outside the academy while earning scholarly credit for work often considered to be "only" professional service. A compelling description of a health communication ethnography, incorporating dispersed representations that reflect multiple points on the continuum, is found in Harter's work on the practice of narrative medicine, which includes a documentary film and a book, among other genres (Harter, 2012; Harter & Hayward, 2010).

Promoting Social Justice through Ethnography

The practice of ethnography in health communication also is employed for exposing and addressing injustice that characterized the original Chicago School, many members of which explored marginalized groups in urban settings (see Lindlof & Taylor, 2011; Warren & Karner, 2009). Conquergood (1995) argued that research is always political, and never neutral; researchers "must choose between research that is 'engaged' or 'complicit'" (p. 85). Researchers cannot remain uninvolved—to refuse to advocate or to assist is to reinforce existing power relations, not to remain impartial. Calls to socially engaged work proliferate across the social sciences (e.g., Denzin & Giardina, 2009; Denzin & Lincoln, 2011; Frey & Carragee, 2007), often under the rubric of applied (Frey & Cissna, 2009), translational (Zerhouni, 2005), participatory action (Wang, 1999), or feminist research processes (Hesse-Biber, 2007). We encourage ethnographers to think of their work as *always already political* in its practices and implications and to highlight the material and ideological implications of our research practices and findings (Miller-Day, 2008).

By consciously producing written, oral, and/or visual accounts that meet specific needs and interests of diverse audiences, ethnographers can foster social justice. To reach practitioners, policymakers, and other stakeholders, we must engage in meaningful dialogue—a process that requires us to listen as much as (or more than) we speak. When we bring our ideas and willingness to collaborate to divergent academic disciplines (Parrott, 2008) and to the general public, we act as scholars and as public intellectuals who "embody and enact moral leadership" (Papa & Singhal, 2007, pp. 126–127). When we speak out, we move beyond the important work of knowledge creation and theory building to apply our scholarly resources to benefit publics more directly. The more varied our ethnographic toolbox, the more opportunities we have to creatively address social inequities and work for positive change. Examples of this trend utilize mixed methods research designs (Mertens, 2007; Sosulski & Lawrence, 2008) and visual and participatory methods such as photovoice (Singhal, Harter, Chitnis, & Sharma, 2007).

References

Agar, M. H. (1980). *The professional stranger: An informal introduction to ethnography.* New York, NY: Academic Press.

Arrington, M. I., Grant, C. H., & Vanderford, M. L. (2005). Man to man and side by side, they cope with prostate cancer: Self-help and social support. *Journal of Psychosocial Oncology, 23*(4), 81–102.

Atkinson, P., Coffey, A., Delamont, S., Lofland, J., & Lofland, L. (2001). Editorial introduction. In P. Atkinson, A. Coffey, S. Delamont, J. Lofland, & L. Lofland (Eds.), *Handbook of ethnography* (pp. 160–174). Thousand Oaks, CA: Sage Publications.

Bach, H. (1998). *A visual narrative concerning curriculum, girls, photography, etc.* Walnut Creek, CA: Left Coast Press.

Baxter, L. A., & Montgomery, B. M. (1996). *Relating: Dialogue and dialectics.* New York, NY: Guilford Press.

Behar, R. (1996). *The vulnerable observer: Anthropology that breaks your heart.* Boston, MA: Beacon Press.

Bloor, M. (2001). The ethnography of health and medicine. In P. Atkinson, A. Coffey, S. Delamont, J. Lofland, & L. Lofland (Eds.), *Handbook of ethnography* (pp. 177–187). London, England: Sage Publications.

Bresler, L. (2006). Embodied narrative inquiry: A methodology of connection. *Research Studies in Music Education, 27*(1), 21–43.

Charmaz, K. (2000). Grounded theory: Objectivist and constructivist methods. In N. K. Denzin & Y. S. Lincoln (Eds.), *Handbook of qualitative research* (2nd ed.) (pp. 509–535). Thousand Oaks, CA: Sage Publications.

Charmaz, K. (2006). *Constructing grounded theory: A practical guide through qualitative analysis.* Thousand Oaks, CA: Sage Publications.

Charmaz, K., & Mitchell, R. G. (2001). Grounded theory in ethnography. In P. Atkinson, A. Coffey, S. Delamont, J. Lofland, & L. Lofland (Eds.), *Handbook of ethnography* (pp. 160–174). Thousand Oaks, CA: Sage Publications.

Charon, R. (2006). *Narrative medicine: Honoring the stories of illness.* Oxford, England: Oxford University Press.

Clifford, J. & Marcus, G. E. (Eds.). (1986). *Writing culture: The poetics and politics of ethnography.* Berkeley, CA: University of California Press.

Coffey, A. (1999). *The ethnographic self: Fieldwork and the representation of identity.* London, England: Sage Publications.

Conquergood, D. (1995). Between rigor and relevance: Rethinking applied communication. In K. N. Cissna (Ed.), *Applied communication in the 21st century* (pp. 79–96). Mahwah, NJ: Lawrence Erlbaum Associates.

Considine, J., & Miller, K. (2010). The dialectics of care: Communicative choices at the end of life. *Health Communication, 25*(2), 165–174.

Corbin, J. M., & Strauss, A. L. (2008). *Basics of qualitative research: Techniques and procedures for developing grounded theory* (3rd ed.). Los Angeles, CA: Sage Publications.

Denzin, N. K. (1997) *Interpretive ethnography: Ethnographic practices for the 21st century.* Thousand Oaks, CA: Sage Publications.

Denzin, N. K., & Giardina, M. D. (2009). *Qualitative inquiry and social justice: Toward a politics of hope.* Walnut Creek, CA: Left Coast Press.

Denzin, N. K., & Lincoln, Y. S. (Eds.). (2011). *The SAGE handbook of qualitative research* (4th ed.). Thousand Oaks, CA: Sage Publications.

Du Pré, A. (1998). *Humor and the healing arts: A multimethod analysis of humor use in health care.* Mahwah, NJ: Lawrence Erlbaum Associates.

Ellingson, L. L. (2005). *Communicating in the clinic: Negotiating frontstage and backstage teamwork.* Cresskill, NJ: Hampton Press.

Ellingson, L. L. (2006). Embodied knowledge: Writing researchers' bodies into qualitative health research. *Qualitative Health Research, 16*(2), 298–310.

Ellingson, L. L. (2009). *Engaging crystallization in qualitative research.* Thousand Oaks, CA: Sage Publications.

Ellingson, L. L. (2011). The poetics of professionalism among dialysis technicians. *Health Communication, 26*(1), 1–12.

Ellingson, L. L., & Quinlan, M. M. (2012) Beyond the research/service dichotomy: Claiming ALL research products for hiring, evaluation, tenure, and promotion. *Qualitative Communication Research, 1*(3), 385–399.

Ellis, C. (2004). *The ethnographic I: A methodological novel about autoethnography.* Walnut Creek, CA: AltaMira Press.

Ellis, C., & Bochner, A. P. (2000). Autoethnography, personal narrative, reflexivity: Researcher as subject. In N. K. Denzin & Y. S. Lincoln (Eds.), *Handbook of qualitative research* (2nd ed.) (pp. 733–768). Thousand Oaks, CA: Sage Publications.

Ellis, C., & Ellingson, L. L. (2000). Qualitative methods. In E. F. Borgatta & R. J. V. Montgomery (Eds.), *Encyclopedia of Sociology* (2nd ed.) (Vol. 4; pp. 2287–2296). New York, NY: Macmillan Reference USA.

Emerson, R. M., Fretz, R. I., & Shaw, L. L. (2011). *Writing ethnographic fieldnotes* (2nd ed.). Chicago, IL: University of Chicago Press.

Fitch, K. L. (1994). Criteria for evidence in qualitative research. *Western Journal of Communication, 58*(1), 32–38.

Foster, E. (2007). *Communicating at the end of life: Finding magic in the mundane.* Mahwah, NJ: Lawrence Erlbaum Associates.

Frank, A. W. (1995). *The wounded storyteller: Body, illness, and ethics.* Chicago, IL: University of Chicago Press.

Frank, A. W. (2000). The standpoint of the storyteller. *Qualitative Health Research, 10*(3), 354–365.

Frey, L. R., & Carragee, K. M.. (2007). *Communication activism—Vol. 1: Communication for social change.* Cresskill, NJ: Hampton Press.

Frey, L. R., & Cissna, K. N. (Eds.) (2009). *The Routledge handbook of applied communication research.* New York, NY: Routledge.

Gardezi, F., Lingard, L., Espin, S., Whyte, S., Orser, B., & Baker, G. R. (2009). Silence, power and communication in the operating room. *Journal of Advanced Nursing, 65*(7), 1390–1399.

Geertz, C. (1973). *The interpretation of cultures: Selected essays.* New York, NY: Basic Books.

Glaser, B. G., & Strauss, A. L. (1967). *The discovery of grounded theory: Strategies for qualitative research.* Chicago, IL: Aldine Publishing Company.

Golden, M. A. (2009). Walking with Grandma through cancer and caregiving. *Iowa Journal of Communication, 41*(1), 73–92.

Golden, M. A. (2010). Dialectical contradictions experienced when placing a spouse with dementia in a residential care facility. *Qualitative Research Reports in Communication, 11*(1), 14–20.

Harter, L. M. (2012). *Imagining new normals: A narrative framework for health communication.* Dubuque, IA: Kendall Hunt Publishers.

Harter, L. M. [producer], & Hayward, C [director]. (2010). *The art of the possible* [film]. Athens, Ohio: Ohio University.

Hesse-Biber, S. N. (Ed.) (2007). *Handbook of feminist research: Theory and praxis.* Thousand Oaks, CA: Sage Publications.

Hesse-Biber, S. N. (2010). Qualitative approaches to mixed methods practice. *Qualitative Inquiry, 16*(6), 455–468.

Janesick, V. J. (2000). The choreography of qualitative research design: Minuets, improvisations, and crystallization. In N. K. Denzin & Y. S. Lincoln (Eds.), *Handbook of qualitative research* (2nd ed.) (pp. 379–399). Thousand Oaks, CA: Sage Publications.

Kaplan, A. (1964). *The conduct of inquiry: methodology for behavioral sciences.* Scranton, PA: Chandler Publishing.

Kerr, C., Nixon, A., & Wild, D. (2010). Assessing and demonstrating data saturation in qualitative inquiry supporting patient-reported outcomes research. *Expert Review of Pharmacoeconomics and Outcomes Research, 10*(3), 269–281.

Lather, P. (1986). Issues of validity in openly ideological research: Between a rock and a soft place. *Interchange, 17*(4), 63–84.

Lather, P., & Smithies, C. (1997). *Troubling the angels: Women living with HIV/AIDS.* Boulder, CO: Westview Press.

Lincoln, Y. S., & Guba, E. G. (1985). *Naturalistic inquiry.* Thousand Oaks, CA: Sage Publications.

Lindlof, T. R., & Taylor, B. C. (2011). *Qualitative communication research methods* (3rd ed.). Thousand Oaks, CA: Sage Publications.

López, E., Eng, E., Randall-David, E., & Robinson, N. (2005). Quality-of-life concerns of African American breast cancer survivors within rural North Carolina: Blending the techniques of photovoice and grounded theory. *Qualitative Health Research, 15*(1), 99–115.

Madison, D. S. (2005). *Critical ethnography: Method, ethics, and performance.* Thousand Oaks, CA: Sage Publications.

Mertens, D. M. (2007). Transformative paradigm: Mixed methods and social justice. *Journal of Mixed Methods Research, 1*(3), 212–225.

Miller-Day, M. A. (2008). Performance matters. *Qualitative Inquiry, 14*(8), 1458–1470.

Minge, J. M. (2007). The stained body: A fusion of embodied art on rape and love. *Journal of Contemporary Ethnography, 36*(3), 252–280.

Morgan-Witte, J. M. (2005). Narrative knowledge development among caregivers: Stories from the nurse's station. In L. M. Harter, P. M. Japp, & C. S. Beck (Eds.), *Narratives, health, and healing: Communication theory, research, and practice* (pp. 217–236). Mahwah, NJ: Lawrence Erlbaum Associates.

Opie, A. (2000). *Thinking teams, thinking clients: Knowledge-based teamwork.* New York, NY: Columbia University.

Papa, M. J., & Singhal, A. (2007). Intellectuals searching for publics: Who is out there? *Management Communication Quarterly, 21*(1), 126–136.

Parrott, R. (2008). A multiple discourse approach to health communication: Translational research and ethical practice. *Journal of Applied Communication Research, 36*(1), 1–7.

Potter, W. J. (1996). *An analysis of thinking and research about qualitative methods*. Mahwah, NJ: Lawrence Erlbaum Associates.

Propp, K. M., Apker, J., Zabava Ford, W. S., Wallace, N., Serbenski, M., & Hofmeister, N. (2010). Meeting the complex needs of the health care team: Identification of nurse–team communication practices perceived to enhance patient outcomes. *Qualitative Health Research, 20*(1), 15–28.

Rambo Ronai, C. (1995). Multiple reflections of child sex abuse: An argument for a layered account. *Journal of Contemporary Ethnography, 23*, 395–426.

Rawlins, W. K. (2005). Our family's physician. In L. Harter, P. Japp, & C. Beck (Eds.) *Narratives, health, and healing: Communication theory, research, and practice* (pp. 197–216). Mahwah, NJ: Lawrence Erlbaum Associates.

Rawlins, W. K. (2009). *The compass of friendship: Narratives, identities, and dialogues*. Thousand Oaks, CA: Sage Publications.

Richardson, L. (2000). Writing: A method of inquiry. In N. K. Denzin & Y. S. Lincoln (Eds.), *Handbook of qualitative research* (2nd ed.) (pp. 923–943). Thousand Oaks, CA: Sage Publications.

Saukko, P. (2004). *Doing research in cultural studies: An introduction to classical and new methodological approaches*. Thousand Oaks, CA: Sage Publications.

Sharma, S., Reimer-Kirkham, S., & Cochrane, M. (2009). Practicing the awareness of embodiment in qualitative health research: Methodological reflections. *Qualitative Health Research, 19*(11), 1642–1650.

Singhal, A., Harter, L. M., Chitnis, K., & Sharma, D. (2007). Participatory photography as theory, method and praxis: Analyzing an entertainment–education project in India. *Critical Arts, 21*(1), 212–227.

Sosulski, M. R., & Lawrence, C. (2008). Mixing methods for full-strength results. *Journal of Mixed Methods Research, 2*(2), 121–148.

Spence, D. P. (1982). *Narrative truth and historical truth: Meaning and interpretation in psychoanalysis*. New York, NY: W. W. Norton.

The, A. M., Hak, T., Koëter G., & van der Wal, G. (2001). Collusion in doctor–patient communication about imminent death: An ethnographic study. *Western Journal of Medicine, 174*(4), 247–253.

Thomas, C. (2010). Negotiating the contested terrain of narrative methods in illness contexts. *Sociology of Health & Illness, 32*(4), 647–660.

Vande Berg, L., & Trujillo, N. (2008). *Cancer and death: A love story in two voices*. New York, NY: Hampton Press.

Van Maanen, J. (1989). *Tales of the field: On writing ethnography*. Chicago, IL: University of Chicago.

Ventres, W., Kooienga, S., Vuckovic, N., Marlin, R., Nygren, P., & Stewart, V. (2006). Physicians, patients, and the electronic health record: An ethnographic analysis. *Annals of Family Medicine, 4*(2), 124–131.

Wang, C. C. (1999). Photovoice: A participatory action research strategy applied to women's health. *Journal of Women's Health, 8*(2), 185–192.

Warren, C. A. B., & Karner, T. X. (2009). *Discovering qualitative methods: Field research, interviews, and analysis* (2nd ed.). New York, NY: Oxford University Press.

Wittenberg-Lyles, E. M., Cie' Gee, G., Oliver, D. P., & Demiris, G. (2009). What patients and families don't hear: Backstage communication in hospice interdisciplinary team meetings. *Journal of Housing For the Elderly, 23*(1–2), 92–105.

Zerhouni, E. A. (2005). Translational and clinical science—Time for a new vision. *The New England Journal of Medicine, 353*(15), 1621–1623.

SURVEY RESEARCH METHODOLOGY IN HEALTH COMMUNICATION

Susan E. Morgan and Nick Carcioppolo

There are often many paths that can be taken on a journey toward a single goal, and, while some paths may prove more efficient or interesting, it is nonetheless true that there is usually more than one way to get to a destination. Such is the case with research methods. For example, health communication scholars interested in increasing enrollment in cancer drug clinical trials may need to investigate patients' attitudes toward clinical trials, explore physicians' attitudes about offering clinical trial enrollment opportunities to patients, observe how oncologists communicate with patients about clinical trials, and determine the types of barriers physicians face to enrolling patients in clinical trials. All of these studies will help to answer important questions that might result in more effective interventions, but each yields very different types of information by way of very different types of investigations.

Surveys are tools that are often very useful in generating a wide variety of knowledge that allow researchers to better accomplish their broader goals. In this chapter, we will provide an overview of survey research methods in health communication. This chapter will help you understand when you should (and should not) use this research method. We will also identify the most important factors you should consider in order to create surveys that will yield the most productive, useful, and valid results.

Definitional and Theoretical Issues

Survey research methodology is one of the most popular, if not predominant, methods for investigation in the social sciences. While surveys are often thought to be synonymous with questionnaires, there are some distinctions that are worth mentioning. The word "survey" comes from the French *surveeir*, meaning "to oversee." A questionnaire is a list of questions. Thus, a survey is the task we seek to perform with a particular population, and the questionnaire is one of the most common tools we use to accomplish that task.

The data that result from surveys can be qualitative or quantitative in nature, and they can be collected using a variety of methods (in-person, computer-assisted, paper and pencil), but surveys rely on a set of common theoretical assumptions. Surveys tend to fall within the category of post-positivistic research approaches. This means that researchers using surveys (at least for the moment) believe that respondents have some piece of knowledge that they are able to convey that researchers can then combine with other pieces of knowledge to create new understandings about a phenomenon. For example, researchers may be interested in employees' level of participation in a worksite health promotion program as a way to evaluate the program's effectiveness. An even more common type of survey involves asking a large number of people about their attitudes and health behaviors as a way of increasing general understanding of the correlations between these variables, perhaps as a preliminary step toward creating a carefully targeted intervention to improve health outcomes.

Applications

Researchers use survey research methods when a phenomenon has parameters that are generally well understood. Additionally, surveys are used when large amounts of data are needed from a population in order to test relationships between variables (e.g., the effect of certain attitudes on self-reported behaviors). Surveys are popular because a lot of data about a large population can be collected at a relatively low expense. However, the information gathered can lack depth because of the inability to ask follow-up questions and the difficulty in gathering open-ended data using this format.

Although surveys can be used as part of formative research, they require that researchers at least understand the topic well enough to know which questions to ask. This may seem like a simple task, but the bigger the gap between the desired behavior and current behaviors, and the smaller the effect sizes (impact) of current interventions designed to address a health issue, the less likely it is that a researcher truly understands the reasons why a population has yet to adopt a preferred behavior. A basic level of understanding is best obtained through methodologically sound interpretative investigations, including ethnographies (see Ellingson & Rawlins, this volume), interviews, and focus groups (see Donovan-Kicken, Miller, & Goldsmith, this volume). These are, by design, smaller in scale than most surveys, and usually provide important information that can aid in the design of survey.

Surveys can include qualitative data, although the results are highly dependent on participants' abilities (and willingness) to articulate the responses to open-ended questions. Researchers can expect higher levels of response to these questions if circumstances are highly motivating (i.e., people in the sample are very frustrated about something), and if respondents believe that their responses will result in some desirable outcome, such as a change in policy or practice.

By contrast, survey research methods are unlikely to be used when researchers want to truly understand the (known or unknown) deeply held motivations, attitudes, and beliefs that affect a behavioral outcome of interest. These may constitute key barriers that are inhibiting targeted behavioral change. These are circumstances that call for strong qualitative investigations. Without a thorough understanding of the variables that affect health outcomes, it is unlikely that a campaign or other type of intervention will succeed.

Employing the Method

There are a number of steps involved with the design and execution of survey-based research. These steps will be described, including (a) deciding on a sampling frame, (b) choosing variables to measure, (c) selecting survey research instruments, (d) determining a research design, (e) deciding on a method of data collection, and (f) pilot testing the finished survey.

Decide on a Sampling Frame

Who is your population of interest? It makes little sense to survey the attitudes of the general U.S. population toward cancer screening when you are actually trying to understand why poor, uneducated Whites in Scranton, Pennsylvania, have low rates of participation in free cancer screenings. Be as specific in your targeting as possible, while recognizing that greater specificity often entails increased costs in time, money, and/or the sample size that can be reasonably obtained. Remember that you need to collect enough data to allow for statistical analysis of the results. Understanding why clinical oncologists at several targeted medical centers have a difficult time communicating with patients about cancer clinical trials might entail surveying oncologists nationwide who are in private practice in the hope that the findings extrapolate to the wider population, particularly if you are not able to conduct focus groups with oncologists at these particular medical centers. In survey research, there is often a fundamental trade-off between the specificity of the population you can reach and the costs involved with reaching a hard-to-access population.

Access a random, representative sample. A randomly selected, representative sample is the gold standard for survey research. Because researchers should anticipate a low response rate, a much larger number of people should be selected than the number of returned questionnaires needed. By contrast, going to an oncology conference to distribute your questionnaire to doctors in attendance will yield a sample that is neither random nor representative. Only oncologists attending the conference were selected and these doctors may be systematically different in some important ways from the larger population of oncologists.

However, there are times when a random, representative sample simply cannot be obtained. There are other non-representative, non-random sampling techniques (called *non-probability sampling*) that can be used to obtain valuable information. These techniques are not without their potential compromises to the validity of the resulting information, so great caution should be exercised when interpreting the data. However, if generalization to the population from which the sample was drawn is not one of the goals of the research (which could be the case in pilot studies or surveys for the purposes of formative research), then there are a number of techniques that can allow a researcher to gain helpful information relatively easily. These techniques include convenience sampling, snowball sampling, purposive sampling, and quota sampling.

Convenience sampling is simply sampling people who are most convenient for the researcher. Even if they are members of the population of interest (because they have Type 1 diabetes, for example), they are unlikely to be representative of the population. *Snowball sampling* can be used with hard-to-access populations, such as sex workers or other marginalized populations. In snowball sampling, one research participant refers the researcher to other people who might be interested in helping with the project. *Purposive sampling* involves carefully selecting individuals who represent a particular set of characteristics of special interest to complete a survey. Surveying only directors of public education at nonprofit organizations would be an example of purposive sampling. *Quota sampling* involves surveying a certain number of people who represent a particular group. For example, if a researcher wanted to understand how people of different Christian denominations thought about organ donation, he or she might survey 50 Catholics, 50 Lutherans, 50 Seventh Day Adventists, 50 German Baptists, and so on. (It would behoove the researcher to sample multiple congregations within each denomination, of course.)

Sample size. Determining the number of people needed to complete a survey (i.e., sample size) is a special challenge for researchers. It is too costly and too time consuming to survey every member of a population, so we have to select a subset of people to represent the group as a whole. However, it is also true that we need to survey enough people that we can be sure that we have a truly representative group, and so that we can conduct meaningful and reliable statistical analyses. Determining the number of research participants needed for a study is called power analysis (see Cohen, 1988; Murphy & Myors, 2003).

Special software can be used to perform power analyses to create a "best guess" for the number of subjects needed (not currently available as part of popular statistical software packages such as SPSS). This analysis must be done in advance of launching the survey (known as an *a priori* analysis). These programs include G-Power and SamplePower. In order to conduct a power analysis, you will need to be able to estimate the effect size of the relationship between the variables you are testing, the level of significance you are using (which is almost always set at .05), and your tolerance level for Type II error, which is the level of chance you are willing to allow that you might not be able to detect a true effect where one exists (usually, but not always, set to .80). In the event that you are testing multiple relationships (as is common), input the lowest effect size that appears to exist. The best way to estimate an effect size is to consult previous research studies. Most editors now require authors to report some measure of effect size. If you are evaluating the impact of an intervention, however, be aware that most rarely exceed an effect size of .01–.03, meaning that the intervention accounts for one to three percent of the variation in outcomes among the individuals participating in the survey. In fact, much health communication research suffers from fairly small effect sizes. The number of subjects needed to detect real effects may be depressingly enormous, but it is better to take a longer period of time and devote additional resources to data collection and have something to show for your efforts than to engage in a lengthy project and be virtually unable to publish the results because of non-significant results.

The most common way to increase power is to increase the sample size of the survey. However, it is also possible to increase power by reducing the standard deviation of key variables. The best way to do this (if it is possible at all) is to be very specific about the populations being examined. For example, be sure that you are testing the impact of an intervention on only the population of greatest interest. For example, the effect of an organ donation campaign on pretest versus posttest attitudes and behaviors should be tested only on non-donors, not on the entire group of people who may have been exposed to the campaign, since many people have already registered as donors. Also, improving the reliability of measures can increase effect sizes by reducing variation due to error in resulting scores. You can often increase the reliability of marginally reliable measures (Cronbach's alpha of, say, .70 or below) using Hayes' (2005) "alphamax" macro for SPSS and SAS. Alphamax is a tool that computes the most psychometrically robust subscale from a set of given items, maximizing the Cronbach's alpha for a particular scale.

Response rates. It is likely that you will discover that people of interest to you who refuse to complete your survey may be systematically different from those who do complete your survey. This introduces bias into your sample. If you have a small response rate, you should try to find out who your non-respondents are so you are clear about what you know about which segment of your target population. However, what constitutes a "good" response rate can vary according to the method of data collection. A summary of response rates by data collection method appears in Table 5.1.

What makes people more or less likely to complete a survey? Researchers often hope to invoke the principle of reciprocity (described well by Cialdini, 2008) through a number of common strategies designed to improve response rates by pre-giving a reward for participation. Some researchers use small, novel gifts, such as a $2 bill to increase compliance (Göritz, 2006; Porter, 2004), whereas many charitable organizations will use nickels, address labels, stickers, and cards.

TABLE 5.1 A Look at Typical Response Rates by Survey Type

Survey Type	*Typical Response Rates*
In person—paper/ computer	May be difficult to determine the response rate. Reported response rates for door-to-door surveys: 72.4% for an Australian health survey (Taylor, Wilson, & Wakefield, 1998), 78.1% for a University of Michigan sociology survey (Willimack, Schuman, Pennell, & Lepkowski, 1995). Response rates for types of in-person surveys other than door-to-door surveys are almost certainly not this high.
Remote—mail	The mean response rate for health surveys published in medical journals is 60%. Surveys published by physicians have a mean response rate of 54%; surveys published by social/behavioral researchers have a mean response rate of 68% (Asch, Jedrziewski, & Christakis, 1997). Average response rate to mailed paper surveys is 55.6% (Baruch, 1999), but response rates as high as 70% are achievable (Dillman, 2000).
Remote—computer	Meta-analyses estimate that response rates for Internet-delivered surveys are on average 11–20% lower than other types of surveys (Manfreda, Bosnjak, Berzelak, Haas, & Vehovar, 2008; Shih & Fan, 2009).
Remote—telephone	Currently around 40% on average, but declining about 1.5% each year (Tourangeau, 2010).

Small gifts, cash, redeemable loyalty points, and other prepaid incentives appear to increase response rate whereas post-paid incentives may not (Göritz, 2006; Porter, 2004). In general, gifts are less effective than cash (Singer, 2002). One meta-analysis found that monetary incentives increase response rate to mailed surveys by an average of 19% (Church, 1993). Non-monetary incentives can also prove to be effective. A study in New Zealand used chocolates as an incentive in a mailed survey, and found that it significantly increased participation in the first mailing, but not in the two subsequent mailings (Brennan & Charbonneau, 2009). Lottery drawings, which are often seen as an alternative to a guaranteed monetary incentive by cash-strapped researchers, appear to be ineffective in all but cross-sectional designs and student participants (Göritz & Wolff, 2007; Laguilles, Williams, & Saunders, 2011; Marcus, Bosnjak, Lindner, Pilischenko, & Schutz, 2007). The following factors also appear to play a role in maximizing response rates:

- Advance notification that they will be receiving a survey: People seem to feel less "put upon" when they've been forewarned that a researcher will be requesting their help at some point in the near future (usually, a few days in advance).

- Interest in the topic: People are more likely to complete questionnaires on topics of particular interest to them. Conversely, people are much less likely to participate in surveys on topics that make them feel uncomfortable or for which they feel some dissonance. Organ donation is a good example of a topic that many people feel uneasy thinking about.
- Survey length: Shorter surveys have higher response rates than longer surveys.
- Vocabulary/visual complexity: Any difficulties reading the survey will result in a drop in response rates. Questions should be simple; make sure that they are written at no more than an eighth-grade level for the general population. You can test this using a tool available on the Internet by searching for "readability index." Similarly, your survey should be attractive and easy to read. Do not crowd questions on a page and use ample white space.
- A sense of connection to the person or organization requesting participation is often very helpful. If you have no connection to the population, providing people with a clear idea of the importance of your project and its potential outcomes can help, though be aware that you might skew your respondents toward those who are high in a trait like altruism.
- Surveys usually begin with easy opening questions to increase confidence and trust and to encourage the respondents to continue answering questions. More sensitive questions should be asked toward the end of the survey, according to this same logic.
- Inclusion of a postage-paid return envelope for the questionnaire.
- Follow-up reminders to complete the survey: This also includes re-mailing of the survey with another cover letter reminding them to complete the survey. This can yield duplicate surveys, so it is important to have some kind of respondent identification number or code so you can eliminate these duplicates from the data file. This number can be self-generated by asking respondents to provide the last four digits of their telephone number and their favorite two-digit number, for example.

Choose Variables to be Measured

It may seem at first that this step is too obvious to warrant mention, but there are a couple of important checks that should be performed. First, reference the theoretical model you are using as a blueprint for your research. Convert the variables in the model into a checklist. For example, if you are using the Theory of Reasoned Action as the foundation for your study, you will construct the following list of variables: (a) beliefs about the behavior (and evaluations of those beliefs), (b) how "socially important others" view the behavior, (c) motivations to comply with the views of these socially important others, (d) behavioral intent regarding the behavior, and (e) self-reported behavior. Now, next to each item on your list, write down which instruments or questions address each variable. Most people are surprised by the number of times they construct a survey and forget to include one or more of their important variables.

Second, make a list of your research questions or hypotheses. Double-check the nomological network: break down each question/hypothesis into its component variables. For example, take a research question such as, "Do women who belong to sororities go to tanning salons more frequently than university women who do not belong to sororities?" The list of variables for this research question would be sorority membership/non-membership, and frequency of tanning salon use. Now, double-check your questionnaire. The variables for every question or hypothesis for your study should directly correspond to your questionnaire. Be sure to take the time to physically list the questions, or you may find that you are missing something important.

Select Survey Items

Adapting instruments or special populations. Each variable in a survey must be operationalized by one or more questions. Often, a small (or not-so-small) group of questions that are designed to measure a single variable is called an "instrument." A published instrument is usually one that has been thoroughly tested and found to be both reliable (as indicated by a high value for Cronbach's alpha) and valid (as indicated by its ability to predict appropriate outcomes and its correlation to other related measures).

It cannot be stated strongly enough that researchers, especially newer researchers, should use established measures in their studies. If you cannot find a measure for what you need, you should probably look harder. It may seem easy to write questions for a survey. It is only after the time and money has been spent on data collection that the vast majority of people discover that they were wrong. No amount of sophisticated data analysis can correct problems with measurement. To the degree that there are even subtle issues with item construction, statistical power to detect real effects is damaged; this leads to unsupported hypotheses for your study and greater difficulty in getting results published.

Even when generally valid and reliable measures are available, there may be times when instruments need to be adapted in order to make sure that they are appropriate for particular populations. For example, when respondents are children, vocabulary used in questions must be greatly simplified. For all populations, it is a good idea to use a readability index (one is available in Word) to make sure that the grade level is appropriate for the literacy of the population.

When the language spoken by the population of interest is different from your own first language (or the original language of the instrument), you will want to hire a translation service. At large universities, there are often translators available through departments of modern languages. Otherwise, a quick Google search will yield many options. It is worth paying extra for a translator who specializes in medical communication, particularly if there are any significant differences in how a health concept is understood in a population. For example, diabetes and its attendant physical antecedents and consequences are not comprehended well by people in many cultures. Organ donation researchers had a difficult time figuring out how members of the Haitian community in Miami understood organ donation in part because the Haitian Creole word for "kidney" was the same as the word for "back." Questions asking individuals if they knew of anyone who had ever needed a "back" transplant led to some very confusing interactions. Many issues can be avoided with a combination of high-quality formative research with the population of interest, but an excellent translator (and a separate process of back-translation into English) will catch any remaining errors.

Literacy issues. Related to readability and cultural issues is the health literacy of a population. Because health literacy is highly dependent on basic literacy, the reading level of the survey questionnaire is the first concern that should be addressed. Then, if health literacy is a concern with your population of respondents, be sure that questions are worded in "living room language" (Weiss, 2007). For example, questions about hypertension might be misunderstood, but using the term "high blood pressure" could be helpful. Similarly, "birth control" is likely to be better understood than "contraception." The lower the level of literacy/health literacy, the more you may want to consider using graphics to help illustrate concepts. Also, at a certain point, it may be more productive to conduct the survey face-to-face so that questions can be read aloud. However, be aware that this presents other complications because of a loss of anonymity, the disclosure of what might be confidential health information to a non-health professional, and the greater possibility of response bias with regard to sensitive questions.

Measurement options. There are several different means by which responses to questions can be measured (i.e., measurement options). Response option formats include:

- Multiple choice;
- Rank order;
- Likert-type scales;
- Semantic differential;
- Analog scales;
- Open-ended response.

In response to a *multiple-choice* question, respondents indicate which category is most appropriate. Demographic variables (e.g. gender, ethnicity) are examples. A question about the number of times a person has seen a doctor in the past month would also have multiple-choice response options.

Questions requiring respondents to *rank order* a set of choices work best in a print or computer format, rather than a phone survey or other oral administration. An example of a question that asks respondents to rank order a set of choices would be: "What did you like best about your colonoscopy experience? Please rank from 1 to 10, with 1 being the best part of your experience."

Likert-type scales are perhaps the most commonly used type of survey question in social science research. Items generally offer response options on a scale from 1 to 5 or 1 to 7. Each number is labeled with a corresponding verbal equivalent response to the question or statement presented in the survey. These responses on a 1 to 5 scale, for example, might be: strongly disagree, disagree, neither agree nor disagree, agree, and strongly agree. It is important to keep labels in the same direction for each component of the survey. So, if you are asking about attitudes toward cancer screening and negative responses correspond to lower numbers, be sure that lower numbers also correspond to negative response to behavioral intentions to engage in those screenings. In other words, "strongly agree" should not correspond to a value of "1" in one part of the questionnaire and "5" in another part.

Semantic differential scales use pairs of adjectives as a format for respondents to evaluate something. The survey might ask a question like, "Please fill in the circle at the point between the two adjectives that reflects the extent to which you believe they describe mammograms." A simple example, shown below, comes from Lopez-McKee (2011), who asked Mexican American women how they felt about getting a mammogram (which, it should be noted, might well be a very different question from how the same women might evaluate mammograms as a screening tool).

Although it is much less common to see visual analog scales (VAS) used in survey research, their popularity is growing, particularly in computer-administered surveys. Respondents can use a slider bar (or, with print surveys, make a mark on a continuous line about 10 cm long) to indicate finer degrees of agreement with a statement. A computer is able to provide a definitive numerical equivalent for the response, though paper surveys require a researcher to use a ruler to measure the distance of the mark between the two poles to obtain a numerical value. Perhaps because VAS is still a relatively novel form of measurement, recent studies indicate that response times are longer with VAS than with Likert-type

Attitudes About Mammography Screening

1. My getting a mammogram during the next 12 months would be:
   Very Bad .... Very good
2. My getting a mammogram during the next 12 months would be:
   Harmful .... Beneficial
3. My getting a mammogram during the next 12 months would be:
   Unnecessary ....Necessary
4. My getting a mammogram during the next 12 months would be:
   Futile .... Useful
5. My getting a mammogram during the next 12 months would be:
   Unimportant ....Important

scales (Couper, Tourangeau, Conrad, & Singer, 2006). Another common type of VAS involves pictorial representations of response options. If you have been to a hospital recently, you may have seen the Wong–Baker FACES Pain Rating Scale (Wilson, Hockenberry, & Wong, 2008). This may be a particularly helpful format for people with limited literacy and/or numeracy, including young children.

In cases where it is not possible or desirable to create set response options, a researcher may elect to offer an open-ended response question. Respondents can respond in whatever way they wish to whatever degree of detail they find appropriate. However, these responses must then be coded or otherwise aggregated in order to be able to make sense of the pattern of responses within the sample, which can be time consuming. Also, many participants skip this question because of the time and effort required to respond.

Choose a Type of Design

As with other types of research, there are multiple choices that health researchers can make regarding survey design, each with certain benefits and drawbacks. This section will focus on four different survey designs: (a) cross-sectional, (b) longitudinal, (c) cohort (comparison group), and (d) panel surveys.

Cross-sectional surveys. Cross-sectional surveys are surveys of a cross-section of a population at one specific point in time. Many health researchers, particularly in public health, refer to cross-sectional surveys as retrospective surveys, as they involve asking participants about their past and current attitudes, beliefs, and behaviors; whereas, information about future behavior is unknown or can only be approximated through intentions. The major advantage of cross-sectional surveys is that they are simple and comparatively inexpensive to conduct, as surveys only have to be administered once to each participant. The disadvantage of cross-sectional surveys is that, although researchers can witness associations among variables, causality cannot be empirically confirmed.

Longitudinal surveys. Longitudinal surveys collect data from participants at more than one point in time. Collecting data at multiple points over time allows researchers to infer cause and effect of associations between different variables, which makes longitudinal surveys more analytic than the typically descriptive cross-sectional survey (Bowling & Ebrahim, 2005). Most longitudinal surveys are prospective, in that they track the progression of individuals forward in time. However, when researchers have access to historical data or medical records, it becomes possible to conduct retrospective longitudinal studies. Health researchers often use longitudinal studies as types of naturally occurring experiments, dividing participants into two groups (a treatment condition and a control) and observing these groups over time. For instance, health communication researchers could survey two groups of cancer survivors—those that regularly attend family therapy sessions and those that do not—to assess how therapy affects subsequent survivor outcomes. Disadvantages of longitudinal surveys include the fact that they are much more expensive than cross-sectional surveys, take much more time, and are susceptible to attrition (Bowling & Ebrahim, 2005).

Cohort (comparison group) surveys. Cohort (comparison group) surveys are a particular type of longitudinal survey. Generally speaking, these surveys follow a particular cohort of people over time. Cohorts are often defined as people who experience an event during a specific time period. They are often delineated as people born at a specific point in time. As another example, an Australian study (Wakefield, Spittal, Yong, Durkin, & Borland, 2011) looked at the effects of exposure to a mass media campaign to quit smoking on the durability of quitting attempts. Participants were assigned to cohorts of those who have attempted to quit smoking in the past year and those who had not attempted to quit smoking in the past year. However, when cohort studies are conducted cross-sectionally rather than longitudinally, they are often referred to as *comparison group* surveys, as the people surveyed can no longer be considered a cohort, since they are only being observed at one point in time.

Panel surveys. Panel surveys are another particular type of longitudinal survey in which the researcher follows the same individuals or households over time to determine trends in attitudes, beliefs, and behaviors. One research firm outlined several benefits of conducting panel research: (a) response rates are typically high and attrition rates are low, as people opt to become panel members; (b) samples can be customized and created from panel participants that are demographically representative across any variable in your data set; and (c) respondent demographic information will already be on file after initial measurement, saving space on the survey and time for the participant (Market Facts, 1994). However, one disadvantage to panel surveys is that there is a self-selection bias, as individuals choose to become panel members, which may make them different in some way from the general population of interest (Pollard, 2002).

Decide on a Method of Data Collection

Researchers have a number of choices for method of data collection. The principal methods used by survey researchers are telephone, paper, and computer-assisted/Internet.

Telephone surveys. Historically, telephone surveys are perhaps the most established technique to recruit a geographically diverse, random sample of a particular population. Many telephone surveys rely on pre-existing contact lists or random digit dialing (RDD) practices to recruit survey participants, which increase the likelihood that a truly random sample of the population of interest is recruited. In contrast to this immense benefit, there are some aspects of telephone surveys that may necessitate the exploration of other survey options. Perhaps the greatest difference between telephone surveys and other types of surveys is the introduction of a third party between the researcher and the participant, adding another level of complexity to the data collection (Bourque & Fielder, 2003).

There are two established types of telephone survey recruitment that health researchers can utilize: list-based recruitment and RDD recruitment. *List-based recruitment* involves calling potential participants who are affiliated with a particular group or organization. For instance, if a researcher wanted to recruit oncologists from Indiana to participate in a telephone survey, one option to recruit a representative sample would be to call participants who are members of the Hoosier Oncology Group, a network of oncologists located in the state of Indiana. Recruitment through RDD results in a random sample of all active telephone numbers, giving researchers access to a geographically diverse population-level sample.

Advantages of telephone surveys include the fact that they can cover a much larger geographic area than many other types of surveys. Further, telephone surveys offer a relatively inexpensive way to tailor questions to specific participants by incorporating skip logic into the survey. Telephone surveys can also save the researcher time, especially when the implementation of the survey is outsourced to another company.

Although telephone surveys can offer the opportunity to save money in some circumstances, overall, telephone surveys can be quite expensive. These expenses largely depend on the number of items and the level of restriction on the sampling frame (the narrower the frame, the more difficult and expensive it is to reach participants). Further, it is becoming increasingly difficult to reach potential participants with the proliferation of caller ID, answering machines, and the replacement of land lines with cell phones (Bourque & Fielder, 2003). Still, it should be noted that cell phone numbers can be included in RDD surveys, as some relatively recent epidemiological research advocates (Voigt, Schwartz, Doody, Lee, & Li, 2011).

Paper surveys. Paper surveys can be utilized in a variety of different contexts, including situations in which the researcher is present in some capacity (e.g., door-to-door, mall intercepts) or those in which the researcher is not present (i.e., mail surveys). Each form of paper survey has its benefits and drawbacks, which may influence the type of paper survey a health researcher would choose for a particular research project.

General benefits of paper surveys are that they are easy to produce because no specialized software is necessary to develop a paper survey. However, there are specialized proprietary software packages available (such as Snap Surveys) that allow researchers to scan paper surveys and automatically upload the data into a spreadsheet, which potentially saves time and eliminates errors of manual data entry. When utilizing paper surveys, it is imperative to attend to the layout, colors, and overall aesthetic of the survey questionnaire. Keep in mind that academics are likely more tolerant of big blocks of text than the lay public. Font choice should be conservative and easily legible; be sure to match character size to the population of interest, as elderly participants and those with vision problems may require a larger font size. Colors and images may be added as a background to headings and footers (perhaps to match your university or organization colors to confer credibility), but should be avoided in question text, which should be black to maximize readability.

When administered in person, surveys take on characteristics that are traditionally associated with interviews and focus groups, in that the appearance and demeanor of the researcher can affect people's willingness to participate. Babbie (1991) states that, as a rule, recruiters should be dressed similarly to the participants that they will be interviewing. This is just as important for self-administered surveys where the recruiter is present as it is for interviews, as the perceived similarity between potential participant and recruiter is a crucial factor in recruitment.

In-person paper surveys, such as mall or event intercepts, are a great way for health communication researchers to reach out to various target populations, particularly when a representative random sample is not particularly necessary. For example, company health fairs, malls, and public events often allow researchers to recruit participants. When administering in-person paper surveys, it is important to consider how the personal attributes of the recruiter will influence participation. One recent study of mall intercept surveying found that a female recruiter was more successful in recruiting participants when she was wearing perfume than when she was not (Adenskaya & Dommeyer, 2011; sadly, the researchers did not report the brand of perfume she was wearing).

Unlike paper surveys, computer-based surveys require participants to either own a computer, have access to a computer (and, in many cases, access to an Internet connection), or, in cases where the researcher supplies access, feel comfortable enough using computers that a lack of computer literacy will not impede participation. For instance, common computer interfaces that most researchers take for granted, such as drop-down menus, scroll bars, and even using a mouse to interact with the display, may present serious problems for some participants. Generally, computer-based surveys should only be considered when computer literacy is known to be very high in the target population.

Computer surveys. Computer-based surveys can be administered both in-person and online. This choice largely depends on the availability of the target audience, the type of sample desired by the researcher, and the level of computer literacy among target audience members. If the target audience has a clear online presence, it may be in the researchers' best interests to post the survey online. For instance, media effects researchers may utilize fan forums of different television shows as an opportunity to post surveys and recruit participants. However, some health surveys may be geographically focused; a researcher funded by the state to assess the impact of a vaccination campaign may need to administer surveys in-person, perhaps at mall kiosks, county fairs, or grocery stores. Some surveys require sampling from particular populations, rather than the college-aged samples that are often relied upon for survey research. Recruiting from specific and narrow populations may necessitate conducting in-person computer surveys, whereas some general surveys allow researchers to simply post the survey online and supply participants with the survey link. Finally, the level of computer literacy among members of the target audience should determine whether computer surveys are delivered electronically or in person. For instance, if someone has a question about the survey or how to use the computer generally, it will be helpful if a member of the research team is available to respond.

Researchers who administer surveys online, or in other computer-interface formats where the researcher is not present (e.g., a kiosk in a mall or pharmacy), have a variety of delivery options for those surveys. Online surveys usually require some form of proprietary software, such as Qualtrics or Snap Surveys. However, there are a host of free survey services available (e.g. Survey Monkey) that offer researchers an alternative to their paid counterparts. Generally, the formatting, editing, templates, analysis, and data exportation options will be more extensive if a paid survey service is utilized. Another option for health researchers to pursue to collect data from online populations is the Time-sharing Experiments for the Social Sciences (TESS) program. TESS, funded by the National Science Foundation and contracted with Knowledge Networks, provides (for a fee) the opportunity to conduct Internet-based surveys and experiments that are administered to nationally-representative probability samples. For those who conduct field research without Internet access, Snap Survey offers a variety of mobile survey options that allow researchers to conduct surveys on devices that do not have an Internet connection.

Advantages of online surveys include the access to participants and populations dispersed across large distances. Further, online surveys, and computer-based surveys in general, offer the advantage of having data entered into a database automatically. Also, Internet availability is more widespread than ever—currently estimated at 80% of the adult U.S. population (Pew Research Center, 2012). Although it is a commonly held belief that samples recruited from the Internet will not be as representative of the population than other recruitment methods, recent research suggests that this may not be the case (Farrell & Petersen, 2010). Disadvantages of online surveys include the fact that participants must be computer literate, will not be able to ask the researcher questions if they arise, and the researcher cannot be sure if participants are taking multiple surveys or misrepresenting themselves in some way to acquire the incentives or compensation that the researcher is offering to complete the survey.

Pilot Testing

The final step involved with developing a survey is to pilot test the questions that you intend to ask your population sample. Pilot testing the questionnaire with at least 5 to 10 members of the population is ideal. If this is not possible, the more closely the characteristics of your "test subjects" approximate the population, the better your results will be. For example, academic researchers would be very lucky indeed if the intended study was of university students; it would be very easy in this case to ask a small number of students to provide feedback on the questions and the format of the questionnaire. However, a survey of oncologists may require asking any doctors, nurses, or other health professionals in a researcher's family or circle of friends to take a look at survey questions.

The most basic goal of pilot testing is to determine whether potential respondents understand the instructions, questions, and response options. Equally important, you need to know whether respondents understand the meanings of all of the concepts represented in the survey, and whether these meanings are consistently assigned by members of the population. For example, if highly acculturated members of a minority community have a different understanding of "cancer" or "diabetes" or "organ donation" from less acculturated or newly immigrated members of that population, you will need to know this ahead of time and either revise your questionnaire or your sample frame accordingly.

Although it is tempting to skip this step, particularly when time is tight, you are likely to regret doing so later. Pilot testing has never failed to turn up at least several problems or outright errors in every study we have conducted, even in studies where we were using previously established measures. Sometimes, instructions turn out to be confusing; sometimes, formatting errors would lead to responses being recorded incorrectly. The point is, problems are strangely invisible to the researchers creating the questionnaire, but are readily apparent to members of the intended sample. Clearing up any problems before the survey is administered can mean the difference between valid and significant results and a really significant mess.

New Developments and Controversies in Survey Research Methodology

Although using computers and the Internet for data collection is old news at this point, the degree to which web-based survey data collection is supplanting RDD telephone survey research is increasing rapidly (Frankel, 2004). Telephone survey research is time intensive and therefore quite expensive. By comparison, web surveys can be less expensively administered using programs such as Qualtrics, Snap Surveys, or Survey Monkey, making it possible to collect larger numbers of responses relatively cheaply. Also, as more people move to cell phones over land lines and join Do Not Call lists, the representativeness of telephone survey respondents can be called into question (Presser et al., 2004).

Indeed, the Internet may represent the "new normal" mode for survey data collection. One prominent survey research methodologist has said that we "may be entering a golden age of measurement" because of the increasing use of technology to assist with data collection (Presser et al., 2004). At the same time, although some claim that most adults in the United States are online, it is extremely difficult to survey "random" Internet users, and more difficult still to ensure that samples are representative of the population of interest. Issues of representativeness of Internet responses will certainly be researched and discussed for a long time to come.

One related controversy pertains to the compensation of respondents for their time and efforts. While it may be preferable to have research participants who are intrinsically motivated to help with research, there is no evidence that they are any more or less representative of a population because of their more altruistic tendencies than those who require some type of compensation. Nonetheless, with response rates to even large, well-established national surveys continuing to drop by about 1% per year (Tourangeau, 2010), providing respondents with some type of financial incentive may be necessary in order to ensure sufficient numbers of participants. Indeed, if everyone else is getting paid, including the researchers, the survey research staff, and the organizations that receive some real value as a result of the data collected, many suggest research participants should receive some reward, particularly because they are generating the product that is so highly prized.

In spite of these minor controversies and questions, survey research represents the most commonly used research methodology in the social sciences because of its capacity to distill important information from large numbers of people. The information contained in this chapter allows researchers to maximize the benefits that can be realized from this method.

References

Adenskaya, L., & Dommeyer, C. J. (2011). Can perfume increase the response rate to a face-to-face survey? *International Business & Economics Research Journal, 3*(2), 37–43.

Asch, D. A., Jedrziewski, M. K., & Christakis, N. A. (1997). Response rates to mail surveys published in medical journals. *Journal of Clinical Epidemiology, 50*(10), 1129–1136.

Babbie, E. R. (1991). *Survey research methods* (2nd ed.). Belmont, CA: Wadsworth Publishing Company.

Baruch, Y. (1999). Response rates in academic studies—a comparative analysis. *Human Relations, 52*(4), 421–434.

Bourque, L. B. & Fielder, Eve P. (2003). *How to conduct telephone surveys* (2nd ed.). Thousand Oaks, CA: Sage Publications.

Bowling, A., & Ebrahim, S. (2005). *Handbook of health research methods: Investigation, measurement and analysis*. Maidenhead, Berkshire, England: Open University Press.

Brennan, M., & Charbonneau, J. (2009). Improving mail survey response rates using chocolate and replacement questionnaires. *Public Opinion Quarterly, 73*(2), 368–378.

Church, A. H. (1993). Estimating the effect of incentives on mail survey response rates: A meta-analysis. *Public Opinion Quarterly, 57*(1), 62–79.

Cialdini, R. B. (2008) *Influence: Science and Practice* (5th ed.). Harlow, England: Pearson Education.

Cohen, J. (1988). *Statistical power analysis for the behavioral sciences* (2nd ed.). Hillsdale, NJ: Lawrence Erlbaum Associates.

Couper, M. P., Tourangeau, R., Conrad, F. G., & Singer, E. (2006). Evaluating the effectiveness of visual analog scales: A web experiment. *Social Science Computer Review, 24*(2), 227–245.

Dillman, D. A. (2000). *Mail and Internet surveys: The tailored design method* (2nd ed.). New York, NY: Wiley.

Farrell, D., & Petersen, J. C. (2010). The growth of Internet research methods and the reluctant sociologist. *Sociological Inquiry, 80*(1), 114–125.

Frankel, M. R. (2004). RDD surveys: Past and future. In S. B. Cohen & J. M. Lepkowski (Eds.) *Eighth Conference on Health Survey Research Methods* (pp. 131–135). Hyattsville, MD: National Center for Health Statistics.

Göritz, A. S. (2006). Incentives in web studies: Methodological issues and a review. *International Journal of Internet Science, 1*, 58–70.

Göritz, A. S., & Wolff, H. G. (2007). Lotteries as incentives in longitudinal web studies. *Social Science Computer Review, 25*(1), 99–110.

Hayes, A. F. (2005). A computational tool for survey shortening applicable to composite attitude, opinion, and personality measurement scales. Paper presented at the meeting of the Midwestern Association for Public Opinion Research, Chicago, Illinois, November 2005.

Laguilles, J. S., Williams, E. A., & Saunders, D. B. (2011). Can lottery incentives boost web survey response rates? Findings from four experiments. *Research in Higher Education, 52*(5), 537– 553.

Lopez-McKee, G. (2011). Development of the mammography beliefs and attitudes questionnaire for low-health-literacy Mexican-American women. *The Online Journal of Issues in Nursing, 16*(1). Available from: http://ana.nursingworld.org/MainMenuCategories/ANAMarketplace/ANAPeriodicals/OJIN/TableofContents/Vol-16-2011/No1-Jan-2011/Articles-Previous-Topics/Mammography-Beliefs-and-Mexican-American-Women.aspx

Manfreda, K. L., Bosnjak, M., Berzelak, J., Haas, I., & Vehovar, V. (2008). Web surveys versus other survey modes. *International Journal of Market Research, 50*(1), 79–104.

Marcus, B., Bosnjak, M., Lindner, S., Pilischenko, S., & Schutz, A. (2007). Compensating for low topic interest and long surveys: A field experiment on nonresponse in web surveys. *Social Science Computer Review, 25*(3), 372–383.

Market Facts (1994). Mail panels vs. general samples: How similar and how different? Research on research, report no. 59. Arlington Heights, IL: Market Facts.

Murphy, K. R., & Myors, B. (2003). *Statistical power analysis: A simple and general model for traditional and modern hypothesis tests* (2nd ed.). Mahwah, NJ: Lawrence Erlbaum Associates.

Pew Research Center (2012). Internet & American life project. Retrieved June 22, 2012, from http://www.pewinternet.org/Static-Pages/Trend-Data-(Adults)/Whos-Online.aspx

Pollard, W. E. (2002). Use of consumer panel survey data for public health communication planning: An evaluation of survey results. In *Proceedings of ASA 2002 Joint Statistical Meetings on Statistics in an Era of Technology Change*, New York City, New York, August 11–15, 2002 (Section on Health Policy Statistics, pp. 2720–2724). Alexandria, VA: American Statistical Association.

Porter, S. R. (2004). Raising response rates: What works? *New Directions for Institutional Research, 2004*(121), 5–21.

Presser, S., Rothgeb, J. M., Couper, M. P., Lessler, J. T., Martin, E. A., Martin, J., & Singer, E. (Eds.) (2004). *Methods for testing and evaluating survey questionnaires*. Hoboken, NJ: John Wiley & Sons.

Shih, T.-H., & Fan, X. (2009). Comparing response rates in e-mail and paper surveys: A meta-analysis. *Educational Research Review, 4*(1), 26–40.

Singer, E. (2002). The use of incentives to reduce nonresponse in household surveys. In R. M. Groves, D. A. Dillman, J. L. Eltinge, & R. J. A. Little (Eds.), *Survey nonresponse* (pp. 163–177). Chichester, Sussex, England: Wiley.

Taylor, A. W., Wilson, D. H., & Wakefield, M. (1998). Differences in health estimates using telephone and door-to-door survey methods—a hypothetical exercise. *Australian and New Zealand Journal of Public Health, 22*(2), 223–226.

Tourangeau, R. (2010). Incentives, falling response rates, and the respondent–researcher relationship. In L. A. Aday & M. Cynamon (Eds.), *Ninth Conference on Health Survey Research Methods* (pp. 183–193). Hyattsville, MD: National Center for Health Statistics.

Voigt, L. F., Schwartz, S. M., Doody, D. R., Lee, S. C., & Li, C. I. (2011). Feasibility of including cellular telephone numbers in random digit dialing for epidemiologic case-control studies. *American Journal of Epidemiology, 173*(1), 118–126.

Wakefield, M. A., Spittal, M. J., Yong, H.-H., Durkin, S. J., & Borland, R. (2011). Effects of mass media campaign exposure intensity and durability on quit attempts in a population-based cohort study. *Health Education Research, 26*(6), 988–997.

Weiss, B. D. (2007). *Health literacy and patient safety: Help patients understand*. Chicago, IL: American Medical Association Foundation. Available from: http://www.ama-assn.org/ama1/pub/upload/mm/367/healthlitclinicians.pdf

Willimack, D. K., Schuman, H., Pennell, B.-E., & Lepkowski, J. M. (1995). Effects of a prepaid nonmonetary incentive on response rates and response quality in a face-to-face survey. *Public Opinion Quarterly, 59*(1), 78–92.

Wilson, D., Hockenberry, M. J., & Wong, D. L. (2008). *Wong's clinical manual of pediatric nursing* (7th ed.). St. Louis, MO: Mosby Elsevier.

Examining Messages and Interpersonal Exchanges

NARRATIVE INQUIRY

Attitude, Acts, Artifacts, and Analysis

Jill Yamasaki, Barbara F. Sharf, and Lynn M. Harter

> "I am led to the proposition that there is no fiction or nonfiction as we commonly understand the distinction: there is only narrative."
>
> *E. L. Doctorow (1977, p. 231)*

When Mr. Nelson, an 80-year-old widower, arrived by ambulance at the shock trauma unit, he had a collapsed lung, shattered pelvis, seven broken bones, multiple abrasions—and the remains of a leather leash clenched firmly in his hand. His distraught family explained he was walking his beloved dog, Patch, when a car hit them in the middle of a crosswalk near his home. The car continued forward, dragging Patch and Mr. Nelson, who refused to let go of the leash until, finally, it snapped.

When Dr. Duke, a 30-year veteran of the unit who "lives and breathes medicine and the hospital," met the ambulance, he saw an elderly, physically broken patient in emergent need. Mr. Nelson was alert but largely unresponsive, looking at Dr. Duke and trembling only when they gently pried the leash from his fingers. "What happened to the dog?" Dr. Duke asked the waiting family, later explaining he had a hunch it was worth asking. The family said Patch was alive, having only suffered minor scrapes, and safe with a neighbor who found him at the scene of the accident. "I've got to get this guy into surgery, and we've got to get this dog down to the hospital," Dr. Duke told a nurse.

When Donna, the co-founder of PAWS Houston, met Mr. Nelson's neighbor with Patch in the hospital lobby hours later, she learned that Patch had been inconsolable since the accident. He wouldn't eat, paced nonstop, and let out frequent sorrowful cries. Donna escorted the neighbor and Patch to the hospital's critical care unit, where a still-despondent

> Mr. Nelson was recovering after the first of multiple surgeries. There, Donna watched as Patch, a 55-pound husky, gingerly crawled up the bed and nestled at his master's side. Moments later, Mr. Nelson visibly softened when he saw the companion he thought he'd lost, and he lifted his hand to pat Patch's head. They stayed that way together for an hour, when Dr. Duke returned to see his patient. "There are forces there between people and their dogs that I firmly believe we don't know and will never know," mused Donna out loud. "That may be," replied Dr. Duke, "but I know one thing. Not all caregivers are human."

We feel it particularly fitting to begin a chapter that explains narrative inquiry as a particular approach to health communication research with a story. Not just any story, but one carefully crafted from field notes, detailing informal tales told in ordinary conversations about extraordinary circumstances. It's the kind of material that often comes up in interactions with research participants, that powerfully makes a point, with meanings that remain with readers or listeners.

The initial story of Mr. Nelson and his beloved companion, Patch, as well as additional participant voices, photographs, and research design issues used throughout the chapter to illustrate our explanations come from an ongoing narrative project conducted by Jill (first author) and a team of graduate students in collaboration with PAWS (Pets Are Wonderful Support) Houston[1]. PAWS Houston is a volunteer-driven nonprofit organization dedicated to preserving the human–animal bond between people and their pets during periods of hospitalization for chronic and/or terminal illness. Its unique personal pet visitation program is available to all patients, except those in bone marrow units, through all major hospitals comprising Houston's Texas Medical Center, the largest medical complex in the world. PAWS Houston volunteers facilitate approximately 25 personal pet hospital visits each month, with more than 85 percent of those visits occurring in critical care. Visits require a physician's order, are usually arranged within 24 hours (or in as little as 30 minutes in end-of-life situations), and normally last about an hour.

In this chapter, we provide an overview of narrative inquiry with particular emphasis on the attitude of the analyst and the ubiquity of narrative material in a wide variety of discursive acts and verbal/visual artifacts for narrative analysis. To exemplify narrative inquiry in health communication research, we draw from and highlight the narrative work of multiple scholars (including our own), making sure throughout to acknowledge the method's strengths and challenges. First, we examine narrative as an orientation toward the study of social phenomena and detail the variety of sources available to and co-constructed by narrative scholars. Then, we discuss several alternative ways of anchoring and shaping analyses from a narrative perspective. As part of this discussion, we demonstrate how narrative analysis may proceed, using two brief excerpts from the PAWS

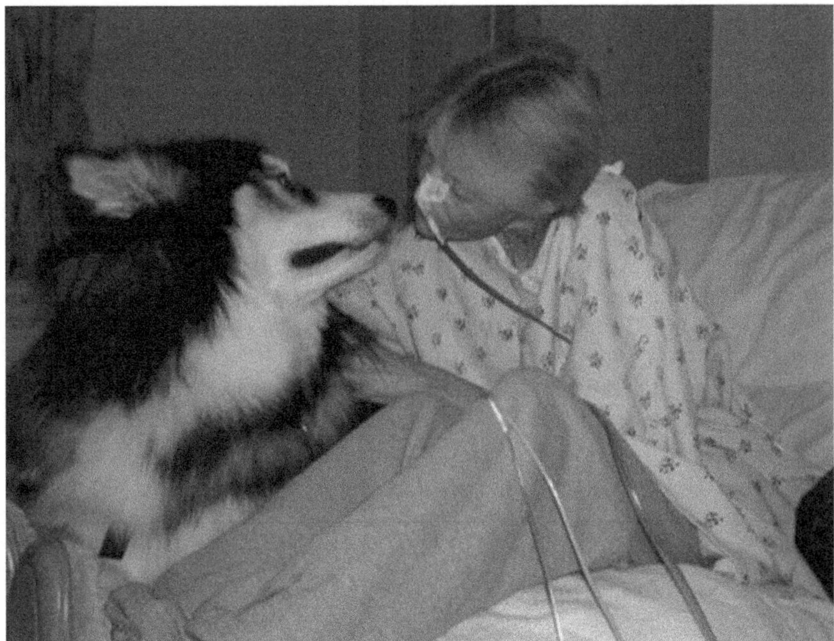

FIGURE 6.1 Patient and Dog

Houston project. We conclude the chapter with an acknowledgment and appreciation of narrative inquiry as an ultimately dialogic practice.

Seeking, Constructing, and Attending to Stories

Narrative inquiry entails a deliberate inclination to seek out and discern the storied elements within human depictions of life events to understand and convey inherent meanings. The search for coherency or sense making in a complex, confusing, ever-evolving, globalized world seems pervasive. References to narratives that frame events, including those that are problematic or discordant, occur in all kinds of commonplace activities—political debates, international diplomacy, cultural gatherings, religious rituals, social and commercial marketing, artistic renderings, family relationships, and, not least among these, interactions pertaining to healthcare, illness, and well-being. Thus, narrative inquiry also requires an aesthetic spirit, or the "boldness of the imagination," which physician and literary critic Rita Charon (2006) describes as "the courage to relinquish one's own coherent experience of the world for another's unexplored, unplumbed, potentially volatile viewpoint" (p. 122).

As an approach to health communication research, narrative inquiry is enacted through study objectives and design, and particularly the ways in which data are elicited. Investigators with an *attitude* open to narrative sensibilities consider both the *acts* of making stories and the resulting textual *artifacts* as important areas of study. While conceptualizing and implementing their research project, this chapter's first author, Jill, and her students purposefully oriented to narrative (i.e., attitude). They recognized the narrative logics guiding the PAWS Houston personal pet hospital visitation program, posited overarching research questions regarding inherent and resulting narrative practices in the medical care that incorporates these visits, and invited stories from patient families, healthcare providers, and volunteers during informal interactions, semi-structured interviews, and participant observation. These relational acts yielded a variety of material artifacts for analysis, including transcribed interviews, field notes, and journals documenting their experiences as trained volunteers who facilitated pet visits and participated in various community outreach events. Additional artifacts collected during the study included PAWS Houston organizational materials, photographs, published articles, and patient reports submitted by volunteers after each visit. Importantly, as we demonstrate with the inclusion of the project in this chapter, narrative inquiry doesn't end with analysis. Our engagement with and representation of these artifacts is itself a narrative act, as is your engagement and understanding as the reader—an ongoing narrative process Arthur Frank calls "thinking with stories" (1995, p. 23).

Fisher (1987; Theory of the Narrative Paradigm) argues that most human communication is inherently organized in story form, but investigators can nonetheless encourage—or, conversely, discourage—participants in field research settings to provide rich, in-depth narrative responses. During interviews conducted for the PAWS Houston narrative project, Jill and her students asked family members, healthcare providers, and volunteers a series of open-ended questions in which they described their own roles and motivations for being involved with PAWS Houston, as well as the ways their views of healthcare have been influenced by participating in the pet visitation program. While several interview questions were aimed at evoking specific memories told in story form (e.g., favorite and least favorite aspects of their involvement, how they became involved with the organization, and typical experiences as part of the pet visitation program), at least one explicit item asked that the respondent share a personal story illustrating the mission of PAWS Houston. Wording interview questions in this way encourages participants to move away from general perceptions and impressionistic accounts to detailed descriptions of defining moments, what Flanagan (1954) aptly termed "critical incidents," often related with deeply felt emotions rekindled through the process of storytelling.

Narrative inquiry in the social sciences is most often associated with gathering data in the form of in-depth interviews; in essence, asking people to tell their stories. Interviews are typically audio- or video-recorded and then transcribed into written text. However, there are myriad other sources for accounts of health-related experiences, including transcriptions of focus group discussions (which, after all, are group interviews); ethnographic field notes that detail the investigator's observations of contexts, interactions, and other phenomena, tending to focus on organizational or community settings (e.g., Ellingson, 2005; Mattingly, 1998); and recorded clinical interactions between health providers and care recipients (e.g., Charon, 2006; Kleinman, 1988; Sharf, 1990). Researchers are also tapping health narratives from less conventional data sources with increasing frequency. These include electronic forms of social media (e.g., Chou, Hunt, Folkers, & Augustson, 2011); photographs, video, art, and other visual formats (e.g., Harter & Hayward, 2010; Makoul, 1999; Radley, 2009; Yamasaki, 2010); television, radio, film, theatre, and other types of performance or entertainment education (e.g., Harter & Japp, 2001; Quinlan & Harter, 2010; Sharf & Freimuth, 1993); creative nonfiction in multiple forms, such as biographical and autobiographical depictions (e.g., Frank, 1991), personal journals (e.g., Tillman-Healey, 1996), and poetry (see Sharf, Harter, Yamasaki, & Haidet, 2011, for a combination of several data sources); and fictional literature that serves as a form of exemplary case study (e.g., Stanford et al., 1995; Yamasaki, 2009).

Narrative inquiry operates on the premise that storied meanings are inherent in human symbolic activities open to the interpretations of research participants and investigator-observers, and herein lies another essential aspect of this approach to scholarship. Narratives that are the focus of study are *necessarily co-constructed* by research participants and investigators; in some situations, the distinctions between these roles may merge into that of collaborators (e.g., Schneider, 2010). Social psychologist Elliott Mishler (1986) observed many years ago that research interviews are as much shaped by the questioner as the respondent, both by the questions asked, as we've previously discussed, as well as how the questioner responds to the informant's comments. The resulting narratives that emerge from these interviews are thus a byproduct of interviewer and interviewee reacting to one another. The process of transforming spoken discourse or field observations into written transcriptions is also a significant form of story editing and co-construction (Mishler, 1991; Riessman, 2008) that is part of the broader undertaking of interpretation (i.e., discerning patterns within and assigning meanings to the various sorts of texts, verbal and visual, selected for a particular research project).

In essence, narrative inquiry requires a sensitivity to attending to discourse and other symbolic forms in terms of their narrative elements, such as plots and characters, accentuated by research designs and questions that encourage participants to provide storied accounts. It also necessitates a realization that stories are related in multiple formats and media, with an openness toward delving into whichever of these may provide ways of understanding queries guiding the investigation.

Approaches to Narrative Analysis

Once data have been identified or elicited, narrative analysis commences. We wish to assert right away that there are many different approaches to analysis, with no one approach especially preferred (for a broad sampling of various narrative analyses, see Harter, Japp, and Beck's 2005 landmark collection); in fact, researchers define what constitutes a narrative in various ways. In her splendid text on narrative methods, sociologist Catherine Riessman (2008) proposes four main analytic categories in which to group several different ways of interpreting narrative texts: thematic, structural, dialogic-performance, and visual. For each category, she delineates certain attributes and chooses exemplars from studies conducted from various social sciences and education to illustrate how investigators have approached their work. In this section, we will briefly allude to those categories, while also elaborating on other issues endemic to conducting narrative analyses that we've learned from our own research experiences.

As a starting point, the analyst must assess the elements of story within the texts under examination. In their most basic forms, these aspects of narrative are not esoteric concepts, but, rather, familiar features recognizable from childhood. Most essential is the idea of *plot*, in which a series of events lead to a tensional situation needing to be resolved. In the words of psychologist Jerome Bruner (1986), a plot is "a plight into which characters have fallen as a result of intentions that have gone awry either because of circumstances, of the 'character of characters,' or most likely of the interaction between the two" (p. 21). Thus, the second necessary narrative feature is that of *characters*, the people or beings implicated within the plot. Other story elements that contribute to our interest and understanding are *motives*, or why characters make certain choices and take particular actions; *scene*, the locale and surroundings in which events transpire; *time or chronology*, the sequence in which the plot is revealed or the temporal orientation of the characters; and *values and life lessons*, the ethical implications and consequences of how the plot is resolved, what rhetorical and literary theorist Kenneth Burke (1984/1935) famously referred to as "equipment for living." Additionally, narrative analysis may take into consideration *context*, the surrounding circumstances in which a narrative is communicated, including the presence of particular audiences; and *storytelling*, the style and means in which the story is conveyed.

As with other kinds of analytic frameworks, it's unlikely that all aspects of narrative will be equally salient in interpreting a particular text or set of texts. While plot and character seem fundamental, other features may not be as compelling or significant, although all should be considered in what Charon (2006) calls a "close reading." Meanwhile, narratives are rarely self-contained and structured linguistic events (i.e., beginning, climax, end), having aptly been referred to as "unruly texts" (Charon & Taylor, 1997). Boje (2001, 2008) argues that stories often unfold, during interviews and in the field settings, as fragments not nearly as tidy or coherent as typically portrayed in academic theorizing.

Boje cautioned researchers against imposing a "counterfeit coherence" (2001, p. 2) on participants' accounts. That said, researchers can still attend to narrative aspects of fragmented accounts—disruption, time, space, characters and their motives. We have reproduced a table of questions inspired by narrative theory initially published in Harter's (2013) articulation of the poetics and politics of storytelling in health contexts.[2]

Depending on their training and perspectives, narrative scholars focus at varying levels of magnitude and specificity in the data. At the broadest level of generality and applicability are master- or meta-narratives. This term refers to

TABLE 6.1 Questions Inspired by Narrative Theory

Characters
• How are characters and actions organized in time and space? • What archetypal characters live in stories (heroes, antagonists)? Who is chosen? Who is barred? Who is not eligible or qualified to enact certain roles?
Setting/Context
• What is the setting(s) of the actions? What is the setting(s) of the storytelling? • How do contexts give rise to particular stories? • How does storytelling reveal conditions of its production? • What sorts of actions or developments does the setting suggest and/or require? • What recurrent patterns of human symbolizing are developed and reinforced by conditions of living? • What narrative conventions are privileged in particular contexts? • What stories are (re)told in particular contexts until they become taken for granted?
Plot/Arrangement and Timing of Events
• How are the past and future envisioned in light of present circumstances? • Why is the succession of events configured in this way? • How did the outcome come about? • What events and actions contributed to the solution? • Are there inconsistencies that suggest alternative narratives? • Where are the gaps in stories? Narrative silences? The unmentioned or unmentionable? Absence of some stories altogether?
Storytelling Activities and Relationships
• Who is narrating? • Who composes the anticipated audience? • To whom are stories told? • How do stories position readers? • What duties are incurred by virtue of witnessing a story? • What does the process of narrating do?

(*Continued*)

TABLE 6.1 (*Continued*)

Consequences of Narratives
• What does the story accomplish? • What are the consequences produced by particular stories? • What social orders are maintained or disrupted through storytelling? • What subjectivities/identities are called into being by stories? • What new possibilities do stories introduce for being in this world? • Under what conditions is storytelling therapeutic? • How do stories evolve and change over time as various constituencies render their experience in alternate stories?
Purposes/Motivations of Narratives
• What worldviews are reflected in stories? • What cultural markers of concern are revealed in narratives? • Whose interests are served (or not) by stories? • What stories are told to justify actions? Relationships? • What motives are assigned to characters through storytelling?

story genres or types characterized by a broad theme or function, often reflective of particular ideologies, assumptions, and values. For instance, Japp and Japp (2005) describe the master narrative of biomedicine, dominant with both experts and the public, as one that explains and treats disease on the basis of scientific validation with measurable, objective evidence. In response, the authors describe the existence of a counter, meta-narrative of "legitimacy" that resists scientific confirmation where it does not exist in favor of individual testimonies of suffering. In a second example, as individuals live longer and with more chronic illness, narrative gerontologists (e.g., Kenyon, Bohlmeijer, & Randall, 2011) have turned attention to the "inside of aging" to counter the longstanding master narrative of aging as decline with a meta-narrative of successful or healthy aging. This perspective moves beyond the biological to a more complex view of aging by focusing instead on the ways in which elderly individuals maintain quality of life and an overall state of well-being by satisfactorily coping with or creatively adapting to age-related challenges. On the basis of examining many individual stories of life-threatening or life-changing illness, Frank (1995), in a third well-known example, developed a typology of master narratives of restoration, chaos, and quest. Informed by Frank and others, Mattingly (2010), drawing on ten years of fieldwork in urban healthcare settings populated by African American families, explored how the practice of hope is connected to and shaped by canonical narratives. Hope, when guided by a quest-like vision of transformation, cannot be reduced to restorative "success" or "cure" often embodied in "clinical hope."

Mid-level analysis accounts for much of the interpretive work on narrative texts done by health communication scholars. Such projects may focus on one exemplary text or sets of texts that are somehow related. Stories may be defined as an entire text, such as an interview, series of interviews, or sets of field notes, or as particularly meaningful episodes within a larger text. One variant of mid-level analysis has a biographical or life-history focus (e.g., de Souza, 2010). More frequently, such studies fall within the category of thematic analyses that are concerned with discursive content. While thematic analyses of various types are common throughout all interpretive work, Riessman (2008) makes the important distinction that "narrative scholars keep a story 'intact' by theorizing from the case rather than from component themes (categories) across cases" (p. 53). The analytic process may be informed and shaped by pre-existing theory (e.g., Adelman & Frey, 1997), or theory may emerge from data immersion (e.g., Geist-Martin, Sharf, & Jeha, 2008). Unlike grounded theory analyses across cases, there is no primary template or series of steps to follow. And, although not required, such analyses frequently consider contextual issues as well as text (e.g., Young & Rodriguez, 2006).

Micro-level analysis is less frequently practiced within health communication research, although used more extensively in other fields of study. While content remains an important concern, microanalysis tends to explore how meaning is derived through examination of structural elements. Much more than thematic analyses, the focus is on the transcribed text, including some paralinguistic elements such as pauses, typically to the exclusion of context. Because of the painstaking attention to detail within transcribed material, the concept of narrative shifts to bounded verbal episodes; in other words, a one-hour interview transcript may be the source of several identifiable stories, each amenable to analysis. Microanalysis generally involves some form of deconstruction of discourse to discover underlying meanings and/or conversation dynamics. Two well-known approaches involve the parsing of narratives into component parts, as described by sociolinguist William Labov, or the rearrangement of story fragments into poetic stanzas, as explained by educational literacy scholar James Gee (for fuller explanation of these techniques, see Riessman, 2008, pp. 77–100). As with every systematized analytic strategy to reveal discursive structure, including more familiar communication methods such as fantasy theme or pentadic analysis, reducing the interpretive process to a set of repetitive steps does not usually lead to rich insights. When used skillfully, however, these frameworks provide a point of departure for in-depth investigations of verbalized narratives, as exemplified by Beach's (2009) study of family conversations about a member experiencing cancer, physician and critical theorist Howard Waitzkin's (1991) detailed examination of the ways patients' attempts to discuss psychosocial concerns with their physicians become marginalized, or Ellingson's (2011) study of the construction and performance of dialysis technicians' professional identity.

Riessman's other two categories of narrative analysis—dialogic-performance and visual—draw attention to particular forms of materials and ways of presenting analyses of stories. It is important to underscore that, for several of the exemplary works cited in this chapter, the analysts themselves use a story-like format to discuss their interpretations of narratives. In other words, this form of scholarship is concerned with artfulness as well as argument, evocation as well as evidence.

What we prefer to call "performative analysis" focuses on the manner in which stories are told, and how the process of telling enhances the meaning of the story's content. Among others, communication scholars who conduct this type of analysis produce autoethnographic and embodied dialogues, reenactments, and performances of lived health and illness experiences. Noteworthy examples include Ellis and Bochner's (1991) reenacted autoethnographic dialogue about personal decision making regarding abortion; Langellier's (2001) dialogue with a breast cancer survivor concerning her decision to tattoo her mastectomy scar as a way of performing her changed identity; Vande Berg and Trujillo's (2008) relational account of cancer as told in two voices; Aleman and Helfrich's (2010) collaborative tale of dementia as narrated by both mother and daughter; Taft-Kaufman and Carilli's (2011) collaborative script about the communication issues surrounding a cancer diagnosis; Defenbaugh's (2011) autoethnographic and embodied performances of life with inflammable bowel disease; and Schneider's (2010) participatory research with adults who have schizophrenia and are homeless, resulting in such autoethnographic collaborations as a readers' theatre, photovoice exhibit, graphic novel, and documentary film.

Although not as prominent in health communication, visual analysis has become increasingly frequent throughout communication studies. In this approach, investigators regard visual artifacts, such as photographs, drawings, film, and video, as narrative media, either alone or, more often, in conjunction with verbal discourse. Researchers may encourage participants to produce visual artifacts as a way of eliciting health narratives, especially from those unaccustomed to giving voice to their experiences and concerns (Makoul, 1999; Wang, 2003; Yamasaki, 2010). The photographs used in this chapter were provided by PAWS Houston, but not taken by participants or correlated with particular interviews. Still, they offer powerful ways of communicating the undeniable bonds and therapeutic impact between very ill patients and their canine companions, neither of whom may have the capacity for speech. Indeed, visual media can serve as a powerful means of conveying the results of narrative analyses, as demonstrated in the award-winning documentary films produced by performance studies scholar Dwight Conquergood (Seigel & Conquergood, 2008/1984) on the health of Hmong immigrants, as well as in the film co-produced by Lynn Harter, one of the authors of the present chapter, on the experiences of families living "new normals" with pediatric cancer (Harter & Haywood, 2010).

In what follows, referring to the above explanation of different analytical approaches, we demonstrate a brief narrative analysis of two excerpts from the PAWS Houston project. Both excerpts are bounded interactions from longer transcripts of interviews conducted with volunteers who facilitate the personal

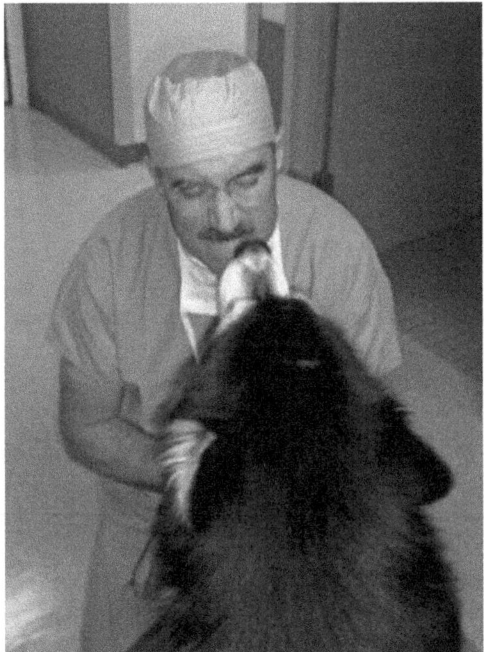

FIGURE 6.2 Doctor and Dog

pet hospital visits. Each exemplar reveals how different types of stories emerge, are encouraged, or are co-constructed through the interview process.

Transcript 1: An Exemplary Story

David (interviewer): You've mentioned the patient in ICU a couple times. What made that visit so meaningful for you?

Vickie (volunteer): Well, she had been in the ICU for a long time. She had a major stroke that had affected her dominant side—her right side—so she couldn't move it very much. She was still on a ventilator after quite a long time because she had a tracheostomy. Her husband just felt it was very important for her to see her dogs. Her dogs were dachshunds. There were two of them, so we needed two volunteers because it's one volunteer for each animal to visit the family. I went in first because I'm an ICU nurse and I wanted to make sure that the other volunteer, who wasn't a nurse, would be okay in this situation.

David: Right. Good.

Vickie: And I went in with the husband and the dog that the lady favored the most. The husband was worried that the dog wouldn't behave properly, so he carried the dog and was really kind of nervous the whole time. I reassured him that usually what the animals do is just lay right down because they understand. They know that this is their human and that they need to be calm.

DAVID: Really!

VICKIE: Yeah, and that is exactly what happened with this dog. He laid him on the bed, and the dog went right to the lady, laid his head on the lady, and stayed there the whole time. The lady, actually, who was right-handed, tried to move her right hand to pet the dog, which was a huge thing. And then, on top of that, the man was telling me stories. Oftentimes, these people just need to talk about their animal, too, but, of course, the lady couldn't talk to me. So the man was telling me how, every morning, she used to wake up and feed this dog a cup of coffee. [*laughs*] And, after she had her stroke and came to the hospital, he had to learn how to make coffee for the dog because the dog was having caffeine withdrawals. [*laughs*] And, as he's telling me all these stories, the lady—the patient—started sticking her tongue out over and over and over. And the man got very nervous and said, "Oh, my gosh, I don't know what's wrong with her. She's never done that before. Maybe she's having a seizure." And I said, "Sir, I think she's missing her coffee." And she looked directly at me. And I said, "I'm so sorry that you're missing your coffee. I'm sure you would like to have some coffee right now." And she nodded her head yes, and I said, "Right now, they can't give you any coffee, but hopefully, eventually, you can have coffee." We were able to ascertain that she understands exactly what we were talking about. So I went to the nurse, and I explained the situation, and I said, "Please let her know anything you are doing to her because she is there. She understands what's going on. She just can't communicate back to you."

DAVID: That's incredible. You made a huge difference.

VICKIE: Yeah, I was able to make a huge difference for that patient because we saw that she could move her affected side when she tried to pet her dog, and we were able to ascertain that she understands what's going on. And, after we switched out dogs and the husband came out, he said, "I can't believe how calm the dog is. He was so crazy and hyper all the way here, but now it's like he understands where she's been and what's going on." And that's exactly what happens over and over again.

DAVID: The animals are wondering what's going on, too.

VICKIE: Yes! They're missing their family member. And they go in, and they see their family member, and they know right away. So, then, all is okay for the animal. The animal benefits so much more than people understand.

The family benefits because they see their family member is still there. And the patient benefits because she loves this animal. This animal is so much a part of her life that she's trying to move part of her body that she thought she couldn't move. And, not only that, we were able to understand that she knew what was going on.

DAVID: And it sounds like you benefit, too.

VICKIE: And I get to witness it all. I'm the lucky party that gets to sit there, and I get nothing but positive out of it because I get to see all these good things happening.

A close reading of the interaction between David and Vickie reveals how various narrative elements combine to create an exemplary story that ties together the therapeutic benefits for everyone involved in a personal pet hospital visit. The plot is both simple and profound: A visit with her favorite dog results in significant breakthroughs for an immobile, nonverbal patient and, by association, her husband and healthcare providers. Because of the dog's presence, the patient attempts to move her right hand, tries to communicate, and indicates comprehension. The patient and her dog are major characters; supporting characters include her husband and the PAWS Houston volunteer, who also happens to be a nurse. As a bounded part of a much longer transcript, the story is a testament to the PAWS Houston program, in particular, and companion animal hospital visits, in general. It also illustrates how David's deft reflections contribute to the ongoing conversation and extend the story, culminating in Vickie's poignant summary of the overarching values exemplified in one especially memorable visit.

Transcript 2: Interlocking Stories

RENEE (INTERVIEWER): Do any visits, in particular, stand out for you as a volunteer?

STACY (VOLUNTEER): Once, I took a pet to visit a young man. He had been in some sort of accident and had multiple fractures, so he was stuck in bed. [Oh.] His friend had actually arranged to bring the dog for him. Clearly, to me, he didn't have that much close family surrounding him. [Oh.] I don't think he was aware the dog was coming to visit. He was just so shocked and surprised, and he started crying. [Aw.] The friend handed her to him, and he was just hugging her and crying. He was so happy to see her.

RENEE: Oh, how sweet.

STACY: Yeah, that one really stands out in my mind because it's not always an emotion you expect from a strong young man. [Right.] For him to show that much emotion just showed me how much that dog meant to him, and it made me feel good that I could help make that happen.

RENEE: It must be very rewarding.

STACY: Yes.

RENEE: What's the best part?

STACY: Far and away, it's the interactions I get to see with patients and their pets. [Yeah.] You know, I work in the hospital so I see therapy dogs come through, but I think it's infinitely better to have the patient's own dog there because it's basically a family member they probably thought they wouldn't get to see while they're in the hospital. [Yeah.] The relationship is already there. [Sure.] And they're often very close to their pets in a different way than they are with their relatives. It's a much more profound experience for them, and they get a lot more out of the visit, because they're connecting with their own family member versus another person's animal.

RENEE: Is that what drew you to PAWS?

STACY: Yes. I worked in a doctor's office before I went to medical school, and I had seen their brochures around, and I thought it sounded interesting and neat. [Yeah.] I hadn't really sought them out. [Sure.] Then, when I went to medical school, one of my professors arranged for PAWS to come give a presentation asking for volunteers, and I got to hear the full story about what they did. [Oh, wow.] Part of why I got into it is because I love animals. I have dogs, and it's something I would definitely want arranged for me if I went into the hospital. [Sure.] And then the fact that I was going into medicine; I hadn't yet been exposed to patients that much yet, and I thought that volunteering would get me into the hospital and interacting with patients.

RENEE: Sure. Wow, I didn't realize you were a doctor. Do you still volunteer?

STACY: Yes. I usually try to facilitate two or three visits a month.

RENEE: That's great. So, do the visits influence what you do as a doctor, too?

STACY: Certainly. [Sure.] For me, as a physician, it gives me a different perspective on some other things we can offer a patient, especially because in the hospital you need a physician order to allow a pet to visit. [Right.] And, at this point in my career, I'm able to write those orders and get it moving. [Yeah.] It's something I know a lot about, and it's something that maybe the physicians I'm working with aren't aware of as an option. [Sure.]

I've had some patients that are in the hospital for up to two months or more. [Oh, wow.] Having that as one of the things we can offer, I think, makes a big difference. It changes their hospital experience, too.

RENEE: How so?

STACY: I mean, seeing patients day to day with their family, yeah they're happy to see them, but you don't see that emotion like you see when you bring their dog in the room. [Sure.] And the fact that they just get so excited and overwhelmed and overjoyed to see their pets, that's the best part of it. [Yeah.] For that brief amount of time—like with that young man who was so broken . . .

RENEE: The one who had multiple fractures from an accident?

STACY: Yes. He was so broken, you know, physically and emotionally, but you can get their mind off the hospital and provide them with that connection and that feeling of unconditional love they can only get from their pet. [Sure.] I see it as soon as I go in the door. I think it's a lot closer to them being at home than just having a family member come visit. It's a little bit more personable.

The interaction between Renee and Stacy demonstrates how the overarching story of PAWS Houston is necessarily enacted through individuals and their stories. In a short space taken from a much longer transcript, three interlocking stories reveal ways the PAWS Houston personal pet visitation program works for different participants. The first story, about a physically and emotionally broken young man's powerful reaction to seeing his dog, illustrates the therapeutic benefits of companion pet visits for hospitalized patients. In the second story, Stacy recounts how the PAWS Houston personal pet visitation program benefited her as a volunteer wanting to interact with patients while studying to become a doctor. The third story reveals how the program provides Stacy, now a doctor, with an additional therapeutic option for her patients. While each story is distinct, larger themes cut across them all, including (a) Stacy's repeated observations that companion pet visits are "infinitely better" than visits from therapy dogs and a "much more profound experience" than visits from family members and (b) the patient-centered care and humanizing medicine that are inherent in the PAWS Houston personal pet visitation program, and endorsed by medical professionals in their educational settings, volunteer efforts, and treatment practices. Finally, Renee's conversation with Stacy demonstrates how narratively sensitive investigators who listen attentively to their participants can move beyond the interview guide to co-construct organic stories that may, ultimately, reveal more than they could have originally anticipated or previously imagined.

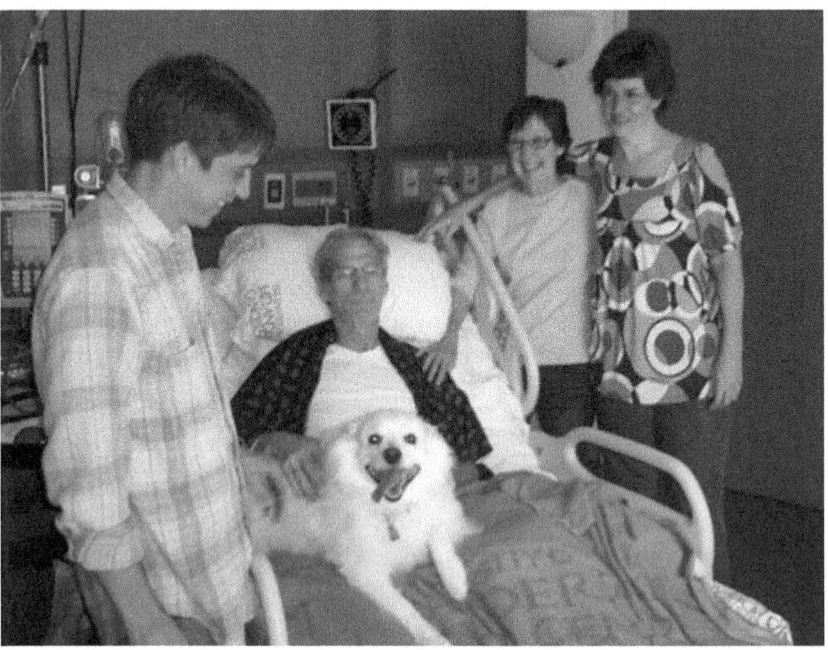

FIGURE 6.3 Family and Dog

Narrative Inquiry as Dialogic Scholarship

> "Thinking *with* stories is a process in which we as thinkers do not so much work on narrative as take the radical step back, almost a return to childhood experience, of allowing narrative to work on us."
>
> *David B. Morris (2001, p. 55, emphasis in original)*

In this chapter, we have defined narrative inquiry with an emphasis on the inclination of the analyst to recognize and attend to the storied elements within human depictions of life events in order to understand and convey inherent meanings. We have delineated the most common qualitative data sources in health communication research that may lend themselves to narrative analysis. Although there is no one favored way of doing narrative analysis, we have explained the elements and perspectives from which narrative studies of field data emanate. To demonstrate, we conducted analyses of two brief examples, applying many of those same features with short narratives excerpted from recently collected data in the ongoing PAWS Houston project. Throughout, we have consciously woven analytic complexity with emotion, description with illustration.

Our chapter both demonstrates and produces the relational ways of knowing inherent in the telling and sharing of stories. As narrative inquiry continues to grow in popularity and prominence, particularly in research concerning issues of health and illness, Frank (2005; 2010) suggests narrative scholars purposefully move beyond the inner workings of the storyteller to understand what stories *do* for story-listeners. What specific capacities do stories have to stretch and expand existing storylines? How do stories work *on* people, affecting what they see as real or possible and shaping their understandings or behaviors in particular ways (e.g., Harter, 2013)? These questions point to the importance of dialogic narrative analysis. Meanwhile, as suggested by Frank (2005), a dialogic standpoint acknowledges the "unfinalizability" of persons and events featured in storytelling and the "perpetual generation" of narrative analysis. "One story *calls forth* another," argued Frank. "The point of any present story is its potential for revision and redistribution in future stories" (p. 967, emphasis in original). From this perspective, narrative analysis ought not claim a final word, but, instead, stimulate ongoing sense making.

Just as the PAWS Houston personal pet visitation program shapes the lived experiences of its participants and the stories elicited by and co-constructed with the research team, we interpret and share stories from the PAWS Houston narrative project with you, the reader, who then constructs your own interpretations in context with the chapter and your own lived experiences. Toward that end, we close with a reflection from Lisa's journal, written after an afternoon of volunteering in the PAWS Houston booth at a community outreach event.

> Working with PAWS Houston this semester has opened my eyes to what it would mean if I couldn't have Murphy, if I couldn't reach for her when I felt pain or needed comfort or knew I was stuck in the hospital or realized I wasn't coming home. That's what I told people visiting the booth today, and everyone instantly agreed. People love the PAWS pet visitation program because it's what they'd want, too. And then one woman came up to the booth and said the most amazing thing. She told me she was waiting for a liver, and she panicked when they put her on the waiting list. "They told me I would be away from home for 60 days!" she said. She didn't worry about her family because she knew they would be with her, but she panicked because she wouldn't see her dog. She actually told me it was a bigger relief to make contact with PAWS Houston and know they'd arrange a visit when the time comes than it will be when she gets the call from the registry. I'll never forget hearing her say that. Before she walked away, I gave her a hug and wished her well and said her story could be mine. If I were in her shoes, I'd feel the same way.

Notes

1. For their cooperation, efforts, and enthusiasm throughout the research project, we warmly thank Priyanka Agarwal, Renee Aiello, Lisa Gregory, Rakhee Sharma, and

David Smith from the Valenti School of Communication at the University of Houston, as well as Donna Dishman, Scott Frank, and all the volunteers, family members, patients, and health-care employees associated with the PAWS Houston program.

2. We gratefully acknowledge Kendall Hunt Publishers for its permission to reproduce this table.

References

Adelman, M. B., & Frey, L. R. (1997). *The fragile community: Living together with AIDS.* Mahwah, NJ: Lawrence Erlbaum Associates.

Aleman, M. W., & Helfrich, K. W. (2010). Inheriting the narratives of dementia: A collaborative tale of a daughter and mother. *Journal of Family Communication, 10*(1), 7–23.

Beach, W. A. (2009). *A natural history of family cancer: Interactional resources for managing illness.* New York, NY: Hampton Press.

Boje, D. M. (2001). *Narrative methods for organizational and communication research.* Thousand Oaks, CA: Sage Publications.

Boje, D. M. (2008). *Storytelling organizations.* Thousand Oaks, CA: Sage Publications.

Bruner, J. S. (1986). *Actual minds, possible worlds.* Cambridge, MA: Harvard University Press.

Burke, K. (1984/1935). *Permanence and change: an anatomy of purpose* (3rd ed.). Berkeley, CA: University of California Press.

Charon, R. (2006). *Narrative medicine: Honoring the stories of illness.* New York, NY: Oxford University Press.

Charon, R., & Taylor, N. D. (1997). Editors' introduction—The unruly mise-en-corps: Body, text, and healing. *Literature and Medicine, 16*(1), vii–xi.

Chou, W.-Y. S., Hunt, Y., Folkers, A., & Augustson, E. (2011). Cancer survivorship in the age of YouTube and social media: A narrative analysis. *Journal of Medical Internet Research, 13*(1), e7: http://www.jmir.org/2011/1/e7/

Defenbaugh, N. L. (2011). *Dirty tale: A narrative journey of the IBD body.* Cresskill, NJ: Hampton Press.

de Souza, R. (2010). Women living with HIV: Stories of powerlessness and agency. *Women's Studies International Forum, 33*(3), 244–252.

Doctorow, E. L. (1977). False documents. *American Review, 26*, 215–232.

Ellingson, L. L. (2005). *Communicating in the clinic: Negotiating frontstage and backstage teamwork.* New York, NY: Hampton Press.

Ellingson, L. L. (2011). The poetics of professionalism among dialysis technicians. *Health Communication, 26*(1), 1–12.

Ellis, C., & Bochner, A. (1991). Telling and performing personal stories: The constraints of choice in abortion. In C. Ellis & M. G. Flaherty (Eds.), *Investigating subjectivity: Research on lived experience* (pp. 79–101). Thousand Oaks, CA: Sage Publications.

Fisher, W. R. (1987). *Human communication as narration: Toward a philosophy of reason, value, and action.* Columbia, SC: University of South Carolina Press.

Flanagan, J. C. (1954). The critical incident technique. *Psychological Bulletin, 51*(4), 327–358.

Frank, A. W. (1991). *At the will of the body: Reflections on illness.* Boston, MA: Houghton Mifflin.

Frank, A. W. (1995). *The wounded storyteller: Body, illness, and ethics.* Chicago, IL: University of Chicago Press.

Frank, A. W. (2005). What is dialogical research, and why should we do it? *Qualitative Health Research*, *15*(7), 964–974.

Frank, A. W. (2010). *Letting stories breathe: A socio-narratology*. Chicago, IL: University of Chicago Press.

Geist-Martin, P., Sharf, B. F., & Jeha, N. (2008). Communicating healing holistically. In H. M. Zoller & M. J. Dutta (Eds.), *Emerging perspectives in health communication: Meaning, culture, and power* (pp. 83–112). New York, NY: Routledge.

Harter, L. M. (2012). The poetics and politics of storytelling in health contexts. In L. M. Harter & Associates (Ed.), *Imagining new normals: A narrative framework for health communication* (pp. 3–27). Dubuque, IA: Kendall Hunt.

Harter, L. M. & Associates (Ed.). (2013). *Imagining new normals: A narrative framework for health communication*. Dubuque, IA: Kendall Hunt.

Harter, L. M., & Japp, P. M. (2001). Technology as the representative anecdote in popular discourses of health and medicine. *Health Communication*, *13*(4), 409–425.

Harter, L. M. [producer], & Hayward, C. [producer, director] (Eds.). (2010). *The art of the possible* [film]. Athens, Ohio: Ohio University Scripps College of Communication.

Harter, L. M., Japp, P. M., & Beck, C. S. (Eds.) (2005). *Narratives, health, and healing: Communication theory, research, and practice*. Mahwah, NJ: Lawrence Erlbaum Associates.

Japp, P. M., & Japp, D. K. (2005). Desperately seeking legitimacy: Narratives of a biomedically invisible disease. In L. M. Harter, P. M. Japp, & C. S. Beck (Eds.), *Narratives, health, and healing: Communication theory, research, and practice* (pp. 107–130). Mahwah, NJ: Lawrence Erlbaum Associates.

Kenyon, G. M., Bohlmeijer, E., & Randall, W. L. (Eds.) (2011). *Storying later life: Issues, investigations, and interventions in narrative gerontology*. New York, NY: Oxford University Press.

Kleinman, A. (1988). *The illness narratives: Suffering, healing, and the human condition*. New York, NY: Basic Books.

Langellier, K. M. (2001). "You're marked": Breast cancer, tattoo and the narrative performance of identity. In J. Brockmeier & D. Carbaugh (Eds.), *Narrative identity: Studies in autobiography, self, and culture* (pp. 145–184). Philadelphia, PA: John Benjamins Publishing Company.

Makoul, G. (1999). Using patient narrative videos for better understanding the illness experience. *Academic Medicine*, 74(5), 580–581.

Mattingly, C. (1998). *Healing dramas and clinical plots: The narrative structure of experience*. Cambridge, England: Cambridge University Press.

Mattingly, C. (2010). *The paradox of hope: Journeys through a clinical borderland*. Berkeley, CA: University of California Press.

Mishler, E. G. (1986). *Research interviewing: Context and narrative*. Cambridge, MA: Harvard University Press.

Mishler, E. G. (1991). Representing discourse: The rhetoric of transcription. *Journal of Narrative and Life History/Narrative Inquiry*, *1*, 255–280.

Morris, D. B. (2001). Narrative, ethics, and pain: Thinking *with* stories. *Narrative*, *9* (Pt. 1), 55–77.

Quinlan, M. M., & Harter, L. M. (2010). Meaning in motion: The embodied poetics and politics of Dancing Wheels. *Text and Performance Quarterly*, *30*(4), 374–395.

Radley, A. (2009). *Works of illness: Narrative, picturing, and the social response to serious disease*. Ashby-de-la-Zouch, England: InkerMen Press.

Riessman, C. K. (2008). *Narrative methods for the human sciences*. Los Angeles, CA: Sage Publications.

Schneider, B. (2010). *Hearing (our) voices: Involving service users in mental health research*. Toronto, Ontario, Canada: University of Toronto Press.

Seigel, T. [director], & Conquergood, D. [producers]. (2008/1984). *Between two worlds: the Hmong shaman in America* [film]. Portland, OR: Collective Eye Films.

Sharf, B. F. (1990). Physician–patient communication as interpersonal rhetoric: A narrative approach. *Health Communication*, *2*(4), 217–231.

Sharf, B. F., & Freimuth, V. S. (1993). The construction of illness on entertainment television: Coping with cancer on *thirtysomething*. *Health Communication*, *5*(3), 141–160.

Sharf, B. F., Harter, L. M., Yamasaki, J., & Haidet, P. (2011). Narrative turns epic: Continuing developments in health narrative scholarship. In T. L. Thompson, R. Parrott, & J. F. Nussbaum (Eds.), *Handbook of health communication* (2nd ed.) (pp. 36–51). Mahwah, NJ: Routledge.

Stanford, A. F., Brauner, D. J., Chambers, T. S., Donnelly, W. J., Hunter, K. M., Poirier, S., & Sharf, B. F. (1995). Reading literary theory, reading *Ivan Ilych*: Old wine in new wineskins. *Caduceus*, *10*(3), 161–178.

Taft-Kaufman, J., & Carilli, T. (2011). Excerpts from *The Waiting Room*. *Text and Performance Quarterly*, *31*(4), 418–429.

Tillman-Healey, L. M. (1996). A secret life in a culture of thinness: Reflections on body, food, and bulimia. In C. Ellis & A. P. Bochner (Eds.), *Composing ethnography: Alternative forms of qualitative writing* (pp. 76–108). Walnut Creek, CA: AltaMira Press.

Vande Berg, L., & Trujillo, N. (2008). *Cancer and death: A love story in two voices*. Cresskill, NJ: Hampton Press.

Waitzkin, H. (1991). *The politics of medical encounters: How patients and doctors deal with social problems*. New Haven, CT: Yale University Press.

Wang, C. C. (2003). Using photovoice as a participatory assessment and issue selection tool. In M. Minkler & N. Wallerstein (Eds.), *Community-based participatory health research* (pp. 179–195). San Francisco, CA: Jossey-Bass.

Yamasaki, J. (2009). Though much is taken, much abides: The storied world of aging in a fictionalized retirement home. *Health Communication*, *24*(7), 588–596.

Yamasaki, J. (2010). Picturing late life in focus. *Health Communication*, *25*(3), 290–292.

Young, A. J., & Rodriguez, K. L. (2006). The role of narrative in discussing end-of-life care: Eliciting values and goals from text, context, and subtext. *Health Communication*, *19*(1), 49–59.

CONVERSATION ANALYSIS

Understanding the Structure of Health Talk

Christopher J. Koenig and Jeffrey D. Robinson

Conversation analysis (hereafter CA) represents a naturalistic and inductive approach to the study of generalizable patterns of interaction that are ultimately amenable to quantification (Robinson, 2007). CA originated at the University of California during the 1960s and has its roots in the work of Erving Goffman and Harold Garfinkel (for reviews, see Heritage, 1984a). CA is now the dominant, contemporary, and methodological framework for the analysis of social interaction (Heritage, 2009). As Robinson (2012) reviewed, CA primarily deals with three questions that are fundamental to communication research:

1. How do speakers 'make sense' or 'make meaning' when they talk, and, similarly, how do listeners know what speakers 'mean' when they talk;
2. How does an utterance's meaning affect subsequent talk; and
3. How does an utterance's meaning affect speakers' 'relationship' with each other?

An alternative method for studying provider–client interaction is the use of pre-existing coding schemata (Roter & Larson, 2002) to divide interaction into component speech acts and place them into mutually exclusive categories, which allows for the generation of frequency counts that can be statistically associated with other variables (for review, see Heritage & Maynard, 2006). However, coding is not itself a method for describing and explaining the social organization of interaction, per se, which is the purview of CA. As Robinson (2011) argued, there has been a social-scientifically pragmatic and symbiotic relationship between CA and traditional coding methods, the former bringing validity to the latter, and the latter empowering the former.

Core Assumptions

CA has at least three core assumptions: (a) talk is a form of social action; (b) meaning making is a product of the *interaction order*, and (c) analysts prioritize members' meanings.

Talk is a Form of Social Action

In contrast to approaches that treat communication as a process of information transmission driven by social-cognitive variables (LeBaron, Mandelbaum, & Glenn, 2003), CA assumes that people produce and understand communication primarily in terms of the social action(s) it accomplishes (Schegloff, 1995). When we communicate, we do not intend to produce behavior (e.g., words, sounds, gestures, etc.), nor is communication interpreted as behavior in and of itself. Rather, we communicate to perform actions, which not only includes "informing," but also delivering bad news, reassuring, recommending, criticizing, complimenting, and the like. Behavior is responded to both in terms of the action it performs, which is publicly available to participants and analysts. Some of the most primary goals of CA involve describing and explaining: (a) how people produce recognizable actions; (b) how people understand others' actions; and (c) the orderly consequences of current actions for the production and understanding of next actions. Although members of a society tend to have non-technical or "common" understandings of the nature of actions—as physicians might have of delivering a diagnosis or recommending a treatment—CA has demonstrated that such vernacular understandings of actions frequently do not represent, and sometimes misrepresent, the richly technical nature of actions, their meanings for participants, and their effects on subsequent interaction and relationships.

Meaning Making is a Product of the Interaction Order

CA assumes that the production and understanding of action are not only influenced by traditional forms of context, such as sex, race/ethnicity, or age, but also by interactional forms of context. Erving Goffman (1983) established that, in interaction with others, we become accountable (i.e., socially responsible) for knowing, and acting in accordance with, a host of norms that are unique to interaction itself. Goffman called this the *interaction order*, because interaction involves a multitude of contexts that "order" our behavior and understanding. He posited this ordering is independent from traditional forms of context, such as sex, age, or ethnicity. One major goal of CA, then, is to describe and explain these interaction orders, and how they affect the production, understanding, and consequences of social action.

Analysts Prioritize Members' Meanings

CA is guided by a particular epistemology that involves a methodological commitment to *prioritizing members' meanings* (Blumer, 1969). The term "member" refers to the person being studied and the term "meaning" refers to how members understand communication behavior. CA has unique methodological and analytic tools to defend claims about the meaning of communication and its "effect" on the production and understanding of subsequent communication. In particular, CA prioritizes participants' meanings in a very practical way—turn-by-turn and action-by-action. What participants say to one another is both a resource for participants to show one another their orientations toward the definition of the situation, as well as evidence to validate such claims based on a data-internal metric; namely, the participant's own orientations to the definition of the situation. The technology participants use for one another is the same technology used by overhearing analysts to ground claims about how language use enacts one or more social actions in real time.

Applications

CA is widely used to study communication in healthcare settings. Much of this research focuses on communication between healthcare and patients (or clients), including physicians (Beach & LeBaron, 2002; Gill, 1998), nurses (Chatwin, 2008; Gordon, Ellis-Hill, & Ashburn, 2009; Pillet-Shore, 2006), pharmacists (John & Housley, 2001; Pilnick, 1998), physical therapists (Parry, 2004a, 2004b), and psychologists (Antaki & Rapley, 2007; Maynard, 1989), among others.

By contrast, the majority of research on communication behavior relies on participants' *self-reports*. Self-reported data involves people reporting what they said or did in a prior conversation, such as in an interview or through a questionnaire survey. Although self-report data is more straightforward and less expensive to collect relative to audiovisual materials, the detail and nuance of communication as it occurs in real time are commonly overlooked and attempts to document communication behavior are frequently inaccurate. Further, self-reports are distorted by limitations associated with memory, self-deception, and social desirability. For example, both patients' and doctors' reports of what they said during medical visits are rarely significantly correlated with what they actually said (DiMatteo, Robinson, Heritage, Tabbarah, & Fox, 2003).

CA data are audio or video recordings of *naturally occurring interaction*. By "interaction," CA refers to two or more people (a) who are physically (or vocally) co-present (e.g., two people standing in front of each other, on the phone with each other, conducting a video conference together, etc.), (b) who have organized themselves as potential conversational participants relative to each other as a potential conversational partner, and (c) whose communication occurs in "real time." By "naturally occurring," CA refers to interaction that has *not* been manipulated by researchers and which occurs in its natural context. For example, in the context of healthcare, CA focuses on actual visits by actual patients and providers without the presence of researchers and without participants being told where to sit, how to act, or what to talk about.

Exemplars

CA has demonstrated that social actions are different from grammatical forms. For instance, the grammatical form of an "interrogative"—or, more vernacularly, a "question"—can implement actions other than "seeking information" (Schegloff, 1984). Furthermore, even when interrogatives do primarily seek information, they can nonetheless embody different action agendas that differentially constrain responses. For example, take the case of primary-care physicians soliciting patients' chief medical concerns (Heritage & Robinson, 2006), represented in Extracts 1 and 2.

Extract 1
01 DOC: what can I do for you today.

Extract 2
01 DOC: sounds like you're uncomfortable.

Heritage and Robinson (2006) demonstrated that these questions embody different action agendas, which have dramatically different consequences for patients' responses. In Extract 1, the general inquiry question "what can I do for you today" is a *Wh*-interrogative that encourages patients, as a first order of business, to present their main health problem. Furthermore, this question tacitly claims that the physician lacks information about the patient's concerns, which encourages an expanded problem presentation. In contrast, the question in Extract 2, "sounds like you're uncomfortable", is a request for confirmation that encourages patients, as a first order of business, to produce tokens of either confirmation or disconfirmation. Requests for confirmation tacitly claim that physicians possess at least some information about the patients' concerns, such as information previously solicited and documented by nurses, which discourages expanded problem presentation and can affect the temporal duration of this part of the visit.

Controlling for patients' age, sex, race, education, and problem type, for urban versus rural practice setting, Heritage and Robinson (2006) found that, when comparing requests for confirmation (e.g., Extract 2), general inquiry questions (e.g., Extract 1) resulted in patients producing significantly longer problem presentations (27 seconds vs. 12 seconds) that included significantly more discrete symptoms. Additionally, they found that, compared to requests for confirmation, when physicians solicited patients' problem presentations with general inquiry questions, immediately after visits patients reported significantly greater satisfaction with physicians' listening behavior and positive affect with regard to relational communication.

CA contrasts with code-category infrastructures that are largely dominated by grammatical form at the expense of function. Code categories frequently exclude actions that are meaningful for participants, and sometimes misrepresent the actions they are designed to capture (Patton, 1989; Stiles & Putnam, 1995). For example, in Extracts 1 and 2, traditional coding may conflate grammatical form and action by coding the questions as a "direct question" or an "open-ended question." While these descriptions may be true on a general level, neither code meaningfully differentiates the function of each question nor differentiates the social actions each question embodies.

The discovery of action has been the forte of inductive studies of social interaction, such as those guided by discourse and CA and ethnography (Heritage & Maynard, 2006). One exemplary discovery of social action is what Heritage and Stivers (1999) termed physicians' "online commentary," or communication that is produced while examining patients and that "describes or evaluates what the physician is seeing, feeling or hearing" (p. 1501). Online commentary affords patients at least some access to physicians' diagnostic reasoning. As such, online commentary has the capacity to foreshadow the existence of medical problems (or lack thereof) and thus, ultimately, whether or not physicians provide treatment. For example, in Extract 3 (Heritage & Stivers, 1999) a patient presents an upper-respiratory problem, and, during the physical examination, the physician provides online commentary about the patient's reported symptoms.

Extract 3

01 DOC: an:' we're gonna have you look s:traight ahea:d,=h
02 (0.5)
03 DOC: J's gonna check yer thyroid right no:w,
04 (9.5) ((physician examines patient))
05 DOC: -> .hh that feels normal?
06 (0.8)
07 DOC: -> I don't feel any: lymph node: swelling, .hh in yer
08 neck area,
09 DOC: .hh now what I'd like ya tuh do I wantchu tuh
10 breath: with yer mouth open. . . .

Instructing the patient to "look s:traight ahea:d," (line 01), the physician explains the imminent examination procedure: "J's gonna check yer thyroid" (line 03). After examining the patient (line 4), the physician produces online commentary: "that feels normal? . . . I don't feel any: lymph node: swelling, .hh in yer neck area," (lines 05–08). Insofar as lymph-node swelling is commonly recognized as a sign of a medical problem, such as an infection, the physician's online commentary contributes to foreshadowing, minimally, a "non-treatable problem" and, maximally, a "no problem at all."

Online commentary can be generally categorized as that which foreshadows "no problems," including utterances such as "that feels normal" (Extract 3, line 05), versus that which foreshadows "problems," including utterances such as "*There's inflammation there*" and "*That ear looks terrible*" (Mangione-Smith et al., 2002). Heritage and Stivers (1999) argue that online commentary has at least three functions. First, it is used to reassure patients about their health status. Next, "problem" commentary can be used to legitimize patients' decisions to seek medical treatment. Third, "no-problem" commentary can be used to tacitly build a case, prior to physicians' official diagnoses, that patients' medical problems are not in need of medical treatment such as antibiotics. Heritage, Elliott, Stivers, Richardson, and Mangione-Smith (2010) found that, compared to physicians' provision of "problem" online commentary, the provision of exclusively "no problem" commentary significantly reduced the likelihood of patients subsequently resisting or challenging physicians' treatment recommendations. This is important because patient resistance can lead to physicians' inappropriate prescription of antibiotics.

Procedures

Transcribing Audiovisual Data

CA assumes that "there is order at all points" in interaction (Sacks, 1984a), and that "no order of detail . . . can be dismissed a priori as disorderly, accidental or irrelevant" (Heritage, 1989, p. 22). Patients respond differently to providers' questions when they contain apparently insignificant differences in speech behaviors. For example, one study showed a difference between the words "some" and "any" in the question, "Are there *some* other issues you would like to discuss?" and "Are there *any* other issues you would like to discuss?" (Heritage, Robinson, Elliot, Beckett, & Wilkes, 2007; Heritage & Robinson, 2011). Ruusuvuori (2001) showed differences in the social actions when providers speak "fluently" versus when they cut themselves off—that is, stop speaking in the middle of a word—when coordinating verbal and nonverbal activities. To capture these minute differences in talk, CA requires transforming talk and other behavior into a detailed textual representation though the process of *transcription*.

Transcription is not a mechanical forerunner to analysis, but an essential part of analysis itself. While transcribing, CA analysts engage in what Sacks (1984a) called "unmotivated looking," where observations about data can be noticed inductively, unmotivated by literature-inspired conceptual frameworks, theories, hypotheses, or research questions. However, CA understands that transcripts are at least a third-generation version of data (Roberts & Robinson, 2004); the first being the in vivo interaction itself, and the second being the perspective-bound audiovisual recordings of the interaction (Atkinson & Heritage, 1984; Ochs,

TABLE 7.1 Basic Transcription Symbols

DOC: PAT:	Speaker identifications are for physician (DOC) and patient (PAT).
[word]	Square brackets indicate onset and offset of overlapping talk.
word=	Equal signs indicate utterances are run together with no gap of silence.
wor-	Hyphens indicate a preceding sound is cut off or self-interrupted.
°word°	Degree signs indicate decreased volume relative to surrounding talk.
(0.8)	Numbers in parentheses measure silences in seconds, by tenths of a second.
(.)	Parenthesis with period indicates a "micropause" less than 2/10 of a second.
wo:rd	Colons represent prolongation or stretching of the preceding sound.
word.	Periods represent falling or turn-final intonation contours.
word,	Commas represent continuing or turn-continuative intonation contours.
word¿	Inverted question marks represent intonation rising higher than comma.
word?	Question marks represent rising intonation contours.
word	Underlining represents emphasis relative to surrounding talk.
<slow>	Less than-greater than symbols indicate decreased pace relative to surrounding talk.
>fast<	Greater than-less than symbols indicate increased pace relative to surrounding talk.
.hh	Period followed by h's indicate in-breaths; the more h's, the longer the inhalation.
hh	H's alone indicate out-breaths or laughter; the more h's, the longer the exhalation.
wo(h)rd	Single parenthesis filled with h's indicate breathy delivery of talk.
(word)	Single parenthesis filled indicates transcriptionist doubt.
((word))	Double parenthesis filled indicates transcriber's description or characterization of some event.

1979). For this reason, analysis is optimally conducted with the audiovisual data in conjunction with the resulting transcript.

While a detailed description of CA transcription is beyond the scope of this chapter, readers are referred to Hepburn and Bolden (2012), who describe procedures for doing CA transcription, as well as to a comprehensive summary of CA transcription conventions as composed by its originator, Gail Jefferson (Jefferson, 2004). See Table 7.1 for the transcription symbols used in this chapter. Emanuel Schegloff has an introductory online tutorial for CA transcription (Schegloff, 2003).

Overall Structural Organization: Describing the Context of Social Activities

The *activity* in which participants are engaged is one significant type of interactional context (Goffman, 1983) that shapes the production and understanding of talk and other behavior (Levinson, 1983). For example, consider the primary care activity of a patient presenting an acute medical problem to her or his physician, such as a new rash. This activity embodies normatively ordered sub-activities, such as opening the visit (e.g., greetings), patients presenting the problem, physicians gathering information about the problem (i.e., history taking), diagnosing, and treating the problem, and, finally, closing the visit (Robinson, 2003). *When* the activity occurs within the visit is also significant: Physicians' diagnosis-related talk is produced and understood differently if it is produced "early," such as during the subactivity of history taking (Heritage & Stivers, 1999). In fact, the exact same words, such as a physician's *How are you?*, frequently embody a different action if uttered early in the opening phase versus at the beginning of the problem-presentation phase (Robinson & Heritage, 2006). It should be noted that the nuanced positioning of social actions within particular activities has consequences beyond interaction itself to medical outcomes. For example, in post-surgical visits, cancer specialists' psychosocial information giving, which is otherwise positively associated with patients' satisfaction, is negatively associated with satisfaction when it occurs during the phase of physical examination (Eide, Graugaard, Holgersen, & Finset, 2003).

Activities are achieved across more than one sequence of action, "which are nonetheless being managed as a coordinated [or coherent] series that overarches its component" parts (Heritage & Sorjonen, 1994, p. 4). According to Levinson (1992), activities are associated with particular sets of inferential schemata that inform the nature and organization of their sub-parts (i.e. sub-courses of action), which are "goal-defined … events with *constraints* on participants, setting, and so on, but above all on the kinds of allowable contributions" (p. 69). Within CA, the organization of an activity—including its sub-parts and their normative ordering—is referred to as an *overall structural organization* (Robinson, 2012). Because such an organization shapes and constrains the production and understanding of social action, when attempting to describe a particular action, one of the first things that conversation analysts do is describe the overall structural organization in which that action occurs.

Turn Design: Constructing Individual Turns at Talk

After describing the overall structural organization of medical interactions, analysts might focus on another common building block of social action: turn design. The proposal that speaking turns are *designed* is tied to the understanding that social actions are finely tuned to be recognized by others according to the norms of the immediate, local context, as well as the overall structural organization of the interaction itself. Turn design can be summed up with the maxim: turn composition matters. That is, the particular ordering of the compositional components to build an action matters for what it "does" or "accomplishes," and thus for the consequences that action has for the subsequent interactional behavior.

For our purposes, we will focus in on the activity of a medical recommendation within the acute medical visit. Physicians typically make recommendations immediately after diagnosing the patient's problem, thereby confirming the presence of a legitimate medical condition. When physicians make a medical recommendation, they are doing a type of social action that is precisely fit to be responsive to patients' presented medical problems. Medical recommendations can take many forms, including recommending a particular type of treatment, such as a prescription medication, an over-the-counter remedy, or even recommending no treatment at all. Extract 4 shows a physician recommending a treatment:

Extract 4. PCT 21–05 Bad cough

01 DOC: I- I would recommend an asthma type inhaler

By using the phrase "I would recommend" (line 01), the physician names the action he is doing—recommending a treatment—which is followed by a type of treatment (line 01). This turn design frames the action as a *recommendation* for the patient's medical problem; in this case, difficulty breathing. While the physician in Extract 4 explicitly recommends a treatment, physicians can enact a similar action using a different turn design. Compare Extract 4 with the following:

Extract 5. PCT 11–04 Seborrhea

01 DOC: alright. what I'm going to do is I'm
02 going to give you some cream to try
03 on your face.

Extract 6. PP 10–10 Throat infection

01 DOC: so I'm gonna give you antibiotics to take.

Extract 7. PCT 14–03 Urinary tract infection

01 DOC: okay. so, (.) uhm:, (1.0) >I'm going to<
02 start you on Bactrim.

In these extracts, physicians use the phrases "What I'm going to do is . . .," "I'm gonna give you . . .," and "I'm going to start you on . . ." to announce a treatment. While both recommending a treatment and announcing a treatment propose treatments for patients' medical problems, compared to the recommendation format in Extract 4, the announcement format in Extracts 5 to 7 are more "direct" (Brown & Levinson, 1987), in that the physician asserts medical authority to treat the patient's problem. This turn design may have the capacity to promote patients' acquiescence to physicians' recommendations, perhaps at the expense of patients' agency (Koenig, 2011). These claims can be supported by collecting and comparing treatment recommendation turn designs across extracts, including how patients respond and ensuing patient–provider treatment-related negotiations.

Comparing Extracts 4 to 7, we can further note that physicians have alternative choices for how they refer to, or formulate, different types of treatment. For example, physicians can use relatively general formulations, such as "some cream" (Extract 5) and "asthma type inhaler" (Extract 4), or more specific formulations, such as "antibiotics" (Extract 6), or even medical-technical formulations, such as "Bactrim" (Extract 7), which is the brand name of a specific antibiotic medication. Research has shown that differences in formulation have significant consequences for action construction, and thus for subsequent talk (Antaki, Barnes, & Leudar, 2005; Bolden, 2010; Garfinkel & Sacks, 1970; Schegloff, 2004).

A final and brief observation about Extracts 5 to 7 is that physicians are recommending prescription medication. However, physicians can recommend other things, such as referrals to specialists, as shown in Extract 8:

Extract 8. PCT 19–07 Ankle sprain

01 DOC: u:m. (1.5) thee uh, typically:: if you have
02 a fracture I send you to see an orthopedist.

Not all recommendations are equal, and it is highly likely that "what is being recommended" (e.g., medicines vs. referrals) matters for the social action being constructed.

In this section, we have focused on turn design to examine how providers make medical recommendations. Turn design examines how turns are constructed—through verbal, vocal, and nonvocal behavior—to enact a particular social action. Turn design is a powerful analytic resource that enables both participants and analysts to consider how individual turns at talk are simultaneously shaped by immediately previous actions, shape current actions, and constrain what kind of actions can follow next. How physicians design turns may be tied to perceived health literacy, presumed knowledge about the treatment, and even familiarity between physician and patient, and can influence how the recommendation may be understood and responded to in context, which we will elaborate in the next section.

Sequence Organization: Collaboratively Building Social Actions and Activities

CA is interested in turn design because small differences in how a turn is produced can result in large differences in the ensuing talk. However, turns at talk do not occur in isolation, but as part of larger chains of social action called *sequences*. Sequence organization seeks to establish the regularities of how turns relate to one another in the local context (Schegloff, 2007). Sequence organization can be summed up with the maxim: turn position matters. The main premise of sequence organization is that each turn is governed by normative rules for what counts as a contextually appropriate response (Sacks, Schegloff, & Jefferson, 1974). The primary way to establish what may be a contextually appropriate response is to look at the position of each current turn in relation to the immediately next turn.

For example, CA research has demonstrated that, as actions, medical recommendations generally pressure recipients to accept, rather than reject, the recommendation. In the context of medicine, patients regularly respond to physicians' recommendations by accepting them, without delay, in the immediately next turn with *okay* or *alright* (Costello & Roberts, 2001; Koenig, 2011; Stivers, 2005a, 2005b), as demonstrated by Extracts 9 and 10:

Extract 9. PCT 11–04 Seborrhea

01 DOC: alright. what I'm going to do is I'm
02 going to give you some cream to try
03 on [your face.
04 PAT: [o:kay.
05 DOC: Twice a day.

Extract 10. PP 10–10 Throat infection

01 DOC: so I'm gonna give you antibiotics to take.
02 PAT: okay.
03 DOC: uhm and I'll give you something called
04 Zithromax.

In both cases, patients accept physicians' announced treatments with "okay" (Extract 9, line 04, and Extract 10, line 02). The fact that patients respond by *accepting* is evidence that they orient to physicians' immediately prior turns as accomplishing the action of recommending a treatment for their medical problems. The paired action sequence of recommendation–acceptance, is collaboratively enacted by physician and patient, respectively.

Once the patient accepts the recommendation, physicians treat the sequence as complete. Evidence for this claim can be supported by looking at the turn after the acceptance. After patients accept the proposed treatment, physicians routinely move onto next activities, such as treatment counseling, where the medication frequency (Extract 9) or the name of the medication (Extract 10) is provided. From a sequence organizational perspective, acceptance is one interactional outcome—but it is not the only outcome possible. By showing how physicians and patients coordinate the medical recommendation sequence, we can begin to make the argument that physicians' recommendations for medicine normatively solicit acceptance more generally.

One way to support the claim that physicians' recommendations for treatment normatively solicit acceptance is to examine cases where patients do something other than respond with an acceptance. For example, see Extract 11 overleaf.

After the physician completes her announcement for the treatment (lines 01 to 02), rather than immediately accepting the recommendation in the next turn, the patient remains silent (line 03):

Extract 11. PCT 14–03 Urinary tract infection

01 DOC:	okay. so, (.) uhm:, (1.0) >I'm going to<
02	start you on Bactrim.
03	(.)
04 DOC:	we can do a three day course of Bactrim.
05 PAT:	[unkay.]((simultaneous head nod))
06 DOC:	[uhm:,]=and uh, (0.2) I need to
07	know how you're feeling=.hh=>uh<

In response to the patient's silence, rather than moving on to new or next matters, the physician reissues her original recommendation using a slightly different turn design: "we can do a three day course of Bactrim." (line 04). The physician orients to the patient's non-acceptance through a shift in format of the initial (lines 01 and 02) and subsequent (line 04) medical recommendations. Initially, the physician announces a recommendation using the first-person singular pronoun I (line 01). After the patient delays acceptance, the physician subsequently modifies the medical recommendation using a proposal format, which uses the first-person plural pronoun "we" (line 04). The shift from announcement to proposal formats simultaneously mitigates the physician's authority and ratifies the patient as an active participant in the medical recommendation, who has, ultimately, veto power over the physician's recommendation. In response, the patient accepts the second turn with "[unkay]" (line 05), produced with a simultaneous head nod. From this extract, we can see that the physician treats the patient's silence (line 03) as doing something other than accepting, which the physician pursues and ultimately receives. With the patient verbally onboard with the proposed treatment, the physician moves to a next activity: planning for possible side effects of the medication (lines 06 and 07).

Another way to support the claim that physicians' recommendations for treatment normatively solicit acceptance is to examine cases where patients do not immediately respond with acceptance; that is, cases where patients accept in a late, or delayed, fashion. For example, in Extract 12 (an extended version of Extract 4), after the physician completes his recommendation (line 01), the patient initially remains silent (line 02), and then produces "°okay°." (line 03) in sotto voce:

Extract 12. PCT 21–05 Bad cough

01 DOC:	I-I would recommend an asthma type inhaler.
02	(0.2)
03 PAT:	°okay.°

04 DOC: tuh help keep your air ways open an'
05 decrease your chance of uh pneumonia.
06 PAT: okay.
07 DOC: okay? .HHhh enh- you've never used that
08 type of medicine?=
09 PAT: no.=huh uh.
10 DOC: okay. well, inhalers deliver a fine mist
11 of medication. ((continues explanation))

The physician treats the patient's delayed acceptance very differently than the physician treated the non-delayed, full-voiced "okay" in Extracts 6 and 7. Here, rather than moving on to next matters, the physician extends his original recommendation by justifying its medical basis: "tuh help keep your air ways open an' decrease your chance of uh pneumonia." (lines 04 and 05). This is evidence that the physician orients to the patient's delayed acceptance as projecting upcoming trouble and a possible rejection. In response to the physician's justification, the patient immediately responds with a full-voiced acceptance: "okay." (line 06). Once the patient accepts the recommendation, the physician moves to a next activity, securing her familiarity with this type of treatment (lines 07–08). Note that the physician uses the patient's two responses (lines 02–03 and line 06) to guess the reason for her initial non-acceptance—the patient lacks familiarity with inhalers as a treatment technology. Once the patient endorses not being familiar with the medication (line 09), the physician calibrates the next activity as one of explaining how inhalers work to deliver medication (lines 10–11) and, later, demonstrating how to use them. Overall, this extract shows that physicians treat patients' delayed acceptances (lines 02–03) as possible non-acceptance, which here is pursued by expanding the recommendation to a second turn (lines 04–05).

In this section, we showed how sequence organization can be used to understand how physicians' recommendations for treatment and patients' responses can be used to jointly construct the medical recommendation as an activity. This section offers insight into the different social actions and activities participants enact in and through their talk. These examples demonstrate how differences in turn design impact the interactional outcomes of the treatment phase of the acute medical visit and help understand the dynamic interplay between turns, social actions, and activities when discussing treatment.

Reliability and Validity

One fundamental premise of CA is that meaning arises out of social interaction and realized in real-time. The goal of analysis is to document how participants produce shared meanings for one another according to the contingencies of the social situation. CA uses empirical audio- and video-recorded interaction and transcripts to investigate and prioritize participants' endogenous meanings as they are produced moment by moment, one turn at a time. To discover these processes, conversation analysts adopt a naive orientation data by investigating and prioritizing participants' meanings as they are produced for one another. One source of validity in CA is derived via the degree to which speaker's practices are shown to be systematic.

CA employs two different, but interrelated analytic procedures: the analysis of single cases and the analysis of practices (Schegloff, 1987). The integrity of single-case analysis is grounded in Sacks' (1984b) assumption of order-at-all-points. In single-case analyses, analysts attempt to demonstrate, from participants' communicative conduct, that participants understand particular features of interaction in ways that are unique to a specific interaction. These data-internal, or *emic*, understandings are assumed to reflect orderly processes, and thus are used to make claims about rule-based structures of interaction (Goodwin, 1984; Schegloff, 1987). For example, in both Extracts 6 and 7 (above), the patient responds to the physician's prior action (at lines 1–3 and 1–2, respectively) with *okay*. There are a variety of other types of tokens or responses that the patient might have given, each of which would have taken up a different stance toward, and thus displayed a different understanding of, the physician's prior action. For example, the patient might have alternatively said uh huh, which would have at least oriented to the physician as not yet being done with his action (Schegloff, 1982). Further, the patient might have said oh, which would have oriented to the physician as having informed the patient; for example, by delivering news (Heritage, 1984b). However, the patient actually responds with "okay," which communicates 'acceptance' (Beach, 1993). This type of response is one, but only one, piece of evidence that patients orient to physicians' *medical recommendations* as a social action that patients can either accept or reject. The response patients deliver may depend on whether the medical recommendation is formatted as a recommendation or announcement.

Simultaneously, CA is also interested in the systematic identification practices of social action that are intersubjectively understood and normatively binding across a range of contexts and participants more generally. A practice-based analysis is a structured orchestration of multiple aspects of conduct that is regularly produced and understood as implementing a particular action. Because CA is only secondarily concerned with idiosyncratic rules (Sigman, 1980), or those shared uniquely by a single dyad, analysts carry the burden of exposing the regularities of practices, and this cannot be achieved with a single case. As Schegloff (1988) noted, although single cases can serve "to launch a proposal" (p. 442) about a practice of action, this proposal is just "a conjecture" (p. 442) until "a substantial number of occurrences" (p. 451) can be assembled.

Practices of action are discovered after engaging in many—perhaps hundreds—of single-case analyses. Through the assembly of many single-case analyses that exhibit the same set of structural features can constitute evidence for a set of rules more generally. Arguments generated by this "core" collection of cases, all of which support a particular set of analytic claims (Schegloff, 1996, 1997) will be complimented by arguments generated by (1) "boundary cases" that contain most, but not all, of the core structural features, and thus that operate slightly differently (Schegloff, 1997); and (2) "deviant cases," or otherwise "core" cases, in which rules are violated, but in which participants somehow orient to such violations, thereby exposing and documenting the existence of the rules being claimed (Have, 2000).

Reliability refers to the degree in which research findings can be produced consistently within and across data. Several scholars have argued, from a radical interpretation of social constructionism, that reliability is not a relevant issue for interpretative research. However, this position has been reviewed and strongly refuted by scholars who employ interpretative methods (Kirk & Miller, 1986; Silverman, 2001). Using a traditional measure of inter-coder reliability (i.e., Cohen's Kappa), Roberts and Robinson (2004) demonstrated that CA methods of transcription are, for the most part (i.e., excepting nuanced features of intonation, pitch, pace, and amplitude), acceptably reliable. Furthermore, once practices of medical action have been documented using CA, they can be reliably identified by trained coders. For example, again documented with the Cohen's Kappa statistic, coders are able to reliably identify different turn formats that physicians use to solicit patients presenting concerns, and that patients use to present such concerns (Mangione-Smith, Elliott, Stivers, McDonald, & Heritage, 2006; Robinson & Heritage, 2006).

Strengths and Limitations of CA

CA has two unique strengths. First, CA emphasizes use of audiovisual data to investigate the details of how participants actively manage and negotiate meaning interactively. Audiovisual data enable the recording and repeated inspection of minute details of the communication process, including inbreath, laughter, gaze, and body orientation, to establish what is meaningful from participants' perspectives in managing meaning. Because audiovisual recordings empirically capture the interactive communication process, they can be used effectively to answer primary research questions, secondary analyses, and pilot preliminary data for future projects.

Second, CA is unique among interpretative research methods because its methodological and analytic strategies are tightly knit into a cohesive whole (Heritage, 2008). Methodologically, CA is highly generative methodology that can lead to unexpected findings that are systematically comparable across data and research findings over time, and can simultaneously build on and incorporate previous findings into new insights about social and communicative practices. CA employs a diverse set of flexible analytic tools of varying complexity and bridging various orders of organization, including overall structural organization, turn design, and sequence organization, among others.

As a research method, CA also has limitations. First, CA uses a unique form of empirical data, audiovisual recordings of naturally occurring interaction, to ground its claims about the ways in which participants manage and coordinate meaning in real-time. CA has been critiqued on the grounds that audiovisual recordings could be supplemented with interviews with participants or ethnographic participant observation that may help contextualize the recordings. From a conversation analytic standpoint, these techniques are problematic on several accounts. Ethnographic and psychological research over the past 40 years has definitively shown participants' perceptions of their own and others' behavior are different from their actual behavior. As a result, asking participants to recall and interpret their own and others' behavior elicits attitudes and beliefs that may be reported in a more favorable light.

Another limitation of CA research is that data collection and analysis is time intensive and requires multiple competences. When planning a project, the analyst must research, acquire, and test various types of technology, including audiovisual equipment, software packages, and secure storage and archival systems. Securing ethical permission and finding sites take time. Once data are collected, the analyst must manage and analyze the data as we describe above. While this general working procedure is easily summarized, the process is highly variable due to the frequency and complexity of the phenomena under investigation. However, even a small number of high-quality recordings can be analyzed in multiple ways.

Challenges

There are several misconceptions about collecting audiovisual data in health environments. One of the most common challenges is the idea that the recording device will somehow change the nature of the interaction, the so-called "Observer's paradox" (Labov, 1972). However, in an elaborately conceived and executed controlled experiment, Penner et al. (2007) show that the effects of recording devices have a minimal effect on actual conversational behavior. However, for CA, this question is somewhat more straightforward. Because CA is interested in how participants coordinate meaning interactively in any given interaction, even if participants are aware of the presence of a recording device, they will still operate according to the principles of conversational behavior, including taking turns and enacting activities and social actions. While participants may suppress certain words, topics, or activities, what they discuss will still yield valid data for analytic purposes. Thus, the possible impact of a recording device is largely a moot point in conversation analytic circles.

One of the common mistakes in collecting and analyzing physician–patient interactions is to define the health context too broadly. For example, researchers that focus only on primary care or family medicine practices can more easily justify research to ethical review boards and prospective data collection sites. Further, the more specific the context and health condition, the more likely an analyst will notice recurrent patterns in which meaning is interactively managed and negotiated. For example, we recommend collecting data in primary care settings with patients presenting new medical problems. Alternatively, researchers could collect specialist visits with people who have a chronic medical problem, such as diabetes or rheumatoid arthritis. Narrowing the context provides the opportunity to develop expertise in a particular setting and/or illness type while learning about important variations in communication in the management of these conditions. Finally, focus on particular action types, such as past medical history, treatment recommendation, or physical examination, that are recurrent across settings can help analysts narrow research even further to enable research have significant and potentially generalizable findings.

The most significant ethical concern about conducting a CA study in health and medical settings involves the collection of audiovisual data. Collecting audiovisual data in healthcare settings can be difficult for various reasons. Many healthcare organizations may have reservations about approving audiovisual data collection due to the Health Insurance Portability and Accountability Act (HIPAA), which enforces stringent rules of privacy and confidentiality. Privacy is the idea that what happens in a healthcare setting will be protected, keeping others from finding out potentially sensitive information about a patient's health. Confidentiality is the idea that information entrusted to someone will be kept in secret and will not be revealed to others. Privacy and confidentiality are at the core of the relationship between providers and patients. When a medical visit is recorded audiovisually, both of these conditions may be put at risk. As a result, CA researchers typically devise elaborate protocols to ensure the privacy and confidentiality of the medical visit. This can be done in various ways. When transcribing, people's names are typically replaced by similar-sounding pseudonyms or by speakership designations to indicate role identities, such as DOC and PAT for a physician and patient. When video is shown to a class or at a research conference, care is taken to ensure that sensitive moments are selected only as needed to demonstrate essential analytic points.

Informed consent is one of the most important aspects of collecting audiovisual data. Informed consent is the process in which a research participant agrees to participate in a research study with adequate knowledge of the potential risks, benefits, and rights of participation and data use. Because many institutional review boards (IRBs) are inexperienced at handling study protocols involving the collection, processing, and archiving of audiovisual data, careful thought about research design and enrollment procedures will help convince IRBs that the research is based on sound ethical principles. When designing a study to collect audiovisual data, one of the ways to incorporate informed consent into the process of data collection is to offer participants several opportunities to opt out of the data-collection process. For example, most research asks participants to sign informed consent documents only *before* beginning a research study. This approach treats informed consent as a one-time event. One way to convince IRBs that patients are comfortable with study procedures may be to ask participants to sign a second, post-visit consent form to confirm they are comfortable with the recording being used for research purposes. Additionally, the post-visit consent can be used for participants to place limitations on the data, such as who may or may not see the data and what purposes it may be used for, such as presentation at scientific meetings or for training and educational purposes. By incorporating additional consent procedures, informed consent is treated as an on-going process in which the research participants have a say not only in whether the data can be used for research but also in how that data may be used.

Conclusion

CA is a comprehensive interpretative research methodology that studies how language is used in actual social situations to understand the process of communication. With its roots in symbolic interactionism and ethnomethodology, CA is part of an empirically descriptive, analytically grounded interpretive research tradition. Empirically, CA uses actual audio- or video-recordings of naturally occurring interaction to examine participants' interactive communicative behavior. Analytically, CA takes the perspective that conversational interaction is taken for granted and only appears to be simple. Talk is simultaneously embedded in situational, cultural, and social contexts, and participants have multiple competing (goal) orientations. One of CA's strengths is the emphasis on communication as an unfolding process to show that the act of speaking has demonstrable consequences in subsequent talk. When using language to communicate, CA shows that participants are not simply representing something inside their own minds, they are doing social action in collaboration with others. They are creating and negotiating identities and enacting activities within their personal and professional lives. CA takes a members' perspective to show how the details of interactional patterns can document the fundamental communication patterns through which we live our lives.

References

Antaki, C., & Rapley, M. (2007). Questions and answers to psychological assessment schedules: Hidden troubles in 'quality of life' interviews. *Journal of Intellectual Disability Research, 40*(5), 421–437.

Antaki, C., Barnes, R., & Leudar, I. (2005). Diagnostic formulations in psychotherapy. *Discourse Studies,* 7(6), 627–647.

Atkinson, J. M., & Heritage, J. (1984). *Structures of social action: Studies in conversation analysis.* Cambridge, England: Cambridge University Press.

Beach, W. A. (1993). Transitional regularities for casual "okay" usages. *Journal of Pragmatics, 19*(4), 325–352.

Beach, W. A., & LeBaron, C. D. (2002). Body disclosures: Attending to personal problems and reported sexual abuse during a medical encounter. *Journal of Communication, 52*(3), 617–639.

Blumer, H. (1969). *Symbolic interactionism: Perspective and method.* Englewood Cliffs, NJ: Prentice-Hall.

Bolden, G. (2010). "Articulating the unsaid" via and-prefaced formulations of others' talk. *Discourse Studies, 12*(1), 5–32.

Brown, P., & Levinson, S. C. (1987). *Politeness: Some universals in language usage* (Studies in international sociolinguistics, Vol. 4). Cambridge, England: Cambridge University Press.

Chatwin, J. (2008). Hidden dimensions: The analysis of interaction in nurse–patient encounters. *Quality in Primary Care, 16*(2), 109–115.

Costello, B. A., & Roberts, F. (2001). Medical recommendations as joint social practice. *Health Communication, 13*(3), 241–260.

DiMatteo, M. R., Robinson, J. D., Heritage, J., Tabbarah, M., & Fox, S. A. (2003). Correspondence among patients' self-reports, chart records, and audio/videotapes of medical visits. *Health Communication, 15*(4), 393–413.

Eide, H, Graugaard, P, Holgersen, K, & Finset, A. (2003). Physician communication in different phases of a consultation at an oncology outpatient clinic related to patient satisfaction. *Patient Education & Counseling, 51*(3), 259–266.

Garfinkel, H., & Sacks, H. (1970). On formal structures of practical actions. In J. C. McKinney & E. A. Tiryakian (Eds.), *Theoretical sociology: Perspectives and developments* (pp. 337–366). New York, NY: Appleton-Century Crofts.

Gill, V. (1998). Doing attributions in medical interaction: Patients' explanations for illness and doctors' responses. *Social Psychology Quarterly, 61*(4), 342–360.

Goffman, E. (1983). The interaction order: American Sociological Association, 1982 presidential address. *American Sociological Review, 48*(1), 1–17.

Goodwin, C. (1984). Notes on story structure and the organization of participation. In J. Maxwell Atkinson & J. Heritage (Eds.), *Structures of social action: Studies in conversation analysis* (pp. 225–246). Cambridge, England: Cambridge University Press.

Gordon, C, Ellis-Hill, C, & Ashburn, A. (2009). The use of conversational analysis: Nurse–patient interaction in communication disability after stroke. *Journal of Advanced Nursing, 65*(3), 544–553.

Have, P. T. (2000). *Doing conversation analysis: A practical guide.* London, England: Sage Publications.

Hepburn, A, & Bolden, G. B. (2012). The conversation analytic approach to transcription. In J. Sidnell & T. Stivers (Eds.), *The handbook of conversation analysis.* Chichester, West Sussex, England: Wiley-Blackwell.

Heritage, J. (1984a). *Garfinkel and ethnomethodology.* Cambridge, England: Polity Press.

Heritage, J. (1984b). A change-of-state token and aspects of its sequential placement. In J. Maxwell Atkinson & J. Heritage (Eds.), *Structures of social action: Studies in conversation analysis* (pp. 299–345). Cambridge, England: Cambridge University Press.

Heritage, J. (1989). Current developments in conversation analysis. In D. Roger & P. Bull (Eds.), *Conversation: An interdisciplinary perspective* (pp. 21–47). Clevedon, Somerset, England: Multilingual Matters.

Heritage, J. (2008). Conversation analysis as social theory. In B. S. Turner (Ed.), *The new Blackwell companion to social theory* (pp. 300–320). New York, NY: Wiley-Blackwell.

Heritage, J. (2009). Conversation analysis as an approach to the medical encounter. In J. B. McKinlay (Ed.), *e-source: Behavioral and social science research.* Watertown,

MA: New England Research Institute; Washington, D.C.: Office of Behavioral and Social Sciences Research, Department of Health and Human Services. Retrieved from http://www.esourceresearch.org/

Heritage, J., & Sorjonen, M.-L. (1994). Constituting and maintaining activities across sequences: And-prefacing as a feature of question design. *Language in Society, 23*(1), 1–29.

Heritage, J., & Stivers, T. (1999). Online commentary in acute medical visits: A method of shaping patient expectations. *Social Science & Medicine, 49*(11), 1501–1517.

Heritage, J., & Maynard, D. W. (Eds.). (2006). *Communication in medical care: Interaction between physicians and patients.* Cambridge, England: Cambridge University Press.

Heritage, J., & Robinson, J. D. (2006). The structure of patients' presenting concerns: physicians' opening questions. *Health Communication, 19*(2), 89–102.

Heritage, J., & Robinson, J. D. (2011). "Some" vs. "any" medical worries: Encouraging patients to reveal their unmet concerns. In C. Antaki (Ed.), *Applied conversation analysis: Changing institutional practices* (pp. 15–30). Basingstoke, Hampshire, England: Palgrave Macmillan.

Heritage, J., Robinson, J. D., Elliot, M. N., Beckett, M., & Wilkes, M. (2007). Reducing patients' unmet concerns in primary care: The difference one word can make. *Journal of General Internal Medicine, 22*(10), 1429–1433.

Heritage, J., Elliott, M. N., Stivers, T., Richardson, A., & Mangione-Smith, R. (2010). Reducing inappropriate antibiotics prescribing: The role of online commentary on physical examination findings. *Patient Education and Counseling, 81*(1), 119–125.

Jefferson, G. (2004). Glossary of transcript symbols with an introduction. In G. H. Lerner (Ed.), *Conversation analysis: Studies from the first generation* (pp. 13–31). Philadelphia, PA: John Benjamins Publishing Company.

John, D. N., & Housley, W. (2001). Talk-in-interaction in the community pharmacy setting: A conversation analytic approach. *International Journal of Pharmacy Practice, 9*(S1): 45.

Kirk, J., & Miller, M. L. (1985). *Reliability and validity in qualitative research.* Beverly Hills, CA: Sage Publications.

Koenig, C. J. (2011). Patient resistance as agency in treatment decisions. *Social Science and Medicine, 72*(7), 1105–1114.

Labov, W. (1972). *Sociolinguistic patterns.* Philadelphia, PA: University of Pennsylvania Press.

LeBaron, C. D., Mandelbaum, J., & Glenn, P. J. (2003). An overview of language and social interaction research. In P. J. Glenn, C. D. LeBaron, & J. Mandelbaum (Eds.), *Studies in language and social interaction: In honor of Robert Hopper.* Mahwah, NJ: Lawrence Erlbaum Associates.

Levinson, S. C. (1983). *Pragmatics.* Cambridge, England: Cambridge University Press.

Levinson, S. C. (1992). Activity types and language. In P. Drew & J. Heritage (Eds.), *Talk at work: Interaction in institutional settings* (pp. 66–99). Cambridge: Cambridge University Press.

Mangione-Smith, R., Elliott, M. N., Stivers, T., McDonald, L. L., & Heritage, J. (2006). Ruling out the need for antibiotics: Are we sending the right message? *Archives of Pediatrics and Adolescent Medicine, 160*(9), 945–952.

Mangione-Smith, R., Stivers, T., Elliott, M. N., McDonald, L., Heritage, J., & McGlynn, E. A. (2002). Parent expectations for antibiotics: Who are the public health campaigns failing to reach? *Pediatric Research, 51*(4), 15A.

Maynard, D. (1989). Notes on the delivery and reception of diagnostic news regarding mental disabilities. In D. T. Helm, W. T. Anderson, A. J. Meehan, & A. W. Rawls (Eds.), *The interactional order: New directions in the study of social order* (pp. 54–67). New York, NY: Irvington Publishers.

Ochs, E. (1979). Transcription as theory. In E. S. Ochs & B. B. Schieffelin (Eds.), *Developmental pragmatics* (pp. 43–72). New York, NY: Academic Press.

Parry, R. H. (2004a). Communication during goal-setting in physiotherapy treatment sessions. *Clinical Rehabilitation, 18*(6), 668–682.

Parry, R. H. (2004b). The interactional management of patients' physical incompetence: A conversation analytic study of physiotherapy interactions. *Sociology of Health and Illness, 26*(7), 976–1007.

Patton, M. Q. (1990). *Qualitative evaluation methods*. Newbury Park, CA: Sage Publications.

Penner, L. A., Orom, H., Albrecht, T. L., Franks, M. M., Foster, T. S., & Ruckdeschel, J. C. (2007). Camera-related behaviors during video recorded medical interactions. *Journal of Nonverbal Behavior, 31*(2), 99–117.

Pillet-Shore, D. (2006). Weighing in primary-care nurse–patient interactions. *Social Science & Medicine, 62*(2), 407–421.

Pilnick, A. (1998). "Why didn't you just say that?" Dealing with issues of symmetry, knowledge, and competence in the pharmacist/client encounter. *Sociology of Health and Illness, 20*(1), 29–51.

Roberts, F., & Robinson, J. D. (2004). Interobserver agreement on first-stage conversation analytic transcription. *Human Communication Research, 30*(3), 376–410.

Robinson, J. D. (2003). An interactional structure of medical activities during acute visits and its implications for patients' participation. *Health Communication, 15*(1), 27–57.

Robinson, J. D. (2007). The role of numbers and statistics within conversation analysis. *Communication Methods and Measures, 1*(1), 65–75.

Robinson, J. D. (2011). Conversation analysis and health communication. In T. L. Thompson, R. Parrott, & Jon F. Nussbaum (Eds.), *The Routledge handbook of health communication* (2nd ed.) (pp. 501–518). New York, NY: Routledge.

Robinson, J. D. (2012). Overall structural organization. In J. Sidnell & T. Stivers (Eds.), *Handbook of conversation analysis*. Chichester, West Sussex, England: Wiley-Blackwell.

Robinson, J. D., & Heritage, J. (2006). Physicians' opening questions and patients' satisfaction. *Patient Education and Counseling, 60*(3), 279–285.

Roter, D., & Larson, S. (2002). The Roter interaction analysis system (RIAS): Utility and flexibility for analysis of medical interactions. *Patient Education and Counseling, 46*(4), 243–251.

Ruusuvuori, J. (2001). Looking means listening: Coordinating displays of engagement in doctor–patient interaction. *Social Science & Medicine, 52*(7), 1093–1108.

Sacks, H. (1984a). Notes on methodology. In J. Maxwell Atkinson & J. Heritage (Eds.), *Structures of social action: Studies in conversation analysis* (pp. 21–27). Cambridge, England: Cambridge University Press.

Sacks, H. (1984b). On doing "being ordinary." In J. Maxwell Atkinson & J. Heritage (Eds.), *Structures of social action: Studies in conversation analysis* (pp. 413–429). Cambridge: Cambridge University Press.

Sacks, H., Schegloff, E. A., & Jefferson, G. (1974). A simplest systematics for the organization of turn-taking for conversation. *Language, 50*(4)(Pt. 1), 696–735.

Schegloff, E. A. (1982). Discourse as an interactional achievement: Some uses of "uh huh" and other things that come between sentences. In D. E. Tannen (Ed.), *Analyzing discourse:*

Text and talk (32nd annual round table on languages and linguistics, School of Languages and Linguistics, Georgetown University, Washington, D.C., 1981) (pp. 71–93). Washington D.C.: Georgetown University Press.

Schegloff, E. A. (1984). On some questions and ambiguities in conversation. In J. Maxwell Atkinson & J. Heritage (Eds.), *Structures of social action: Studies in conversation analysis* (pp. 266–298). Cambridge, England: Cambridge University Press.

Schegloff, E. A. (1987). Analyzing single episodes of interaction: An exercise in conversation analysis. *Social Psychology Quarterly, 50*(2), 101–114.

Schegloff, E. A. (1988). Description in the social sciences I: Talk-in-interaction. *IPRA Papers in Pragmatics, 2(1)*, 1–24.

Schegloff, E. A. (1995). Discourse as an interactional achievement III: The omnirelevance of action. *Research on Language and Social Interaction, 28*(2), 185–211.

Schegloff, E. A. (1996). Some practices for referring to persons in talk-in-interaction: A partial sketch of a systematics. In B. A. Fox (Ed.), *Studies in anaphora* (pp. 437–485). Philadelphia, PA: John Benjamins Publishing Company.

Schegloff, E. A. (1997). Practices and actions: Boundary cases of other-initiated repair. *Discourse Processes, 23*(3), 499–546.

Schegloff, E. A. (2003). Transcription project. Retrieved July 4, 2012, from http://www.sscnet.ucla.edu/soc/faculty/schegloff/TranscriptionProject/index.html

Schegloff, E. A. (2004). On dispensability. *Research on Language and Social Interaction, 37*(2), 95–149.

Schegloff, E. A. (2007). *Sequence organization in interaction: A primer in conversation analysis* (Vol. 1). Cambridge, England: Cambridge University Press.

Sigman, S. J. (1980). On communication rules from a social perspective. *Human Communication Research*, 7(1), 37–51.

Silverman, D. (2001). *Interpreting qualitative data: Methods for analyzing talk, text, and interaction* (2nd ed.). Thousand Oaks, CA: Sage Publications.

Stiles, W. B., & Putnam, S. M. (1995). Coding categories for investigating medical interviews: A meta classification. In M. Lipkin, S. M. Putnam, A. Lazare, J. G. Carroll, & R. M. Frankel, *The medical interview: Clinical care, education, and research* (pp. 489–494). New York, NY: Springer.

Stivers, T. (2005a). Non-antibiotic treatment recommendations: delivery formats and implications for parent resistance. *Social Science & Medicine, 60*(5), 949–964.

Stivers, T. (2005b). Parent resistance to physicians' treatment recommendations: One resource for initiating a negotiation of the treatment decision. *Health Communication, 18*(1), 41–74.

DIRECT OBSERVATION AND CODING OF PHYSICIAN–PATIENT INTERACTIONS

Robert A. Bell and Richard L. Kravitz

Communication is the glue that binds physicians and patients, establishing rapport, facilitating information exchange, and promoting patient education and counseling (Ong, de Haes, Hoos, & Lammes, 1995). Effective communication is not only a fundamental clinical skill but has been shown to enhance patient outcomes (Street, Makoul, Arora, & Epstein, 2009). For this reason, there has been growing interest in developing valid methods for describing communication in clinical settings. This chapter focuses on one such method, interaction analysis (IA), which entails the direct observation, systematic coding, and quantitative analysis of physician–patient interaction.

IA is one of several ways in which communication between physicians and patients can be studied. For example, clinical communication can be investigated via ethnographic methods (e.g., McCoy, 2005), grounded theory (e.g., Julliard, Vivar, Delgado, Cruz, Kabak, & Sabers, 2008), and conversation analysis (see chapter by Koenig and Robinson in this volume). These approaches can complement traditional IA. In the first section of this chapter, we describe the essential features and assumptions underlying IA of encounters between doctors and patients. In the next section, we outline the steps involved in this kind of research. In the final section, we review recent developments and controversies in the application of IA to clinical communication.

Nature of the Method

Description of Method

By way of overview, we will briefly introduce the IA investigative process here; we elaborate on these steps in the next section. The prototypical study is outlined

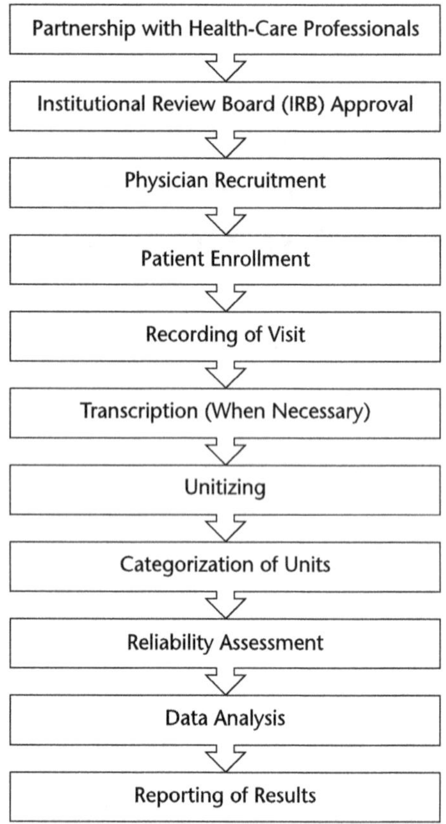

FIGURE 8.1 Investigative Process in IA Studies of Physician–Patient Interaction

in Figure 8.1. Researchers typically begin by partnering with one or more healthcare practices, clinics, or systems. Once administrators of the system(s) approached agree to provide access to their clinical sites, the investigator will usually have sufficient information to prepare the human subjects review protocol to the governing institutional review board (IRB). Upon IRB approval, physicians working at those locations are recruited based on the study's eligibility requirements. Thereafter, patients are recruited from participating physicians' practices. Recruitment is usually limited to patients having a scheduled visit within a specified time period. The visit is then audiotaped or videotaped; depending on study requirements, transcriptions of those tapes may be prepared. Patient and physician questionnaires may be administered before and after the visit to obtain additional information related to the investigator's research purposes.

The next step is unitizing the recorded discourse. "Unitizing" is the process of segmenting the interaction into units, such as utterances or idea units. Each unit is classified using categories that reflect the investigator's research interests. Reliability is assessed throughout the coding process by having two or more coders independently categorize the same units to measure intercoder agreement. Once reliability has been established, indexes can be computed that describe the extent to which particular communication behaviors were exhibited in the interaction. These indexes are analyzed descriptively and in conjunction with other variables about the physician, patient, or setting to answer the study's research questions and hypotheses. These results are presented in a scholarly article or other research outlet.

Theoretical Assumptions

Observational studies of patient–physician interaction have been primarily descriptive, focusing on what doctors and patients do rather than testing theory-based hypotheses (Roter & Hall, 1989). When theories have been referenced, their purpose has been to frame research questions generally and guide post hoc interpretation of results. In recent years, efforts have been made to more tightly couple theory and research. Examples include applications of accommodation theory (Street, 1991) and theories of relational communication (Siminoff & Step, 2011), as well as the development of models based on principles of reciprocity (Roter, 1988), emotion regulation (Finset & Mjaaland, 2009), partnership (Street & Millay, 2001), and communication functions (Street & Epstein, 2008).

Applications

IA can address many questions about communication between doctors and their patients. At the most basic level, researchers can describe the distribution of communication acts in clinical settings. A European research team provides a good example of this use of IA (Deveugele, Derese, De Bacquer, van den Brink-Muinen, Bensing, De Maeseneer, 2004). These investigators analyzed videotaped medical visits between 183 general practitioners representing six different nations and 2,801 of their patients. They found that the standard visit consisted predominantly of instrumental behaviors (59% of statements), such as giving information, agreeing, asking questions, and giving directions. Socioemotional behaviors, such as partnership- and rapport-building, were less common (37% of statements).

Second, measures of communication behavior derived from IA can be used as dependent (outcome) variables. For example, researchers have sought to determine if communication differs as a function of patient and physician gender (Bertakis & Azari, 2007), and patient age (Callahan, Bertakis, Azari, Robbins, Helms, & Chang, 2000), race (Oliver, Goodwin, Gotler, Gregory, & Stange, 2001), and socioeconomic status (Fiscella, Goodwin, & Stange, 2002). Coded communication has also served as a dependent variable in studies of the effects of context. For example, researchers have explored how interaction is affected by the presence of a patient companion (Wolff & Roter, 2011) and have examined differences in how family practice and internal medicine physicians communicate with patients (Paasche-Orlow & Roter, 2003). Communication behaviors have also been used as dependent variables to test the effects of interventions, especially communication training programs (Helitzer, LaNoue, Wilson, de Hernandez, Warner, & Roter, 2011).

Communication variables generated through IA can also be used as independent variables to predict visit outcomes. For example, one research team asked if physician self-disclosure increases patient satisfaction (Beach, Roter, Rubin, Frankel, Levinson, & Ford, 2004). Other investigators have studied the effect of patient and physician expressions of tension on patient satisfaction (Carter, Inui, Kukull, & Haigh, 1982). In our own work, we demonstrated that patients' requests for physician action predicted provision of tests, medication prescriptions, and referrals to other providers (Kravitz, Bell, Azari, Kelly-Reif, Krupat, & Thom, 2003).

Exemplars

As we have seen, IA is a flexible method that can address many types of questions about physician–patient communication. The value and nature of the method can be understood further by briefly examining two recently published exemplars.

Is Patient-Centered Care Associated with Lower Health-Care Costs?

This question was posed by Bertakis and Azari (2011) in a study that took place over a 12-month period. Each of 509 new adult patients without a provider preference was randomly assigned to receive care from one of 108 primary care physicians. Visits were videotaped and coded using the "Davis Observation Code (DOC)," which is discussed later. After controlling for patient characteristics and risk behaviors, it was found that the patients of doctors who exhibited more patient-centered communication had fewer visits to specialists, lower hospitalization rates, fewer laboratory and diagnostic tests, and lower medical charges overall.

Are Black and White Patients with Hypertension Treated Differently?

Hypertension (high blood pressure (BP)) contributes to cardiovascular morbidity and mortality, especially for Blacks. Cené and her colleagues sought to determine if physicians communicate differently with Black and White patients with hypertension (Cené, Roter, Carson, Miller, & Cooper, 2009). Patients from each race were classified as having controlled or uncontrolled BP. Audiotapes of their interactions with their doctors were coded using the Roter Interaction Analysis System (RIAS), described later. The investigators found that Blacks with uncontrolled BP, in comparison with Whites with controlled BP, had shorter visits characterized by less biomedical, psychosocial, and rapport-building communication. Similar deficits were observed when comparing Black and White patients with controlled BP. The authors conclude that race is associated with the quality of communication between patients and physicians.

Employing the Method

Procedures

We will now return to Figure 8.1. The steps depicted in the model describe the prototypical IA study; some steps may be omitted, depending on the nature of the investigation. For example, researchers can sometimes address their research questions using a sample of interactions previously recorded. Likewise, an investigator may opt for a coding strategy that does not require transcription.

Partnership with Healthcare Professionals

The first step is to partner with healthcare professionals who can provide access to clinical settings. In a perfect world, a researcher would sample healthcare systems from a sampling frame of all healthcare systems in operation within a region of interest (for example, the United States). In reality, resource constraints force clinical communication researchers to take a more local approach. Most published studies involve data collection within a single healthcare system, and often at a limited number of sites therein. For some projects, funding may be available for multicenter studies. The research setting is usually selected for its close proximity to the research team or based on the investigators' system affiliations.

IRB Approval

For all studies involving human research participants, researchers must obtain the approval of their institution's IRB. Patients enjoy special protections and legal rights, including privacy rights protected by the Health Insurance Portability and Accountability Act (HIPAA). A discussion of these protections is beyond the scope of this chapter. Protocols are usually prepared after access to a research site has been negotiated and before physicians and patients have been contacted.

Recruiting Physicians

Even when a healthcare system eagerly provides access to its clinical settings, its physicians may be less enthusiastic. Physicians, like patients, are research participants who must give their informed consent to be in the study. Some physicians will be more likely than others to consider the research burdensome and to be threatened by having their clinical behaviors come under study. Thus, the sample of participating physicians will not necessarily be representative of all physicians in the settings studied. It is thus useful to obtain demographic and practice characteristics of participating and nonparticipating physicians and adjust statistically for any bias in the sample.

The researcher can attempt to increase the willingness of physicians to participate in several ways. First, the investigator can emphasize the importance of the research to the medical profession. To avoid biasing physician behavior, this case must be made without revealing the specific study hypotheses. Next, the investigator can ask system administrators to encourage participation. Third, a monetary token of appreciation can be offered to physicians to demonstrate respect for their time. For example, we are currently carrying out an evaluation of two interventions intended to encourage patients with depressive symptoms to seek the help of their doctors. The physicians in this study are being given a $20 gift certificate for each enrolled patient, up to a maximum of $240. Finally, we note that IA studies can burden the doctor's staff. It is a kind gesture to offer staff a token of appreciation, such as money or a gift card.

Patient Recruitment

Once physicians have been recruited, enrollment of patients can begin. The patients under the care of a physician collectively constitute that physician's "panel." Only those patients who have a scheduled appointment within the data collection time period will be eligible to participate in the study. Other eligibility requirements might need to be established, based on study objectives. In some studies, efforts are made to solicit the participation of all eligible patients with scheduled appointments during the duration of the study. Depending on one's objectives, this approach could be questionable because it will overrepresent the kinds of patients who see their doctor more often, such as women, the elderly, the insured, and people with chronic conditions. As a result, the researcher should consider the value of stratifying patients based on gender, age, and other criteria. The voluntary nature of research participation presents a further challenge to patient sample representativeness. Patients consenting to participate may differ from non-volunteers along both measured and unmeasured characteristics, including demographics, attitudes, values, health status, and other qualities. When data are available, one should compare participating patients with aggregated profiles of the healthcare systems' patient population and make statistical adjustments for any biases.

Recording Visits

Audio recording has never been easier, as recording systems are now quite small and inconspicuous; filter out some noise; and record on high-capacity devices. The recording of visits must always be carried out with the informed, written consent of the patient. Furthermore, patients may halt recording at any time for any reason; in our experience, they rarely exercise this right.

Transcription

Coding interactions directly from an audio or video recording will not always be feasible. For example, when intricate coding of verbal behavior will be carried out, reliance on transcripts may be preferable to repeated reviews of the tapes. When coding involves identification of broad units, such as topics discussed, transcription is usually not needed. A transcript resembles a script, reporting what was said, and by whom. Noticeable events, such as laughter and crying, might also be noted in brackets. At times, the transcriber may be unsure of what was said and would indicate this by using a notation, such as [inaudible].

Here is an example of a portion of a transcript, from one of our earlier studies, that involves a patient with chronic back issues and the patient's primary care physician:

> PATIENT: For the last two to three months, I have just sat and just cried. I can't sleep, I have a hard time sitting. My back hurts so bad, I am just going crazy.
>
> DOCTOR: What part, the same area as usual?
>
> PATIENT: I think it must be, because it hurt so bad last night when I went to bed, and now across my shoulders and all the way down my spine and mainly right down, down into through here.
>
> DOCTOR: Right here. I can take a look?

This simple transcription emphasizes the verbal exchange of information, unlike the transcription procedures used in conversation analysis, which include notations for overlapping talk, silence, stress, amplitude changes, prolongation of sounds, and other features of speech (Atkinson & Heritage, 1984).

Unitizing

Audio or video recordings, or transcripts of those recordings, need to be unitized—broken down into "nuggets" that can be categorized. There is no standard approach to unitizing, but parceling participants' speech into units must be based on a set of explicit decision rules. For example, when using the Verona Medical Interview Classification System (VR-MICS), the process of creating speech units is as follows:

> "[A] speech unit begins when the person (physician or patient): (1) starts talking; (2) introduces some new content into what s/he is saying (change

> of content), or (3) changes their way of saying something (change in formulation). [T]he unit ends when (1) the person (physician or patient) stops talking either spontaneously or following interruption, or a pause is indicated in the transcription; or (2) when coded speech units are followed by changes in content or formulation indicating the beginning of a new unit."
>
> *(Del Piccolo, Mead, Gask, Mazzi, Goss, Rimondini, & Zimmermann, 2005, p. 254)*

An investigator wishing to profile what doctors and patients say in their visits will usually find it necessary to unitize and code every patient and physician utterance. Since communicators can express multiple ideas in a single statement, a given utterance can contain two or more units that will need to be identified and independently coded. In our studies of patient requests, we found that patients often made compound requests (usually linked by "and") that needed to be separated before coding. For example, the patient who says, "I need a refill for Tiazac and a referral to see the eye doctor" has made two requests, one for a medication refill and one for a referral.

Utterance-by-utterance unitizing is not always necessary. For example, investigators who are interested in a specific kind of communicative act or function would simply need to extract relevant instances from the visit recordings or transcripts. In some instances, a researcher only cares to know whether or not certain communication behaviors were exhibited in each visit studied. In such situations, the visit is considered in its entirety and the task of the coders is to check off those behaviors present anywhere in the visit. We took this approach in a study of the counseling that physicians provide to help patients with hypertension manage their condition (Bell & Kravitz, 2008). When coded behaviors are common and the investigator wishes to know *how often* they are present in a visit, it may be necessary to identify the presence/absence or frequency of the behaviors in question within successive time frames. For example, with the DOC coding scheme (described below), visits are segmented into 15-second frames for analysis.

Categorization of Units

The set of categories used to classify each unit is the defining feature of the coding scheme. These categories must be *mutually exclusive* (each unit placed in only one category) and *exhaustive* (every unit can be categorized). The mutual exclusivity criterion can be challenging because communicators often accomplish multiple goals in a single utterance. Consider the patient who anxiously says, "Doctor, I have a lump in my neck!" The patient is both providing information and expressing concern. For these kinds of statements, the coder must make a judgment about the primary objective of the utterance based on established guidelines. The exhaustiveness criterion can be met by including an "Other" or "Not Clinically Relevant" category for problematic units.

Many coding schemes have been advanced over the years. The scheme selected should reflect the study's research objectives. Most of the coding systems used in physician–patient interaction research vary along two dimensions: comprehensive versus focused; and process versus content. Comprehensive coding schemes seek to classify every patient and physician utterance. Other researchers take a more focused approach to coding by examining a particular type of communication, such as participation behaviors, requests, or acts of shared decision making. The process versus content coding dimension refers to the distinction between classifying units based on abstract features of communication versus classifying based on topic. Examples of process codes include "asking for information," "expressing concern," and "giving reassurance." Content codes could include "therapeutic regimes," "biomedical information," "lifestyle behavior," and so on. Hybrid systems that categorize units based on both process and content considerations have also been developed, as noted below.

The placement of discourse units into categories sounds easy—like sorting coins into containers based on denomination. Realistically, this process can be extremely difficult, for natural talk is messy. It is checkered with pauses, interruptions, false starts, overlapping talk, incomplete ideas, and indirectness. As a result, coders must make inferences when choosing the appropriate category for each unit. The inferences coders make should be guided by clear definitions and formal rules of application that are delineated in a coding manual. The manual needs to define the nature of the unit to be coded and provide clear instructions about how coders should parse the stream of talk. The categories into which these units will be placed must be clearly defined. Problematic types of utterances need to be identified in advance and rules need to be developed to ensure that coders handle such units in a standard fashion. The detailed instructions required in IA necessitate preparation of a lengthy document. For example, the coding manuals for the Taxonomy of Requests by Patients (TORP) and RIAS systems (described below) are 34 and 56 pages long, respectively. Training coders how to follow these instructions can take several days or longer.

Dozens of coding systems have been used in studies of clinical communication over the years. We briefly describe, below, several of the most commonly used systems to illustrate the method. Excluded from this review are older schemes that have fallen out of favor or been subsumed in newer systems. These include Bale's (1950) Interaction Process Analysis and the Relational Communication Control coding approach (O'Hair, 1989; Rogers & Farace, 1975). Also excluded are coding approaches developed to assess interaction in a single specialty, such as oncology (e.g., Dent, Brown, Dowsett, Tattersall, & Butow, 2005; Ford, Hall, Ratcliffe, & Fallowfield, 2000), and newer schemes that have not yet received extensive use, such as MEDICODE (Richard & Lussier, 2006) and the Siminoff Communication Content and Affect Program (SCCAP) (Siminoff & Step, 2011).

Roter's Interaction Analysis System

RIAS is based on Bale's (1950) scheme for coding small group decision making and has been used in more than 250 published studies of doctor–patient communication (RIASWorks, 2011). Each "communication unit," defined as "the smallest discriminable speech segment to which a classification may be assigned" (Roter, 2012, p. 4), is assigned to a single category. RIAS categories have been grouped into two sets: Socioemotional Exchange and Task-focused Exchange codes (see Table 8.1). Coding is carried out directly from audiotapes or videotapes

TABLE 8.1 Socioemotional Exchange and Task-Focused Exchange Categories in RIAS

Socioemotional Exchange Categories	*Task-Focused Exchange Categories*

• Personal Remarks, Social Conversation
• Laughs, Tells Jokes
• Shows Concern or Worry
• Reassures, Encourages, or Shows Optimism
• Shows Approval—Direct
• Gives Compliment—General
• Shows Disapproval—Direct
• Shows Criticism—General
• Empathy Statements
• Legitimizing Statements
• Partnership Statements
• Self-Disclosure Statements
• Asks For Reassurance
• Shows Agreement or Understanding
• Back-Channel Responses
	• Transition Words
	• Gives Orientation, Instructions
	• Paraphrase/Checks For Understanding
	• Asks For Understanding
	• Bid For Repetition
	• Asks For Opinion
	• Asks For Permission
	• Medical Condition
	  • Gives Information
	  • Asks Closed-Ended Questions
	  • Asks Open-Ended Questions
	• Therapeutic Regimen
	  • Gives Information
	  • Asks Closed-Ended Questions
	  • Asks Open-Ended Questions
	• Lifestyle Information
	  • Gives Information
	  • Asks Closed-Ended Questions
	  • Asks Open-Ended Questions
	• Psychosocial Information
	  • Gives Information
	  • Asks Closed-Ended Questions
	  • Asks Open-Ended Questions
	• Other Information
	  • Gives Information
	  • Asks Closed-Ended Questions
	  • Asks Open-Ended Questions
	• Counsels Or Directs Behavior
	  • Medical Condition/Therapeutic Regimen
	  • Lifestyle & Psychosocial
	• Requests for Services or Medication

Note: Operational definitions, coding instructions, and examples can be found in the RIAS coding manual (Roter, 2012).

of the interactions, obviating the need for transcripts. All Socioemotional categories are process oriented and include codes such as "laughs/tells jokes" and "empathy statements." Examples of Task-Focused categories are "gives orientation/instructions" and "asks for permission." The categories "gives information," "asks closed-ended questions," and "asks open-ended questions" appear five times in the scheme, under each of five topic categories (e.g., medical condition), making RIAS a hybrid scheme that encompasses process and content coding. Scoring rules have been developed to combine specific categories to create more general measures (e.g., patient-centeredness and verbal dominance). Impressive evidence of the reliability and validity of RIAS has been reviewed by Roter and Larson (2002).

Verbal Response Mode

Stile's (1979) Verbal Response Mode (VRM) was originally developed to examine communication in psychotherapy contexts, but has since been used in studies of the medical interview (e.g., Shaikh, Knobloch, & Stiles, 2001). The unit of analysis is the sentence or any part thereof that has meaning, such as an independent clause. The analyst examines each unit in context and makes three determinations:

1. Source of Experience—Does the unit refer to the experience of the speaker or the listener?
2. Frame of Reference—Is the frame of reference that of the speaker or other person?
3. Presupposition—Does the speaker presume to have specific knowledge about the listener or not?

Crossing these three dichotomous decisions produces eight verbal response modes (see Table 8.2). For example, the mode "disclosure" is based on the experience and frame of reference of the speaker and makes no specific presumption about the knowledge of the listener.

The investigator will typically compute the proportion of utterances that fall within each mode, and will do so separately for patient and physician. These eight VRM codes can also be used to measure three role dimensions in the interaction: attentive–informative, acquiescence–directiveness, and presumptuous–unassuming. As noted in Table 8.3, below, all eight VRM codes are used in the calculation of each role dimension. For example, four modes are used to assess attentiveness and the remaining four modes are used to measure Informativeness; this pattern is repeated for the other two role dimensions. The VRM has been applied reliably to medical interaction data (e.g., Meeuwesen, Schaap, & van der Staak, 1991; Shaikh et al., 2001), but evidence of validity is limited (see Carter et al., 1982).

TABLE 8.2 Stiles' VRM

Verbal Response Mode	*Brief Definition*	*Classification Principles*		
		Source of Experience	*Frame of Reference*	*Presupposition*
Disclosure	Revelation of subjective information about the speaker, such as thoughts, feelings, and intentions.	speaker	speaker	no
Edification	Provision of objective information.	speaker	other	no
Advisement	Communications that seek to guide the other's behavior through advice, commands, persuasion, and other means.	speaker	speaker	yes
Confirmation	Communications that compare the speaker's experience with the experience of the listener to uncover agreement or disagreement, shared experiences, shared intentions, and so forth.	speaker	other	yes
Question	A communication that requests information or guidance.	other	speaker	no
Acknowledgment	Utterances that let the listener know that his or her communication was received by the speaker.	other	other	no
Interpretation	Verbalizations that explain the listener to himself/herself through judgment, evaluation, or labeling.	other	speaker	yes
Reflection	Use of repetition, clarification, or restatement to put the other person's experiences into words.	other	other	yes

TABLE 8.3 VRM Components that Compose Each of Six Role Dimensions

	VRM Components							
Role Dimension	*Disclosure*	*Edification*	*Advisement*	*Confirmation*	*Question*	*Acknowledgment*	*Interpretation*	*Reflection*
Attentiveness					√	√	√	√
Informativeness	√	√	√	√				
Acquiescence		√		√		√		√
Directiveness	√		√		√		√	
Presumptuous			√	√			√	√
Unassuming	√	√			√	√		

TABLE 8.4 Modified DOC Clusters and Corresponding Codes

Cluster	*No. of Codes*	*Code(s)**
Technical	*8*	*Structuring Interaction, History Taking, Family Information, Physical Examination, Evaluation Feedback, Planning Treatment, Treatment Effects, Procedure*
Health Behavior	*5*	*Compliance, Health Education, Health Promotion, Nutrition, Exercise*
Addiction	*2*	*Substance Use, Smoking Behavior*
Patient Activation	*3*	*Health Knowledge, Patient Question, Chatting*
Preventive Service	*1*	*Preventive Service*
Counseling	*1*	*Counseling*

Note: Refer to Bertakis and Azari (2011, Table 1, p. 231) for brief definitions of each code.

Davis Observation Code

DOC was developed at University of California, Davis (Callahan & Bertakis, 1991), and was subsequently modified to include measures of patient-centered care (Bertakis & Azari, 2011). This scheme has been used widely in physician–patient interaction research. Coding is carried out on successive 15-second segments of the medical visit. For each segment, coders note the occurrence of each of 20 clinical behaviors that cluster into 6 broader groups, as described in Table 8.4. Solid evidence of reliability and validity has accumulated over the past 20 years.

Street's Patient Participation Coding System

Street and his colleagues have proposed that during patient–clinician encounters, patients participate in their medical care primarily by asking questions, expressing their concerns, and asserting their preferences and views (Street & Millay, 2001) (see Table 8.5). Trained coders review tapes of the medical visits to be analyzed, pulling out instances of patient participation for transcription and coding. Over several studies, Street and his colleagues have demonstrated that these three codes parsimoniously capture key aspects of what it means to be a participating patient.

Taxonomy of Requests by Patients

The TORP (Kravitz, Bell, & Franz, 1999; Kravitz, Bell, Franz, Elliott, Amsterdam, Willis, & Silverio, 2002) was developed as part of a project examining mutual influence in clinical care, and has since been used in about a dozen published studies. Request units are initially identified using definitions and decision rules that are represented in a flow chart, as depicted in Figure 8.2. Thereafter, each

TABLE 8.5 Street's Patient Participation Coding System—Process Categories, Operational Definitions, and Examples

Process Category	*Operational Definition**	*Example*
Asking Questions	*Utterances in interrogative form intended to seek information and clarification.*	*"What is hypertension?"*
Expressions of Concern	*Utterances in which the patient expresses worry, anxiety, fear, anger, frustration, and other forms of negative affect or emotions.*	*"I'm worried about what this could be."*
Assertive Responses	*Utterances in which the patient expresses his or her rights, beliefs, interests, and desires, as in offering an opinion, stating preferences, making suggestions or recommendations, disagreeing, or interrupting.*	*"I would rather not take medication for this if there is another option."*

**Note*: Operational definitions are taken verbatim from Street and Millay (2001, Table 1, p. 63).

request is classified as an information request or an action request. Each request for information is further classified into 1 of 12 topical categories (e.g., physical problem, drug therapy, preventive care). Likewise, action requests are more precisely classified into 1 of 8 resource categories (e.g., diagnostic testing,

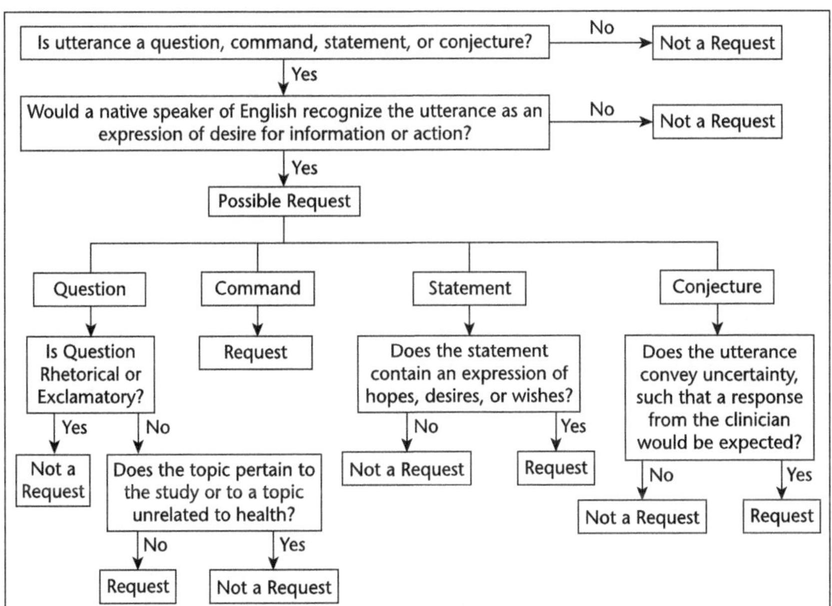

FIGURE 8.2 Decision Flowchart Used to Identify Request Units in Research Employing the TORP

new medication, medication refill). TORP thus represents the content coding of a single type of communication act—the patient request. This scheme also includes codes for assessing other features of each request, as well as physicians' responses to their patients' requests.

Assessing Performance of Prescribed Communication

Coding schemes have been developed to evaluate the extent to which physicians communicate in prescribed ways. Krupat, Frankel, Stein, and Irish (2006), for example, developed the Four Habits Coding Scheme (FHCS) to evaluate the outcomes of physician training in the Four Habits approach to clinical communication. In the realm of smoking cessation, Lawson, Flocke, and Casucci (2009) developed the 5A's Direct Observation Coding (5A-DOC) scheme to assess physician performance of five tasks—Ask, Advise, Assess, Assist, Arrange—for identifying and treating smokers in primary care.

Ratings as Coding

Up to this point, we have focused on coding schemes that place discourse units into *nominal* (unordered) categories that have been given labels descriptive of a shared feature of the classified units. We would be remiss if we did not acknowledge that physician–patient communication researchers also use ordered categories on occasion. For example, the RIAS approach augments nominal category coding with global affective ratings. Specifically, the physician and patient is each rated on a set of six-point Likert scales to assess "overall affective impressions" of their levels of anger, anxiety, depression, emotional distress, dominance, and other affective states.

Reliability Assessment

The data generated from the coding of interactions has no value if it is not reliable. Reliability is established by demonstrating that two or more coders, working independently, exhibit a high level of agreement in their coding decisions. We will revisit this topic in a later section on reliability and validity.

Data Analysis

Once data have been reliably coded, the investigator can generate results using descriptive and inferential statistics. Here, we will briefly discuss two data analysis issues that are likely to confront investigators using IA methods: computing indexes and adjusting for correlated (clustered) data.

Computation of Indexes

Once coding has been completed, the investigator will create behavioral indexes to summarize the communication in each physician–patient visit. The simplest indexes are tallies of the frequency with which each category was present in the visit. As we have already seen, investigators will often compute more general indexes by summarizing across the tallies of two or more categories. For example, with TORP we have many "information request" and "action request" categories that can be analyzed separately, but we also collapse across these to create summary "information request" and "action request" indexes. Likewise, investigators using RIAS have often combined the Socioemotional and Task category sets listed in Table 8.1 to create two broad indexes.

Researchers will need to decide whether to use frequencies, which are raw counts of the occurrence of a particular behavioral code (e.g., "patients asked questions an average of 12 times per visit"); percentages and proportions, which express the frequency of the code in terms of its "share" of the whole (e.g., "17 percent [or 0.17] of patients' utterances involved question-asking"; or rates, which express the average frequency of occurrence of the behavioral code for a standard period of time (e.g., "on average, patients asked 2.2 questions per minute"). It is also possible to create indexes that represent the ratio of two frequencies. For example, for RIAS, verbal dominance is operationalized as the ratio of patient utterances to doctor utterances (Paasche-Orlow & Roter, 2003). When absolute frequencies are used, it is often desirable to control for the effects of visit length (cf. Street & Millay, 2001, p. 65). Percentages, proportions, and ratios are especially useful when trying to assess the relative contributions of physicians and patients to the medical interaction and other questions related to "balance," "equilibrium," "dominance," and so forth.

Analyzing Correlated (Clustered) Data

The typical IA study in medical settings involves the recruitment of physicians, followed by the recruitment of >1 patient within each physician panel. It is possible that a physician's patients will be more similar to one another than to the patients of other physicians in the study. This is a problem because many statistical tests assume that our observations are independent, not "clustered." Clustered data typically results in larger sampling variability than what would have been obtained had patients been sampled directly. This must be taken into account in our standard error estimates and our tests of hypotheses. Our team does so with the "svy" commands in Stata (Stata Corporation, 2011), which also incorporate weighting and stratification options. Other software packages have similar features. Generalized estimating equations (GEE) provide another option for analyzing correlated data (Hardin & Hilbe, 2007).

Reporting Results

Once data analysis has been completed, results can be written up for presentation or publication. The introduction of the report should describe the issue that motivated the study; review relevant literature; describe the specific objectives of the project, including hypotheses and research questions; and explain why IA was the chosen method. We have found that social science journal editors are usually more concerned about the theoretical framing of articles and expect a more extensive review of the literature, whereas nursing and medical journal editors are more concerned about the clinical significance of the research. One would be wise to select a target journal before commencing with writing.

Reporting of methods and results will be very similar for communication, nursing, public health, and medical journals. Editors and reviewers will expect to find details about the study setting and the sampling of physicians and patients. When data are available, the profile of participating physicians and patients should be compared to the population of physicians and patients from the system(s) studied. Reports should also describe the coding process, including training of coders, and report unitizing and category-specific reliability coefficients. Details should be provided about the computation of indexes, adjustments for clustered data, and use of case weighting and stratification. The discussion section should examine the theoretical and/or clinical significance of findings, consider potential policy implications, acknowledge study limitations, and offer avenues for future research.

Reliability and Validity

Interaction coding is a process of measurement. The quality of data produced through this process is evaluated with regard to the principles of reliability and validity.

Reliability

Coding reliability is established by providing evidence that our scheme, if applied repeatedly to the same interactions, produces the same result. Evidence of the reliability (intercoder agreement) of IA data requires a duplication of coding activities. Two or more coders need to independently code all or a sample of representative interactions. The data are reliable if these coders independently come to the same conclusion in most of their coding decisions. A number of factors can lower levels of intercoder agreement, including inadequate coder training, poorly defined categories, ambiguous data, and even poor quality audiotapes or videotapes. Ideally, investigators would assess the reliability of unitizing and categorization. With few exceptions (Kravitz et al., 2002), unitizing reliability has rarely been reported.

Investigators have many different ways to measure intercoder agreement (Popping, 2010), but Cohen's (1960) kappa (κ) has emerged as the standard approach. Percent agreement continues to be reported as well, but this is an inadequate measure of reliability because it does not correct for chance agreement between coders. Reporting of one kappa value for "overall coding agreement" is not acceptable; a separate κ coefficient should be reported for every variable in the coding scheme. Landis and Koch (1977) offer guidelines for evaluating the kappa values obtained. In recent years, Krippendorff's (2004) alpha (α) coefficient has gained popularity as a measure of agreement. His approach can accommodate any number of coders; can assess reliability at all levels of measurement, from nominal to ratio; and can be augmented with coefficients that assess the extent to which coding disagreements were random (Krippendorff, 2008).

Validity

Because IA is a process of measurement, this discussion of validity is grounded in the language of measurement validity. When developing a coding scheme, investigators will typically begin by identifying a set of codes to measure behaviors that, on its face, appears to capture the essential elements of the communication process of interest. This judgment call is sometimes referred to as "face validity." However, believing that one's coding scheme is valid does not make it so. Empirical evidence of validity is needed. When possible, evidence should be collected for three types of validity: criterion-related, construct, and content validity.

Criterion-related validity refers to the extent to which variables generated from interaction coding are associated with concrete, real-world criteria. A criterion can be assessed at the same time (concurrent validity) that the scheme is being employed, as is the case in cross-sectional research designs. For example, a system to code physicians' use of medical jargon should be strongly associated with their patients' level of misunderstanding in the visits studied. Alternatively, in longitudinal designs, the coding scheme under study can be validated by using it to predict a criterion measured in the future (predictive validity). For instance, a coding scheme developed to assess physicians' provision of information about a newly prescribed medication should predict patient adherence to their new drug regimen in the weeks following the visit.

Construct validity concerns the degree to which the codes in our coding scheme correlate with other constructs in logical ways. Specifically, we should expect the constructs we have measured to be strongly correlated with other measures of the same (or very similar) constructs. Strong correlations among different operationalizations of the same construct provide evidence of convergent construct validity. We should also expect weak correlations between the constructs we have coded and other constructs that are theoretically distinct (discriminant construct validity). Suppose, for example, that we want to code interactions to devise a measure "physician verbal dominance." We could measure dominance by dividing physician talk time in a visit by total visit talk time. To demonstrate the construct validity of this measure, we would need to show that it is strongly correlated (converges) with other measures of verbal dominance, such as the global ratings of the participants or third parties. We would also need to demonstrate that it has little or no relationship with unrelated constructs, such as physician friendliness or verbal aggression.

Content validity refers to the degree to which coding categories represent the full range of the construct they are intended to operationalize. Consider, for example, a coding scheme designed to assess physician empathic communication. If this scheme included a category for "verbal acknowledgment of patient distress," but did not code for physicians' "expression of appropriate emotion" in response to the patient distress, we might feel that an important facet of empathy has been ignored. Likewise, we would doubt the content validity of any scheme designed to measure patient participation if it excluded a code for patient question-asking.

Tradeoffs Between Reliability and Validity

Reliability is a necessary but not sufficient condition for validity. Ironically, however, there can be a tension between reliability and validity (Krippendorff, 2004). For example, researchers know that they are expected to report their coding reliability, and may opt to increase reliability by making the definitions of their categories overly specific. In doing so, coding disagreements will be reduced, but cases that fall within the intended meaning of the category might not be placed within it under the restrictive (but more reliable) definition. One way to strike a balance between reliability and validity is to compare units placed within each category with one another, and then again with the units assigned to different categories. Do the observed differences between units within and across categories make sense? If not, then category definitions need to be reconsidered, even if intercoder agreement was high.

Strengths and Limitations of Method

Strengths

The primary strength of IA is that it generates data grounded in *direct observation*. Using survey data or electronic medical records as proxy measures of communication in medical encounters is suspect. Patient and physician post-visit reports of the nature and content of their communication often do not agree with each other or with tape recordings of the actual visit (e.g., DesHarnais, Carter, Hennessy, Kurent, & Carter, 2007; Gilchrist, Stange, Flocke, McCord, & Bourguet, 2004;

Shaikh, Nettiksimmons, Bell, Tancredi, & Romano, 2012). A related strength is that IA offers the opportunity to study clinical communication *naturalistically*. The medical visits studied exist independent of the research. This is in sharp contrast with most experimental studies of social interaction, in which independent variables are manipulated to create the situations studied.

Limitations

IA fails to provide a strong basis for causal inference. In experimental research, investigators create equivalent experimental and control groups by randomly assigning research participants to contrasting conditions. This allows for the control of confounding variables that would otherwise make it difficult to isolate cause and effect. Suppose, for example, that we want to know the effects of the variable "primary care specialty" on clinical communication. Let us assume that this variable has two levels: family practice and internal medicine. We will not be able to carry out a true experiment because we cannot randomly assign physicians to be in the family practice or internal medicine group. Physicians come to us already "assigned" by virtue of their professional training. As a result, any differences we observe between family practice and internal medicine doctors could be due to other variables on which the two doctor groups differ. The most we can do is rely on statistical controls to try to remove the effects of confounding variables—and hope for the best. (We do not wish to leave the reader with the impression that IA methods can never be used in conjunction with true experiments. In fact, such experiments are sometimes possible, as when doctors are randomly assigned to receive or not receive training, and their subsequent interactions are coded to assess the effects of the training.)

A second limitation deals with the generalizability of results. Clinical communication researchers will never have the resources to take a national sample of patients, fly to each patient's city or town, and record their next visit with their doctor. Instead, we must hope that our local doctors and patients are representative of the general population, or, perhaps, carry out our study in two or three diverse locations (multi-center research). Ultimately, this weakness can be managed through the replication of research by investigators across diverse settings, followed by a meta-analysis of those studies (see Noar's chapter in this volume).

A third potential weakness is the possibility of reactivity. This is the concern that doctors and patients may alter their communication behavior because they know their visit is being recorded. In our experience, physicians and patients quickly forget that they are being recorded and get down to business.

Challenges

Researchers wishing to analyze clinical communication face challenges. First, IA is an expensive, labor-intensive endeavor that cannot easily be carried out on a sample of interactions of sufficient size without funding support. In our recent experience, it costs $50 to $200 per medical visit to undertake the kinds of analyses we have described in this chapter, not including investigator time.

Next, social scientists may find it difficult to gain access to clinical settings because they are not usually known to the administrators at their local healthcare system. Access will be less of an issue for the physician-researcher, who may be practicing in the healthcare system and know the administrators who could grant access. We believe it is often best for social scientists (the PhDs) and physician researchers (the MDs) to team up. The MDs in interdisciplinary research teams can help secure access to research settings, understand better the constraints that shape physician behavior, and have a keener sense of how research findings can improve clinical practice. The PhDs, on the other hand, tend to be more comfortable thinking in theoretical terms, and often (though not always) have more training in research methods and statistics.

Third, although nonverbal communication is important in clinical communication (Mast, 2007), it is understudied (Gorawara-Bhat & Cook, 2011). Many patients who are willing to be audiotaped may balk at the idea of being videotaped due to privacy or modesty concerns. Although audiotapes can provide some information through vocalic cues, videotapes are needed to code for most nonverbal signs of involvement, affiliation, emotional states, and other unspoken aspects of the interaction. Even when permission to videotape can be obtained, the logistics of video recording are challenging (Roter, Frankel, Hall, & Sluyter, 2006).

Finally, investigators may find it difficult to link visit communication to the most meaningful outcomes—changes in patient health. Distal outcomes related to morbidity and mortality play out over the course of weeks, months, and even years. Tracking patients for such an extended period of time is prohibitively expensive. For this reason, much of the research reported to date links interaction to proximal outcomes that can be measured at the conclusion of the visit, such as patient satisfaction, trust, and medical adherence intentions.

Recent Developments and Controversies

IA methods continue to undergo refinement. In this final section, we will focus on two issues: efforts to improve the efficiency of the approach in clinical contexts, and calls to take "process" more seriously.

Enhancing Efficiency

One strategy being developed to increase the coding efficiency is "interaction sampling." Could "thin slice" samples of physician–patient visits be used in observational studies of medical encounters to represent the full session? Roter and her colleagues believe so (Roter, Hall, Blanch-Hartigan, Larson, & Frankel,

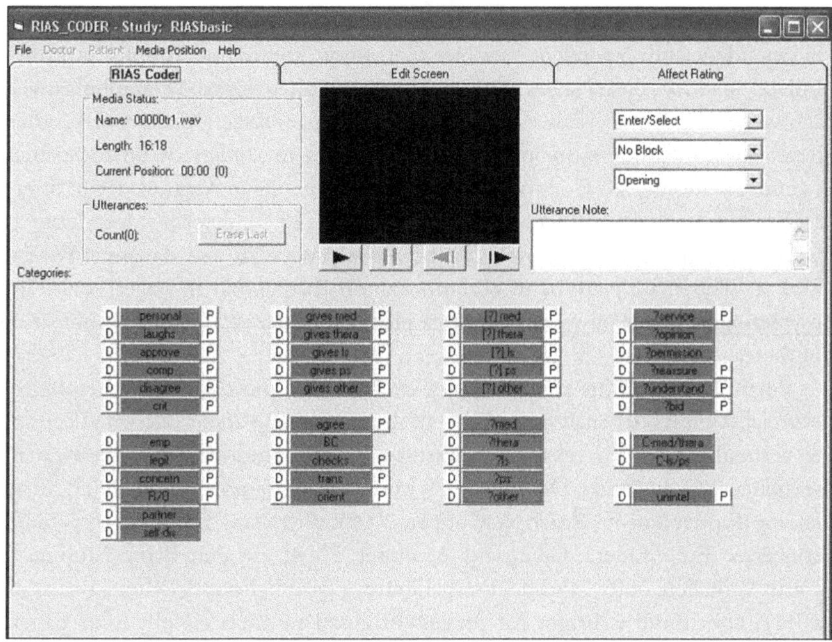

FIGURE 8.3 Screenshot of the RIAS Software Used to Aid Coding and Analysis of Interaction Between Providers and Patients

Note: Coding can be based on audiotaped, videotaped, or transcribed interactions. This application can be used to record information about sequencing of communication acts. It can also accommodate communication between multiple dyads in the same interaction (e.g., physician–patient, physician–third party, medical assistant–patient).

2011). They coded the full duration of 253 medical visits and then extracted three 1-minute-long "slices," finding strong correlations between each segment and the full session data on key variables. More research is needed, but this approach is promising.

Efficiency can also be enhanced with coding software applications. For example, the RIAS is supported by software that simplifies coding activities, as illustrated in Figure 8.3 (RIASWorks, 2011). Software is also available for SCCAP (Siminoff & Step, 2011). In our own work, we have found that "off the shelf" qualitative data analysis software, such as NVivo (QSR, 2010), can be adapted to facilitate coding of transcripts.

Putting "Process" into IA

Human communication is invariably defined as a "process" that unfolds over time. Unfortunately, many IA studies of clinical communication have not been true to this notion of process. Instead, studies have often taken what Poole (2007) refers to as a "variance theory" approach by focusing on static associations among independent and dependent variables that ignore the temporal order of events. Indeed, when we create tallies of what patients and physicians did communicatively across the length of a visit, we are not even looking at *inter*action. Of course, others have also called for more processual approaches in studies of doctor–patient communication (e.g., Connor, Fletcher, & Salmon, 2009; Makoul, 1998; Street, 1991), but how do we accomplish this? Poole (2007) describes four ways in which communication research can be more processual and dynamic: We can look at sequences; patterns of communication that unfold in stages; social and psychological mechanisms that drives a process of interest; or some combination of these.

Fortunately, over the past few years, we have seen more processual research—especially sequential analysis studies—of the physician–patient dialogue (Bensing & Verheul, 2009). For example, investigators have studied information-giving sequences (Goss, Mazzi, Del Piccolo, Rimondini, & Zimmermann, 2005), turn-taking (Roter, Larson, Beach, & Cooper, 2008), physicians' responses to patients' concerns (Eide, Quera, Graugaard, & Finset, 2004; van den Brink-Muinen & Caris-Verhallen, 2003), and doctor–patient eye gaze behaviors (Montague, et al., 2011). The future is bright for process-oriented research on physician–patient communication.

Note

Preparation of this chapter was supported by a grant from the National Institute of Mental Health (R01 MH079387 [Kravitz]).

References

Atkinson, J. Maxwell, & Heritage, J. (1984). *Structures of social action: studies in conversation analysis*. Cambridge, England: Cambridge University Press.

Bales, R. F. (1950). *Interactional process analysis: A method for the study of small groups*. Cambridge, England: Addison-Wesley Press.

Beach, M. C., Roter, D., Rubin, H., Frankel, R., Levinson, W., & Ford, D. E. (2004). Is physician self-disclosure related to patient evaluation of office visits? *Journal of General Internal Medicine*, *19*(9), 905–910.

Bell, R. A., & Kravitz, R. L. (2008). Physician counseling for hypertension: What do doctors really do? *Patient Education and Counseling*, *72*(1), 115–121.

Bensing, J., & Verheul, W. (2009). Towards a better understanding of the dynamics of patient provider interaction: The use of sequence analysis. *Patient Education and Counseling*, *75*(2), 145–146.

Bertakis, K. D., & Azari, R. (2007). Patient gender and physician practice style. *Journal of Women's Health*, *16*(6), 859–868.

Bertakis, K. D., & Azari, R. (2011). Patient-centered care is associated with decreased health care utilization. *Journal of the American Board of Family Medicine*, *24*(3), 229–239.

Callahan, E. J., & Bertakis, K. D. (1991). Development and validation of the Davis Observation Code. *Family Medicine, 23*(1), 19–24.

Callahan, E. J., Bertakis, K. D., Azari, R., Robbins, J. A., Helms, L. J., & Chang, D. W. (2000). The influence of patient age on primary care resident physician–patient interaction. *Journal of the American Geriatrics Society, 48*(1), 30–35.

Carter, W. B., Inui, T. S., Kukull, W. A., & Haigh, V. H. (1982). Outcome-based doctor–patient interaction analysis: II. Identifying effective provider and patient behavior. *Medical Care, 20*(6), 550–566.

Cené, C. W., Roter, D., Carson, K. A., Miller, E. R., & Cooper, L. A. (2009). The effect of patient race and blood pressure control on patient–physician communication. *Journal of General Internal Medicine, 24*(9), 1057–1064.

Cohen, J. (1960). A coefficient of agreement for nominal scales. *Educational and Psychological Measurement, 20*(1), 37–46.

Connor, M., Fletcher, I., & Salmon, P. (2009). The analysis of verbal interaction sequences in dyadic clinical communication: A review of methods. *Patient Education and Counseling, 75*(2), 169–177.

Del Piccolo, L., Mead, N., Gask, L., Mazzi, M.A., Goss, C., Rimondini, M., & Zimmermann, C. (2005). The English version of the Verona medical interview classification system (VR-MICS): An assessment of its reliability and a comparative cross-cultural test of its validity. *Patient Education and Counseling, 58*(3), 252–264.

Dent, E., Brown, R., Dowsett, S., Tattersall, M., & Butow, P. (2005). The Cancode interaction analysis system in the oncological setting: Reliability and validity of video and audio tape coding. *Patient Education and Counseling, 56*(1), 35–44.

DesHarnais, S., Carter, R. E., Hennessy, W., Kurent, J. E., & Carter, C. (2007). Lack of concordance between physician and patient: Reports on end-of-life care discussions. *Journal of Palliative Medicine, 10*(3), 728–740.

Deveugele, M., Derese, A., De Bacquer, D., van den Brink-Muinen, A., Bensing, J., & De Maeseneer, J. (2004). Is the communicative behavior of GPs during the consultation related to the diagnosis? A cross-sectional study in six European countries. *Patient Education and Counseling, 54*(3), 283–289.

Eide, H., Quera, V., Graugaard, P., & Finset, A. (2004). Physician–patient dialogue surrounding patients' expression of concern: Applying sequence analysis to RIAS. *Social Science & Medicine, 59*(1), 145–155.

Finset, A., & Mjaaland, T. A. (2009). The medical consultation viewed as a value chain: A neurobehavioral approach to emotion regulation in doctor–patient interaction. *Patient Education and Counseling, 74*(3), 323–330.

Fiscella, K., Goodwin, M. A., & Stange, K. C. (2002). Does patient educational level affect office visits to family physicians? *Journal of the National Medical Association, 94*(3), 157–165.

Ford, S., Hall, A., Ratcliffe, D., & Fallowfield, L. (2000). The Medical Interaction Process System (MIPS): An instrument for analysing interviews of oncologists and patients with cancer. *Social Science & Medicine, 50*(4), 553–566.

Gilchrist, V. J., Stange, K. C., Flocke, S. A., McCord, G., & Bourguet, C. C. (2004). A comparison of the National Ambulatory Medical Care Survey (NAMCS) measurement approach with direct observation of outpatient visits. *Medical Care, 42*(3), 276–280.

Gorawara-Bhat, R., & Cook, M.A. (2011). Eye contact in patient-centered communication. *Patient Education and Counseling, 82*(3), 442–447.

Goss, C., Mazzi, M. A., Del Piccolo, L., Rimondini, M., & Zimmermann, C. (2005). Information-giving sequences in general practice consultations. *Journal of Evaluation in Clinical Practice, 11*(4), 339–349.

Hardin, J. W., & Hilbe, J. M. (2007). *Generalized linear models and extensions*. College Station, TX: Stata Press.

Helitzer, D. L., LaNoue, M., Wilson, B., de Hernandez, B. U., Warner, T., & Roter, D. (2011). A randomized controlled trial of communication training with primary care providers to improve patient-centeredness and health risk communication. *Patient Education and Counseling, 82*(1), 21–29.

Julliard, K., Vivar, J., Delgado, C., Cruz, E., Kabak, J., & Sabers, H. (2008). What Latina patients don't tell their doctors: A qualitative study. *Annals of Family Medicine, 6*(6), 543–549.

Kravitz, R. L., Bell, R. A., & Franz, C. E. (1999). A taxonomy of requests by patients (TORP): A new system for understanding clinical negotiation in office practice. *The Journal of Family Practice, 48*(11), 872–878.

Kravitz, R. L., Bell, R. A., Azari, R., Kelly-Reif, S., Krupat, E., & Thom, D. H. (2003). Direct observation of requests for clinical services in office practice: What do patients want and do they get it? *Archives of Internal Medicine, 163*(14), 1673–1681.

Kravitz, R. L., Bell, R. A., Franz, C. E., Elliott, M. N., Amsterdam, E., Willis, C., & Silverio, L. (2002). Characterizing patient requests and physician responses in office practice. *Health Services Research, 37*(1), 217–238.

Krippendorff, K. (2004). *Content analysis: An introduction to its methodology* (2nd ed.). Thousand Oaks, CA: Sage Publications.

Krippendorff, K. (2008). Systematic and random disagreement and the reliability of nominal data. *Communication Methods and Measures, 2*(4), 323–338.

Krupat, E., Frankel, R., Stein, T., & Irish, J. (2006). The Four Habits Coding Scheme: Validation of an instrument to assess clinicians' communication behavior. *Patient Education and Counseling, 62*(1), 38–45.

Landis, J. R., & Koch, G. G. (1977). The measurement of observer agreement for categorical data. *Biometrics, 33*(1), 159–174.

Lawson, P. J., Flocke, S. A., & Casucci, B. (2009). Development of an instrument to document the 5A's for smoking cessation. *American Journal of Preventive Medicine, 37*(3), 248–254.

MacCoy, L. (2005). HIV-positive patients and the doctor–patient relationship: Perspectives from the margins. *Qualitative Health Research, 15*(6), 791–806.

Makoul, G. (1998). Perpetuating passivity: Reliance and reciprocal determinism in physician–patient interaction. *Journal of Health Communication, 3*(3), 233–259.

Mast, M. S. (2007). On the importance of nonverbal communication in the physician–patient interaction. *Patient Education and Counseling, 67*(3), 315–318.

Meeuwesen, L., Schaap, C., & van der Staak, C. (1991). Verbal analysis of doctor–patient communication. *Social Science & Medicine, 32*(10), 1143–1150.

Montague, E., Xu, J., Chen, P.Y., Asan, O., Barrett, B. P., & Chewning, B. (2011). Modeling eye gaze patterns in clinician-patient interaction with lag sequential analysis. *Human Factors, 53*(5), 502–516.

O'Hair, D. (1989). Dimensions of relational communication and control during physician–patient interactions. *Health Communication, 1*(2), 97–115.

Oliver, M. N., Goodwin, M. A., Gotler, R. S., Gregory, P. M., & Stange, K. C. (2001). Time use in clinical encounters: Are African-American patients treated differently? *Journal of the National Medical Association, 93*(10), 380–385.

Ong, L. M., de Haes, J. C., Hoos, A. M., & Lammes, F. B. (1995). Doctor–patient communication: A review of the literature. *Social Science & Medicine, 40*(7), 903–918.

Paasche-Orlow, M., & Roter, D. (2003). The communication patterns of internal medicine and family practice physicians. *The Journal of the American Board of Family Practice, 16*(6), 485–493.

Poole, M. S. (2007). Generalization in process theories of communication. *Communication Methods and Measures, 1*(3), 181–190.

Popping, R. (2010). Some views on agreement to be used in content analysis studies. *Quality and Quantity: International Journal of Methodology, 44*(6), 1067–1078.

QSR. (2010). *NVivo qualitative data analysis software, Version 9*. Melbourne, Australia: Qualitative Solutions and Research Pty. Ltd.

RIASWorks. (2011). Bibliography and abstracts of RIAS Studies 2011. Retrieved March 8, 2012, from http://www.riasworks.com/resources_a.html

Richard, C., & Lussier, M.T. (2006). MEDICODE: An instrument to describe and evaluate exchanges on medications that occur during medical encounters. *Patient Education and Counseling, 64*(1–3), 197–206.

Rogers, L. E., & Farace, R. V. (1975). Analysis of relational communication in dyads: New measurement procedures. *Human Communication Research, 1*(3), 222–239.

Roter, D. L. (1988). Reciprocity in the medical encounter. In D. S. Gochman (Ed.), *Health behavior: Emerging research perspectives* (pp. 1293–1303). New York, NY: Plenum Press.

Roter, D. L. (2012). *The Roter method of interaction process analysis*. Baltimore, MD: RIASWorks, Johns Hopkins University Bloomberg School of Public Health.

Roter, D. L., & Hall, J. A. (1989). Studies of doctor–patient interaction. *Annual Review Of Public Health, 10*, 163–180.

Roter, D. L., & Larson, S. M. (2002). The Roter interaction analysis system (RIAS): Utility and flexibility for analysis of medical interactions. *Patient Education and Counseling, 46*(4), 243–251.

Roter, D. L., Frankel, R. M., Hall, J. A., & Sluyter, D. (2006). The expression of emotion through nonverbal behavior in medical visits: Mechanisms and outcomes. *Journal of General Internal Medicine, 21*(S1), S28–34.

Roter, D. L., Larson, S. M., Beach, M. C., & Cooper, L. A. (2008). Interactive and evaluative correlates of dialogue sequence: A simulation study applying the RIAS to turn taking structures. *Patient Education and Counseling, 71*(1), 26–33.

Roter, D. L., Hall, J. A., Blanch-Hartigan, D., Larson, S., & Frankel, R. M. (2011). Slicing it thin: New methods for brief sampling analysis using RIAS-coded medical dialogue. *Patient Education and Counseling, 82*(3), 410–419.

Shaikh, A., Knobloch, L. M., & Stiles, W. B. (2001). The use of a verbal response mode coding system in determining patient and physician roles in medical interviews. *Health Communication, 13*(1), 49–60.

Shaikh, U., Nettiksimmons, J., Bell, R. A., Tancredi, D., & Romano, P. S. (2012). Accuracy of parental report and electronic health record documentation as measures of diet and physical activity counseling. *Academic Pediatrics, 12*(2), 81–87.

Siminoff, L. A., & Step, M. M. (2011). A comprehensive observational coding scheme for analyzing instrumental, affective, and relational communication in health care contexts. *Journal of Health Communication, 16*(2), 178–197.

Stata Corporation (2011). *Stata statistical software: Release 12*. College Station, TX: Stata Press.

Stiles, W. B. (1979). Verbal response modes and psychotherapeutic technique. *Psychiatry, 42*(1), 49–62.

Street, R. L. (1991). Accommodation in medical consultations. In H. Giles, J. Coupland, & N. Coupland (Eds.), *Contexts of accommodation: Developments in applied sociolinguistics* (pp. 131–156). New York, NY: Cambridge University Press.

Street, R. L., Jr., & Millay, B. (2001). Analyzing patient participation in medical encounters. *Health Communication, 13*(1), 61–73.

Street, R. L., & Epstein, R. M. (2008). Key interpersonal functions and health outcomes: Lessons from theory and research on clinician-patient communication. In K. Glanz, B. K. Rimer, & K. Viswanath (Eds.), *Health behavior and health education: Theory, research, and practice* (4th ed.) (pp. 237–269). San Francisco, CA: Jossey-Bass.

Street, R. L., Makoul, G., Arora, N. K., & Epstein, R. M. (2009). How does communication heal? Pathways linking clinician-patient communication to health outcomes. *Patient Education and Counseling, 74*(3), 295–301.

van den Brink-Muinen, A., & Caris-Verhallen, W. (2003). Doctors' responses to patients' concerns: Testing the use of sequential analysis. *Epidemiologia e Psichiatria Sociale, 12*(2), 92–97.

Wolff, J. L., & Roter, D. L. (2011). Family presence in routine medical visits: A meta-analytical review. *Social Science & Medicine, 72*(6), 823–831.

IT'S NOT WHAT YOU KNOW . . .

Social Network Analysis and Health Communication

Rachel A. Smith

Humans are a social species. When we are diagnosed with a health condition, we share that news with others. Health professionals work with each other to provide care. Organizations collaborate in order to connect patients with the technologies or experts required for their care. Our communication activities link actors (patients, providers, and organizations) together; our organizational hierarchies can shape with whom we communicate and what we say. Social network analysis is a perspective that focuses on estimating, predicting, and understanding the consequences of patterns in these links (Freeman, 1978). This method includes means by which to uncover links between actors, to estimate an actor's position within the system of links, and to estimate the character of a system based on the links within it. Social network analysis is a method that includes means by which to understand changes within a network over time, to predict its appearance, and to test its influence on actor-level and system-level outcomes. With the attention and excitement about social network analysis, the number of methodological options and analyses continue to grow. This chapter will provide an introduction to social network analysis and its utility to health communication research; readers interested in greater detail should consult one of the many texts now available (Newman, 2010; Scott, 2013; Wasserman & Faust, 1994). As an introduction, this chapter describes the fundamental concepts of social network analysis, its assumptions and applications, and procedures to gather and estimate basic parameters.

The Nature of Social Network Analysis

Background and Definitions

Social network analysis is the study of the pattern of relationships among a set of actors (Freeman, 1978; Wasserman & Faust, 1994). Freeman's (2004) book covering the history of social network analysis from a network perspective describes the long history of social network analysis as a methodology in the social sciences. Work in the 1920s by Moreno and Jennings (reviewed in Freeman, 2004) is marked as a seminal turning point for social network analysis. In their research, people's social problems and mental health concerns were framed within the "psychodrama" of their lives, due, in part, to the "sociatry" (i.e., pathological organization of groups and their members' interactions; Moreno, 1946) in which they lived. This work assumed that people were aware of the pattern of their interactions with others, and their mental health and esteem were shaped by their perceived position within the system. Matrices were used to present information about the relations among actors, such as the patterns within an elementary school classroom based on which students liked and disliked one another. Sociograms were used to depict these relationships. Estimates were created or adopted from graph theory to quantify actors' positions and system structures. Indeed, the therapy produced from these efforts focused on changing people's patterns in order to improve their well-being. From its beginnings, then, visual displays of networks have been an integral component in social network analysis, as has the intent to understand networks in order to adjust them.

A "social network" is defined as a set of dyadic ties, all of the same type, among a set of actors and the dyadic links among them (Wasserman & Faust, 1994). Actors (also called nodes) are discrete social entities, which can be almost anything: people, organizations, events, ideas, or even websites. In social network analysis, the pattern of links among actors (i.e., the structural properties of the network) is emphasized as shaping the actors within it. The links, also referred to as "relations" or "ties," can be anything establishing a connection between pairs of actors: conversations about health news, shared clients, or joint ventures. For example, a cancer-support network may represent the self-reported support (ties) provided between patients going through chemotherapy (actors). A continuum of care network may represent healthcare organizations (actors) with common clients (ties). Of note, actors may be connected in many different ways: healthcare organizations may be connected through shared clients, shared providers, common insurance providers, and so on. Typically, a social network represents one specific type of relation among a set of actors. To complete this last illustration, three different networks could be created for health-care organizations to represent (a) shared clients, (b) shared providers, or (c) shared insurance providers. Social network analysis includes multiple procedures for quantitatively capturing the pattern of relations, typically of one type, among a set of actors.

Theoretical Assumptions

Social network analysis embodies perspectives that may be considered a counterpoint to other social science perspectives, and focuses on patterns of relationships between actors, while most other perspectives focus on the attributes of actors. For example, some theories of social influence attempt to explain why people are able to persuade others to do what they want them to do. Traditionally, we might theorize that people with more credibility and competence are more persuasive. With social network analysis, we might theorize that people with more centrality in a social network are more persuasive. Fundamentally, then, social network analysis prioritizes an inter-dependent view of social processes and effects, over an individualist view. Multiple theories (Monge & Contractor, 2003) embrace these social network perspectives, such as dynamic social impact theory (Nowak, Szamrej, & Latané, 1990), social capital (e.g., Lin, Cook, & Burt, 2001), and organizational field-nets (Kenis & Knoke, 2002).

Regardless of the theory guiding the project, estimates from social network analyses are usually provided at the node-level and the system-level. For example, we might be interested in the diffusion of new evidence-based treatments among a set of healthcare providers. At the node-level, we might ask how providers' position in the healthcare network, such as their centrality in it, shapes their likelihood of prescribing these new treatments. At the system-level, we might ask how the network's structural features, such as density, influence providers' prescriptions.

Applications

Social network analysis has been used in many diverse public health and medical applications. Valente (2010) provides many examples, including the associations between people's interpersonal networks and mortality, organizations' collaboration networks, and patient care. Existing studies consistently show the health benefits of larger, more diverse interpersonal networks (e.g., access to more information about treatment, resources to support health behaviors) and costs associated with poor coordination among providers (Valente, 2010). In addition, many chronic conditions, such as HIV and cancer, involve a diverse set of providers, including in-patient and out-patient care. Providers often refer patients to see other providers, so as to provide comprehensive care. In a study of transfers among organizations serving people living with HIV, organizations reported referring clients to 1 to 29 different organizations in the past month, and yet most clients were referred to only 6 of these organizations (Kwait, Valente, & Celentano, 2001). As providers "share" the care of patients between them, some providers, such as primary care providers, may be more centrally located than others. For example, in a study of care provided to all patients in three US veterans' facilities, primary care physicians' connections to other providers through shared patients was 42% higher than those of general surgeons and 250% higher than cardiologists (Parchman, Scoglio, & Schumm, 2011).

Employing Social Network Analysis: Bare Bones

This chapter limits its description of social network analysis to whole networks, in which all dyadic ties between actors are measured and available for analysis. Two designs are used to collect network data: whole network and egocentric. Whole network designs "examine sets of interrelated objects or actors that are regarded for analytical purposes as bounded social collectives, although in practice network boundaries are often permeable and/or ambiguous" (Marsden, 2005, p. 8). In contrast, egocentric designs focus on "a focal actor or object and the relationships in its locality" (Marsden, 2005, p. 8). At a minimum, whole-network designs measure one set of objects (also called actors or nodes) linked by one set of relationships, observed at one occasion. The following procedures focus primarily on one-mode networks (i.e., one set of actors are involved) from a whole-network design, with a brief discussion of two-mode networks (i.e., with two sets of actors).

Network Data

The primary data for network analysis differs from data traditionally used in social science. Traditional data consists of rows of subjects and columns of variables. A simple example appears in Table 9.1. With the traditional data structure, we can assess the association between two columns of variables, such as correlating height and weight. We can also compare subjects based on a given variable, such as how many men versus women get vaccinated for the flu. Network data needs to capture dyadic ties between actors; the data is presented in a matrix.

In a one-mode network, the data matrix consists of rows and columns representing the actors and cells representing the tie between them. An example appears in Table 9.2.

This matrix includes the names of all actors in the network in the rows and in the columns. Imagine that these actors are residents in an assisted living facility. The cells represent interpersonal communication between two residents for at

TABLE 9.1 Example of a Traditional Data Structure

Name	*Sex*	*Age*	*Flu Vaccine*	*Height*	*Weight*	*Sociability*	*Physical Limits*
Susan Brown	Female	80	No	63	130	10	Low
Mark Clark	Male	76	No	65	160	4	Low
Mary Garcia	Female	83	Yes	60	150	8	Low
Linda Jones	Female	88	No	66	175	4	High
David Moore	Male	75	Yes	70	190	6	Low
Paul Nelson	Male	79	Yes	64	240	5	High
Lisa Peters	Female	78	Yes	58	170	2	Low
Karen Scott	Female	81	No	68	165	5	Low
Joey Turner	Male	79	No	65	225	2	High
Gary Wright	Male	84	No	72	170	8	High

TABLE 9.2 Example Matrix of an Interpersonal Communication Network with Undirected Ties

	Brown	*Clark*	*Garcia*	*Jones*	*Moore*	*Nelson*	*Peters*	*Scott*	*Turner*	*Wright*
Brown	–	1	1	1	0	1	0	0	0	0
Clark	1	–	0	1	1	0	1	0	0	0
Garcia	1	0	–	1	0	1	0	0	0	0
Jones	1	1	1	–	1	1	1	0	0	0
Moore	0	1	0	1	–	0	1	0	0	0
Nelson	1	0	1	1	0	–	1	1	0	0
Peters	0	1	0	1	1	1	–	1	0	0
Scott	0	0	0	0	0	1	1	–	1	0
Turner	0	0	0	0	0	0	0	1	–	1
Wright	0	0	0	0	0	0	0	0	1	–

least 2 minutes in the past 24 hours. The data in the example matrix represent binary measurement: "1" indicates a 2-minute conversation occurred; "0" indicates that it did not. The diagonals are ignored, because we are not concerned about whether the resident talked with him/herself in the past 24 hours. This type of matrix is also called a graph: a social network with undirected, dichotomous (1 or 0) ties between one set of actors (Wasserman & Faust, 1994). It is the most common type of data analyzed in the existing literature. The visual representation of the data in Table 9.2 appears in Figure 9.1.

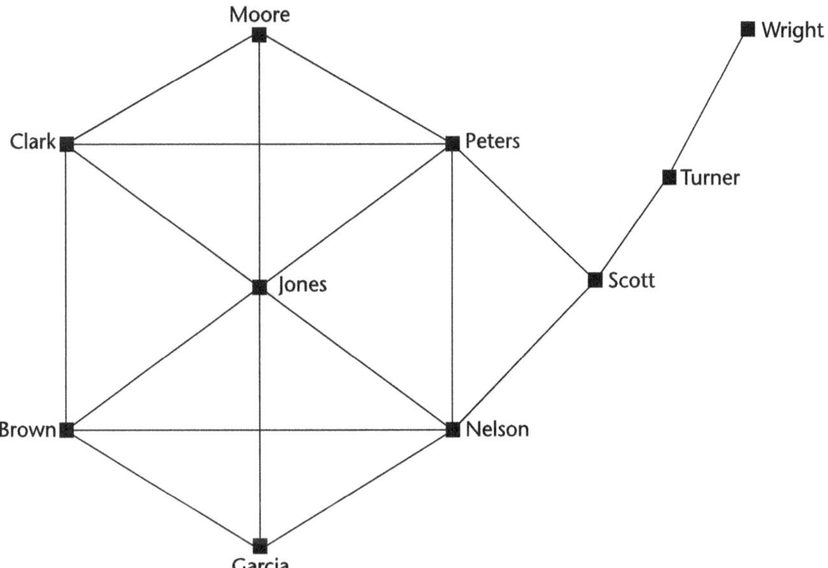

FIGURE 9.1 Sociogram of a Fictitious Interpersonal Communication Network Among Residents Within an Assisted Living Facility (the residents, depicted as black squares, have lines connecting them if they had a face-to-face conversation for longer than 2 minutes within the past 24 hours)

Directed and Undirected Ties

The previous example of a conversation network is composed of undirected ties, which represent only mutual or reciprocal ties. If Susan talked with Mary, then Mary talked with Susan. Sometimes, our interest is in directed relations; that is, when one actor has a connection to another actor that may or may not be reciprocated. For example, Susan could be sick with a viral infection, which is transmitted from Susan to Mary. Mary, on the other hand, may not transmit the virus back to Susan. The sociogram for a network with directed ties now has arrowheads to convey directionality (see Figure 9.2, below, where an arrow starts from Susan Brown and ends with Mary Garcia). As with the conversational network, the matrix of directed ties is square, because the rows and columns represent the same set of actors in the infectious disease network. The data are also binary: a "1" indicates that transmission occurred, while a "0" indicates that it did not. The data is entered by rows, which has substantive meaning for their interpretation. For example, the first row in Table 9.3 indicates that Susan Brown transmitted the virus to Mark Clark, Mary Garcia and Linda Jones. In the third row, Garcia is recorded as transmitting the virus to no one else. The data matrix, then, may not be symmetrical: the data above the diagonal may not be the same as that below it.

The analysis of directed and undirected ties can both provide useful information about the relations among actors in a net. Directed and undirected ties differ in how they are entered into the data matrix. The difference is also reflected in the

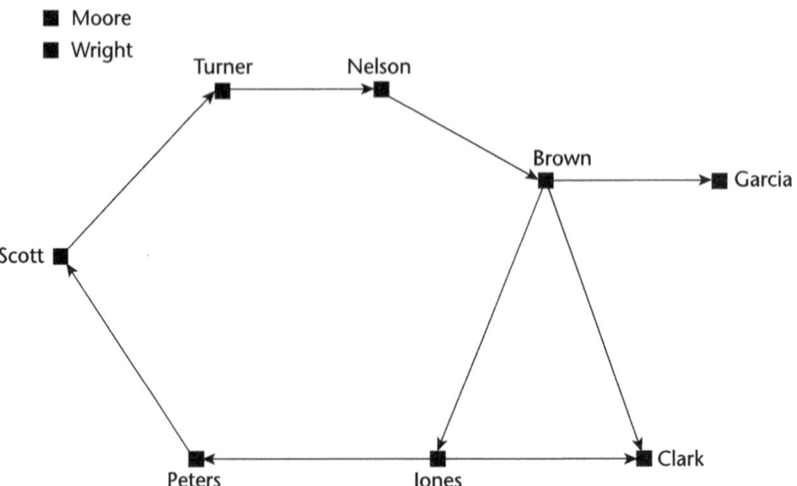

FIGURE 9.2 Sociogram of a Fictitious Infectious Disease Network Among Residents Within an Assisted Living Facility (the residents are depicted as black squares; the arrows indicate disease transmission from one resident to another)

TABLE 9.3 Example Matrix of a Disease Transmission Network with Directed Ties

	Brown	*Clark*	*Garcia*	*Jones*	*Moore*	*Nelson*	*Peters*	*Scott*	*Turner*	*Wright*
Brown	–	1	1	1	0	0	0	0	0	0
Clark	0	–	0	0	0	0	0	0	0	0
Garcia	0	0	–	0	0	0	0	0	0	0
Jones	0	1	0	–	0	0	1	0	0	0
Moore	0	0	0	0	–	0	0	0	0	0
Nelson	1	0	0	0	0	–	0	0	0	0
Peters	0	0	0	0	0	0	–	1	0	0
Scott	0	0	0	0	0	0	0	–	1	0
Turner	0	0	0	0	0	1	0	0	–	0
Wright	0	0	0	0	0	0	0	0	0	–

sociograms of directed ties. Sociograms of undirected ties appear as lines without arrowheads; sociograms of directed ties use arrowheads, showing how an actor's tie is directed from one (at the tail of the arrow) to another (at the arrowhead). Last, the estimates used to analyze directed and undirected data differ as well (more on this in the analysis section, below). Once one has decided on a set of actors, the relation tying them together, and whether the tie is directional or not, one must decide how to collect the data.

Sampling

The task of sampling may appear to be an obvious extension of general principles of sampling in survey research, but this is not the case (Scott, 2013). The general principles of sampling are based on theories of probability and well-established rules for judging the reliability of sample data. There are no such rules for relational data; a representative sample of actors from a larger group may not provide a useful sample of relations in the system (Alba, 1982). There are three common approaches to sampling network data: positional, event-based, and relational (Scott, 2013; Wasserman & Faust, 1994). These approaches help researchers decide on the network's boundary and members. Notably, these decisions are about sample inclusion and exclusion; they are not about drawing a sample. Indeed, as alluded to in the previous section, researchers are encouraged to collect data about all network members. The position-based approach uses information such as employment in an organization to determine the network boundary and members. The event-based approach uses actions, such as participation in an intervention program, to make these decisions, and the relational approach uses the relations themselves, such as friendships. The first two approaches may be chosen without consulting the respondents. The third approach, however, is often respondent based: researchers ask one respondent to identify his or her friends, and research continues to those friends, repeatedly asking the friendship question until a chosen endpoint.

In short, there are at least two sampling challenges. First, even in whole-network designs, participants often list network members who are not included in the sample. Even though the researchers may decide on the boundaries of a whole network by position, events, or relationships, the researchers' boundaries often do not perfectly match those reported by participants. When researchers decide to limit the whole network to only those sampled, their relationships are likely to be underestimated. Further, there is no reason to expect that these relationships are a "random" representation of all the relations of these actors (Scott, 2013). Second, in very large samples, actors are often unrelated. Burt (1983) estimated that the amount of relational data lost through sampling is equal to (100-*k*), in which *k* is the equal to the sample size as a percentage of the population. Thus, a 10% sample would generate a loss of 90% of the data, making the identification of structural features almost impossible. Work into the issues that arise when the entire actor network is not sampled has been considered (Frank, 2005), and greater guidance on respondent-based sampling techniques, such as snowball sampling, is ongoing (Burt, 1983; Scott, 2013).

Data Collection

Data can be collected through surveys, interviews, membership records, observations, and experiments; researchers often use surveys, and many books cover best practices for developing surveys (see Morgan & Carcioppolo, this volume). In this chapter, two issues relevant for social network analysis are discussed: generating actors and limiting choices.

Roster or Free Recall

To collect whole-network data, each actor needs to provide answers about all the other actors in the network. Imagine we were gathering the interpersonal communication data featured in Table 9.2. We need to record the 1s and 0s for each cell; that is, did Susan talk with Mark? Did Mark remember talking with Susan? Researchers can decide to provide each actor (e.g., Susan Brown) with a complete list of all actors in the network (i.e., a "roster"; Mark Clark, Mary Garcia, Linda Jones, and David Moore, etc.) and ask the actor to mark those with whom she or he had at least a 2-minute conversation in the past 24 hours. In contrast, researchers could ask Susan to write down the names of people with whom she talked in the past 24 hours. Susan, then, fills in a blank or many blanks with names. This is referred to as "free recall."

A roster is often the preferred method, because it relies on recognition instead of memory. Humans exhibit both recognition and memory biases when they answer questions, but many of the accuracy and competency issues appear with attempts to recall relevant actors. People often forget some of their own friends when they try to freely recall them (think about movie stars, trained in memorizing lines, who forget to thank someone at an award ceremony, even after practicing their speeches). Pragmatically, freely recalled actors present an additional problem: Susan may write down "Beth," Mark may write down "Betty," and Mary may write down "Elizabeth." Are Beth, Betty, and Elizabeth the same person? Unless you go back and talk to everyone, you may never know, and end up misrepresenting the number of actors in the network. On the other hand, it can be very difficult to get access to rosters, and their accuracy is not perfect. If you get a roster of students enrolled at the beginning of school, but collect data two months later, some students may have left and others may have started school. All techniques have their advantages and disadvantages.

Fixed Choice Versus Free Choice

Researchers may decide to allow actors to report on as many actors as they like (free choice) or we can limit their choices (i.e., fixed choice). For example, in the friendship network in Table 9.2, we could have asked the actors to pick up to three of their closest friends. In this case, we have fixed the maximum number of friends for any given actor to three. On the other hand, we could ask them to mark down anyone they consider a friend.

Fixed-choice designs put artificial constraints on the reported number of ties. For example, if we asked people to provide five friends, then some people constrain their answers to their top five friends, while others try to come up with five when they only have three friends. For this reason, fixed-choice answers may not represent the relationships well. Free-choice designs are affected by memory issues. Humans have a tendency to remember about seven things (plus or minus two; Miller, 1956). In addition, with the option to pick as many actors as one likes, participants will sometimes mark down everyone (i.e., "I'm friends with everyone").

Measurement

For years, scholars (Alba, 1982; Batchelder, 1992; Frank, 2005; Marsden, 2005; Wasserman & Faust, 1994) have issued a call for increased attention to sampling and measurement for social data. Considerable work remains in developing good techniques for sampling, good measures of sampling variability for network concepts, and the overall foundation of measurement. The greatest amount of work in the analysis of social networks has focused on the geometry of binary matrices. It is not surprising that respondents are often asked to make a binary judgment of social data. For example, in a whole-network design, respondents may be presented a roster of members (collected ahead of time), and asked to mark their friends. However, studies show that other types of scales, such as ordinal ratings of relationship strength or rankings, are more reliable than binary judgments (Ferligoj & Hlebec, 1999). When making dichotomous judgments, respondents have differing thresholds for claiming that a relationship exists or not (Feld & Carter, 2002; expansiveness bias, Kashy & Kenny, 1990). Asking respondents to report on more complex social phenomena, such as the size, density, or composition of their networks, has been even more problematic (Burt, 1987; Sudman, 1985).

One way to think about social data is that researchers are asking untrained coders to report on their observations. In observational studies, training coders has always been considered a fundamental concern related to data quality and inference. Research on coder training (see multiple chapters in Krippendorff & Bock, 2009) may guide the biases and communication issues that appear, particularly in gathering data validly and consistently from multiple observers.

Analysis: Centrality Estimates with One-Mode Data of Undirected Ties

One of the most common questions about a network concerns centrality. At the actor and network level, researchers want to learn who is most central and how centralized the network is. With the interpersonal communication network data (Table 9.2, seen in Figure 9.1), one could estimate: (a) which residents are most central, by being in physical proximity of more residents than others; and (b) how centralized the physical proximity network is. The actor-level information could provide important insights into the social functioning of the residents or the unmet needs of some residents to move from their room into another location. The network-level information could provide insights into equity within the residential facility: if only a few residents are very central, this might reveal hidden, institutional segregation. At the network level, we could also estimate the network's density: that is, how many of the residents, of all possible residents in the facility, spend time around one another. The density of the physical proximity network could suggest a connected community within the facility, and highlight concerns about how quickly an infectious disease, such as influenza, could spread throughout the system.

There are many definitions of centrality, with even more estimates available to capture these different definitions. For example, look at the sociogram in Figure 9.1, and consider the following questions. Who do you think is the opinion leader? Who is most "in the know?" Who is best positioned to be a super-diffuser? It is likely that you found yourself picking different people as you considered these different definitions of importance in a network. Indeed, all centrality estimates attempt "to quantify the prominence of an individual actor embedded in a network" (Wasserman & Faust, 1994, p.169). Aggregated scores across a network summarize "how variable or differentiated the set of actors is as a whole with respect to a given measure" (Wasserman & Faust, 1994, p. 169). We will consider three types of centrality: (a) degree, (b) betweenness, and (c) closeness, for the interpersonal-communication network, which is a one-mode, undirected matrix. The data in Table 9.3 (Figure 9.1), referred to a "Krackhardt's kite," provides a terrific opportunity to explore these differences.

Degree Centrality

Centrality can be thought of in terms of connectivity. For example, we may assume that people with more connections have more power within the network (Wasserman & Faust, 1994). Actors with more ties may have greater access to resources and less dependency on any single person for access (Cook & Emerson, 1978). Degree centrality is an estimate of the number of direct ties an actor has with other network actors (Freeman, 1978). From Table 9.3, one simply sums the number of ties across a row or down a column (the data is redundant) for each member. Degree centrality varies from 6 to 1: Jones has the highest degree centrality, and Wright has the lowest.

Betweenness Centrality

Centrality can also be thought of in terms of one's position within the flow of a network. For example, the actor that lies between other actors in the system can find out rumors from different corners more quickly. The person between two others in a network is also in a position of brokerage, in that they have the power to facilitate the connection or not (Wasserman & Faust, 1994). A person with nonredundant contacts, (i.e., one who is between actors who are not directly connected to each other; Burt, 1992; Monge & Contractor, 2003), may have a great deal of power because they control information and its interpretation. Burt (1992) was instrumental in understanding that more connections, even to well-connected others, do not necessarily equal more benefit to the actor. Each network connection has opportunity costs, and energy spent on redundant contacts is inefficient.

Betweenness centrality, then, focuses on measuring the network paths between actors. If equal amounts of information flow between people in a network, and if we assume this information takes the shortest path, betweenness centrality provides a measure of the fraction of that information that will flow through a given person on its way through the network. Betweenness centrality estimates the shortest path (or paths) between every pair of actors in the network and on what fraction of those paths a given actor lays; it is the average number of shortest paths that use a particular actor (Freeman, 1978). In Figure 9.1, the shortest path from Wright to Clark includes Turner, Scott, Peters, and either Moore or Jones. If we continue to work through the shortest paths between actors, we see that Scott appears on more paths than anyone else. Betweenness centrality for the interpersonal communication network varies from 14 (Scott) to 0 (Garcia, Moore, and Wright); Scott has the highest betweenness centrality, while Garcia, Moore, and Wright have the lowest.

Closeness Centrality

Another way to consider centrality is in one actor's ability to reach all other actors quickly. Actors who are closer to other actors can quickly interact with them without many intermediaries (Wasserman & Faust, 1994). Closeness centrality is estimated as the reciprocal sum of the shortest distances (geodesic paths) from one actor to the other actors. In Figure 9.1, if we count the distance from Peters to all the other actors, she can reach everyone in 14 paths: she can reach Moore, Jones, Clark, Scott, and Nelson in 1 path (5*1 = 5); Brown, Garcia, and Turner in 2 paths (2*3 = 6); and Wright in 3 paths (1*3 = 3), thus (5+6+3 = 14). The distances vary from 14 (Nelson and Peters) to Wright (29); Nelson and Peters have the highest closeness centrality, while Wright has the lowest.

Normalized Estimates for Actors' Centrality

While raw numbers may be useful, they are dependent on the number of actors in a network. For this reason, as well as to compare between networks, it can be helpful to normalize the data. Normalization means standardizing the raw information by the network's characteristics. For example, for degree centrality, the estimates are normalized by dividing the sum by the total number of actors minus one. Jones, then, is connected to 67% (or 6/[10–1]) of the actors in the system. Scott's normalized betweenness centrality is 39%, meaning that Scott has 39% of the maximal possible betweenness. Nelson and Peters have normalized closeness centrality scores of 64%; they have 64% of the maximum possible distance to others.

Returning to concepts, Jones may best represent popularity, Scott may be most "in the know," and Nelson and Peters may be best able to spread things through the residential community. As stated earlier, a multitude of centrality estimates are available to best match the nuances of the theoretical question to be tested. Possible questions include the following: Who has control over what flows through the network? Who has the best visibility of what is happening in the network? Who are the peripheral players?

Network Central Tendencies

For every actor estimate of centrality, there is a summary statistic for the network. For degree centrality, two summaries are available to estimate the quality of the network: density and degree centralization. Density (the average standardized degree estimate) reflects how many of the total possible ties are observed. A density of 1 occurs when all nodes are tied; in our situation, when every resident has had at least a 2-minute, face-to-face conversation with each other resident in the past 24 hours. A density of 0 occurs in a completely unconnected system. The density of the interpersonal communication network in our example is .40. "Degree centralization" reflects the distribution of connections within the network. When degree centralization is 1, then all of the ties connect to a few people; when centralization is 0, then the ties are equally distributed. The degree centralization for the interpersonal communication network is 33%, indicating that conversation participation is rather even across the network. Centralization indexes are also available for betweenness centrality and closeness centrality. The centralization index is 30% for betweenness and 27% for closeness, indicating that betweenness is evenly distributed across actors.

Analysis: Centrality Estimates With One-Mode Data of Directed Ties

With undirected data, centrality rests on the notion of involvement. In comparison, directed data places an emphasis on receiving or giving ties. For example, the interpersonal conversation network used in the previous example could have been concerned with who initiates conversation with others. In that case, we would need directed data in which we could differentiate between initiators and their targets. Some estimates created for one-mode, undirected ties can be extended to directed data, while others cannot (Wasserman & Faust, 1994). Of those discussed in the previous section, degree and closeness centrality are easily extended to directional relations; betweenness centrality is not. A brief example of degree centrality for directed ties is presented next.

Degree centrality in directed data has two estimates: outdegree and indegree. Outdegree represents initiating the relational tie (transmitting the virus, in our example), and is the number of ties originating from a particular actor. When the actor's data is entered by rows, outdegree centrality is the sum of non-zero entries within a particular row. For example, the first row shows that Brown transmitted the virus to Clark, Garcia, and Jones, which results in an outdegree centrality of 3. The last row shows that Wright, on the other hand, transmitted the infection to no one, resulting in an outdegree of 0. Indegree, in contrast, represents receiving the relational tie (contracting the virus, in our example), and is the number of ties landing on an actor. When the actor's data is entered by rows, then indegree centrality is the sum of non-zero entries within a particular column. For example, the first column shows that Brown received the virus from Nelson, which results in an indegree centrality of 1.

Outdegree and indegree estimates can be normalized by dividing by the total number of actors minus 1. Brown's normalized centrality estimate is 33%, indicating that Brown transmitted the virus to 33% of the network. Clark has the highest indegree centrality, with a normalized estimate of 22%, indicating that Clark contracted the virus from 22% of the network.

Network centralization indexes are also available for both outdegree and indegree centrality. The estimates indicate that the infectious disease network is not strongly centralized; the network centralized index is 29% for outdegree and 15% for indegree. The network is more centralized by outdegree than indegree, suggesting that one node or a small subset of nodes was more responsible for transmitting the virus, but receiving the virus more equivalent across the system.

Hypothesis Testing

Health communication researchers conducting quantitative analysis often use some kind of inferential statistic and report effect sizes and significance tests. One natural inclination is to incorporate network-based estimates for actors, such as their centrality, into traditional data structures (e.g., adding another column to Table 9.1) and run typical inferential statistics with them. A fundamental issue to understanding hypothesis testing with social network analysis is that, due to the inherent interdependence in network data, many tools of inferential statistics do not apply directly to network data. There are a growing number of alternative approaches to estimating standard errors with network data, such as robust ANOVAs (e.g., Gold et al., 2007), non-parametric methods using bootstrap approaches (e.g., Snijders & Borgatti, 1999), and quadratic assignment procedures (Krackhardt, 1987). Typically, these procedures use bootstrapping techniques to create standard errors, in which the distribution is created by sampling the network with replacement. Before showing an example of such hypothesis testing, let us first review more basic tests of the network.

Let us revisit the finding that the density of the residents' interpersonal conversation network was .40. Originally, we might have started the study with the hypothesis that some of the residents talk with each other. This claim can be represented by a hypothesized prediction that the network's density is different from 0. We can compare the observed density (.4) to the theoretical parameter (0), after providing a number of samples to use in the bootstrap procedure to calculate a bootstrap standard error, a z-score, and a significance test (Snijders & Borgatti, 1999). With 5,000 samples, the estimated $SD = 0.11$, $z = 3.54$, $p < .001$. The findings suggest that the network density differs from zero more than could be expected by chance.

We might have hypothesized that residents with greater sociability (e.g., a measure of how social they are) talk with more residents in a given day. Thus, our claim is that sociability is positively associated with degree centrality. We can regress our dependent variable, degree centrality, on sociability, and then assessing the significance of the association with standard errors from bootstrap procedures can be performed. With 5,000 permutations, the estimated correlation between sociability and degree centrality is –.29, which is not statically significant, $p = .78$.

A Glimpse into Groupings

While centrality is pervasive in research using social network analysis, it is necessary to note the theoretical import of subgroups and the opportunities within social network analysis to consider forces among or processes in subgroups. The concepts of neighborhoods, communities, teams, rivalry, and segregation may be considered and tested as particular patterns of relations. Put differently, we may be able to predict the shape of segregation between two groups as relative cohesion within the two groups and few ties between them. We may be able to predict how particular policies create fractionalizations into smaller subgroups. An actor's position within a subgroup may predict his or her sense of inclusion or ingroup solidarity. Multiple means of defining subgroups within a network exist, each highlighting different aspects of connection—different procedures can provide different answers.

A Glimpse Into Two-Mode Analysis

Before concluding this discussion of analysis, a brief discussion of two-mode networks is provided. To review, in one-mode networks, there is one set of actors. In two-mode analysis, the ties occur between two groups of nodes. For example, an investigator may be interested in people and the events they attend, in customers and the items they purchase, or in patients and their health providers. One way to think of the benefits of two-mode analysis is as a means of revealing why actors in a one-mode network are connected.

Modern medicine puts patients in contact with many providers (Bodenheimer, 2008). The implication is that many diverse resources may be needed to address health conditions, particularly chronic ones such as cancer or HIV. A study using Medicare claims data shows that, between 2000 and 2002, a typical beneficiary with chronic conditions may visit up to 16 different physicians in a year (Pham, Schrag, O'Malley, Wu, & Bach, 2007). A second implication is that coordination is needed among providers in order to avoid a range of negative outcomes, including duplication of services, contradictory care plans, or missing services (e.g., due to misattribution that someone else was covering that part of the patient's care). Studies show that failures in the coordination of care are common and compromise healthcare quality (see Bodenheimer, 2008, for a review) and are an important contributor to readmission of patients within 30 days of hospitalization (Epstein, 2009).

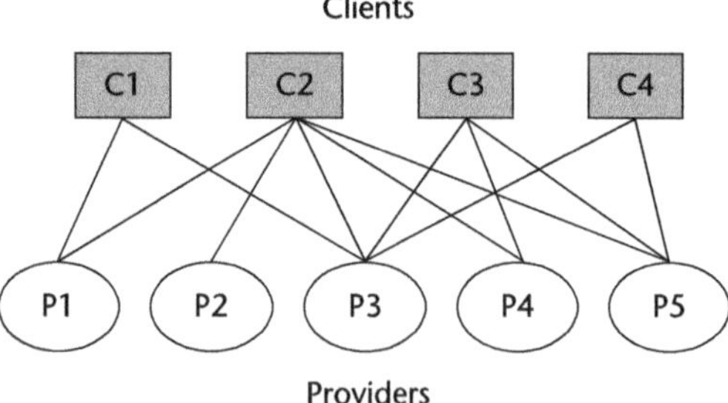

FIGURE 9.3 Hypothetical Two-Mode Network of Clients (C) and Providers (P) (clients, depicted as gray squares, and providers, depicted as white circles, are connected through health encounters; no ties exist between clients or between providers)

One way to conceptualize the healthcare system is as a social network of patients and providers who are connected through health encounters (see Figure 9.3). Framed in this way, we can use social network analysis to quantitatively represent the pattern of relationships between patients and providers as a two-mode network (one mode, patient; the other mode, provider), and to measure their access to positions within it. This framework also allows us to investigate how patients' and providers' characteristics shape the network of care and differences in treatment resulting from it. Said differently, we have an opportunity to investigate a means by which health disparities occur.

The data for two-mode analysis differ from one-mode: in two mode-analysis, one mode is represented in the rows, while the other appears in the columns. To revisit our interpersonal communication network of residents, we may have residents in the rows and the rooms they visited in the columns. With both sets of information, we can re-estimate the centrality of our actors based on where they went. We can estimate not only which actors are central, but which locations are central. This information can be very useful for intervention designs that need to consider where to locate an event or to post information (see Smith, 2009, for this discussion in relation to mass media or group-based interventions).

A recent study used two-mode analysis to investigate Namibians' participation in social groups in one community (Smith & Baker, 2012). Most participants reported membership in at least 1 of the 84 different groups present in that community; most participated in 1 group, but some participated in up to 4 groups, while others did not participate in any of them. From the other perspective, 3 of the groups were churches, and 30% of the participants were members of these churches, affording these groups some of the highest degree and betweenness centrality. This study tested a complex hypothesis about HIV risk and HIV stigma. Facing a chronic condition such as HIV requires support; thus, respondents with higher perceived HIV risk may have more central positions within the community network, as long as they do not perceive HIV as stigmatized. Higher perceptions of HIV risk and HIV stigma may be associated with less central positions, in order to protect oneself from social rejection or because the community pushed them out. The results provided support for the interaction. "The combination of perceptions-risk and stigma . . . is related to structural-level features of the community network, built from participation in community groups" (Smith & Baker, 2012, p. 530).

Strengths and Limitations of Social Network Analysis

The strengths of social network analysis are its ability to quantify structural patterns, and to allow for testing how the structure of a network can influence outcomes at the individual and aggregate level. At the individual level, we might be interested in an actor's capacity to obtain advice, help, or resources. At the aggregate level, we might be interested in how the structure in which people are embedded may shape mobilization, efficiency, and resilience.

Some limitations of social network analysis include its sensitivity to missing data and potential issues with reliability. Network estimates can change—dramatically, in some cases—with the omission or addition of just one node or just one tie. With those dramatic examples in mind, the general reaction has been to question estimates with missing data. Recent work has focused on understanding the effects of data missing at random on network centrality estimates (Costenbader & Valente, 2003), and means by which to generate confidence intervals around the kinds of centrality scores discussed in this chapter (Borgatti, Carley, & Krackhardt, 2006). For reliability, it is not uncommon for the network ties to be measured with single items for a concept, such as "please mark which of these people [on a roster] are your friends." At the same time, even if someone uses multiple items for friendship, there is no guidance on best practices for assessing reliability and creating a composite for use within a network analysis.

Challenges for Researchers

Social network analysis provides a rich perspective and array of procedures to assess patterns of relations among actors in a network. As they are often used by the public, the concepts of social networks and social networking do not necessarily coincide with social network analysis. Asking who goes online to connect with others through Facebook is a question about actors, not about the pattern of relations among actors. Researchers interested in testing how well websites' features predict their centrality in an online network, built by hyperlinks between websites, aligns with social network analysis. One opportunity for health communication research is to reflect on concepts with structural aspects to them, and then to hypothesize about and test their patterns, structures, and shapes. For example, what if there was a shape to social capital?

When conducting research using network analysis, researchers may need to embolden their ethical guidelines and pay careful attention to privacy when presenting findings. Network surveys may ask people to report on their connections to others. This research can make it very challenging to keep respondents anonymous (Borgatti & Molina, 2005). Further, when data are presented in matrix or sociogram form, it may be possible to identify individuals who represent unique positions within a network. Borgatti and Molina (2005) provide a thoughtful conversation on ethical guidelines for organization research using network analysis that could be extended to health communication research. Further attention and guidelines are needed.

Recent Developments, Controversies, and Conclusions

An exciting future topic in network research is the dynamics of networks over time. Specifically, "network processes are series of processes of events that create, sustain and dissolve social structures" (Doreian & Stokman, 1997, p. 3). We can ask questions such as the following: How do networks evolve over time? What factors shape the structure? It is possible that some people have equivalent positions in a healthcare network, but some people arrived at their positions more quickly than others, explaining differences in their outcomes. If some patients navigate healthcare systems more effectively, this may appear not only in the cumulative health network providing care, but in the speed with which one accumulates the network. Network analysis is considered a perspective under a larger umbrella of systems sciences. Other methodologies under the umbrella, such as agent-based modeling, can allow us to forecast and test evolution over time.

One of the controversies within social network analysis is in causal inference. Disagreement about how to draw valid conclusions from observed network data over time is likely to exist for some time. The issues are not trivial. Until these methods are further developed, we should proceed with caution when designing network-based interventions. For example, scholars have called for research into the influence of delivery networks on patient care (Kwait et al., 2001). Such research could be important for understanding the implications of policies aimed at patients' interactions with providers, such as designating primary care providers as medical homes for patients. Kwait et al. (2001) note that an important question (which may be investigated in a prospective experiment) is whether ad hoc relationships between providers through individual patient referrals are more or less effective in providing care in comparison to structured, formalized relationships between providers. While it will not eliminate the problem, the integration of network studies into experimental designs may provide a useful avenue to further refine our research.

Getting Started

Network analysis has the potential to help us understand health communication, to design interventions based on this understanding, and to track the diffusion of interventions. Here is a basic checklist before starting social network research. First, define your actors, ties (including direction), and modality clearly based on your research question(s). Use these definitions and your theoretical rationale to guide your decisions on how to collect these data into a network matrix. Align your decision-making criteria for selecting network estimates with your research questions, and present your reasoning. It is often helpful to use existing software programs, such as UCINET (Borgatti, Everett, & Freeman, 2002) or Pajek (Batagelj & Mrvar, 2003), to correctly execute the calculations, and visualization programs, such as NetDraw, to display your sociogram. One note about sociograms: people make attributions about the actors and groups depicted in a sociogram. Recent research (e.g., Smith & Fink, 2010) showed that people draw inferences about network actors' power from a sociogram based on the actor's centrality within a sociogram. The attributions made from sociograms are not well understood, and are an important avenue for future research.

Note

Preparation of this chapter was supported by a grant from the National Institute on Drug Abuse (P50-DA010075-16). The content is solely the responsibility of the author and does not necessarily represent the official views of the National Institute on Drug Abuse or the National Institutes of Health.

References

Alba, R. D. (1982). Taking stock of network analysis: A decade's results. In S. B. Bacharach (Ed.), *Research in the Sociology of Organizations*, Vol. 1 (pp. 39–74). Greenwich, CT: JAI Press.

Batagelj, V., & Mrvar, A. (2003). Pajek: Analysis and visualization of large networks. In M. Jünger & P. Mutzel (Eds.), *Graph drawing software* (pp. 77–103). Berlin, Germany: Springer.

Batchelder, W. H. (1992). Inferring meaningful global network properties from individual actor's measurement scales. In L. C. Freeman, D. R. White, & A. K. Romney (Eds.), *Research methods in social network analysis* (pp. 88–134). Fairfax, VA: George Mason University Press.

Bodenheimer, T. (2008). Coordinating care—A perilous journey through the health care system. *New England Journal of Medicine*, *358*(10), 1064–1071.

Borgatti, S. P., & Molina, J.-L. (2005). Toward ethical guidelines for network research in organizations. *Social Networks*, *27*(2), 107–117.

Borgatti, S. P., Everett, M. G., & Freeman, L. C. (2002). *UCINET 6 for Windows: Software for social network analysis*. Lexington, KY: Analytic Technologies.

Borgatti, S. P., Carley, K. M., & Krackhardt, D. (2006). On the robustness of centrality measures under conditions of imperfect data. *Social Networks*, *28*(2), 124–136.

Burt, R. S. (1983). Studying status/role-sets using mass surveys. In R. S. Burt & M. J. Minor (Eds.), *Applied network analysis: A methodological introduction* (pp. 100–118). Beverly Hills, CA: Sage Publications.

Burt, R. S. (1987). Social contagion and innovation: Cohesion versus structural equivalence. *American Journal of Sociology, 92*(6), 1287–1335. doi:10.1086/228667

Burt, R. S. (1992). *Structural holes: The social structure of competition.* Cambridge, MA: Harvard University Press.

Cook, K. S., & Emerson, R. M. (1978). Power, equity and commitment in exchange networks. *American Sociological Review, 43*(5), 721–739.

Costenbader, E., & Valente, T. W. (2003). The stability of centrality measures when networks are sampled. *Social Networks, 25*(4), 283–307.

Doreian, P. & Stokman, F. N. (1997). The dynamics and evolution of social networks. In P. Doreian & F. N. Stokman (Eds.), *Evolution of social networks* (pp. 1–18). Amsterdam, Netherlands: Gordon and Breach Publishers.

Epstein, A. M. (2009). Revisiting readmissions—changing the incentives for shared accountability. *The New England Journal of Medicine, 360*(14), 1457–1459.

Feld, S. L., & Carter, W. C. (2002). Detecting measurement bias in respondent reports of personal networks. *Social Networks, 24*(4), 365–383.

Ferligoj, A., & Hlebec, V. (1999). Evaluation of social network measurement instruments. *Social Networks, 21*(2), 111–130.

Frank, O. (2005). Network sampling and model fitting. In P. J. Carrington, J. Scott, & S. Wasserman (Eds.), *Models and methods in social network analysis* (pp. 31–56). New York, NY: Cambridge University Press.

Freeman, L. C. (1978). Centrality in social networks: I. Conceptual clarification. *Social Networks, 1*(3), 215–239.

Freeman, L. C. (2004). *The development of social network analysis: A study in the sociology of science.* Vancouver, BC, Canada: Empirical Press.

Gold, M., Taylor, E. F., Gruene Segersten, K., Doreian, P., Coughlan, J., & Lipson, D. (2007). *Evaluation of a learning collaborative's process and effectiveness to reduce health care disparities among minority populations. Final report prepared for the agency for healthcare research and quality.* Washington, D.C.: Mathematica Policy Research, Inc.

Kashy, D. A., & Kenny, D. A. (1990). Do you know whom you were with a week ago Friday? A re-analysis of the Bernard, Killworth, and Sailer studies. *Social Psychology Quarterly, 53*(1), 55–61.

Kenis, P. N., & Knoke, D. (2002). How organizational field networks shape inter-organizational tie-formation rates. *Academy of Management Review, 27*(2), 275–293.

Krackhardt, D. (1987). QAP partialling as a test of spuriousness. *Social Network, 9*(2), 171–186.

Krippendorff, K., & Bock, M. A. (Eds.). (2009). *The content analysis reader.* Thousand Oaks, CA: Sage Publications.

Kwait, J. L., Valente, T. W., & Celentano, D. D. (2001). Interorganizational relationships among HIV/AIDS service organizations in Baltimore: A network analysis. *Journal of Urban Health, 78*(3), 468–487.

Lin, N., Cook, K. S., & Burt, R. S. (Eds.). (2001). *Social capital: Theory and research.* New York, NY: Aldine de Gruyter.

Marsden, P. V. (2005). Recent developments in network measurement. In P. J. Carrington, J. Scott, & S. Wasserman (Eds.), *Models and methods in social network analysis* (pp. 8–30). New York, NY: Cambridge University Press.

Miller, G. A. (1956). The magical number seven, plus or minus two: Some limits on our capacity for processing information. *Psychological Review, 63*(2), 81–97.

Monge, P. R., & Contractor, N. S. (2003). *Theories of communication networks*. New York, NY: Oxford University Press.

Moreno, J. L. (1946). Psychodrama and group psychotherapy. *Sociometry, 9*(2/3), 249–253.

Newman, M. E. J. (2010). *Networks: An introduction*. Oxford, England: Oxford University Press.

Nowak, A., Szamrej, J., & Latané, B. (1990). From private attitude to public opinion: A dynamic theory of social impact. *Psychological Review, 97*(3), 362–376.

Parchman, M. L., Scoglio, C. M., & Schumm, P. (2011). Understanding the implementation of evidence-based care: A structural network approach. *Implementation Science, 6*(1), 1–10.

Pham, H. H., Schrag, D., O'Malley, A. S., Wu, B., Bach, P. B. (2007). Care patterns in Medicare and their implications for pay for performance. *New England Journal of Medicine, 356*(11), 1130–1139.

Scott, J. (2013). *Social network analysis: A handbook* (3rd ed.). Thousand Oaks, CA: Sage Publications.

Smith, R. A. (2009). Using social network information to design effective health campaigns to address HIV in Namibia. In L. Lagerwerf, H. Boer, & H. Wasserman (Eds.), *Communicating health in emerging countries: Alternative media and appeals in Southern Africa* (pp. 35–54). Leiden, South Africa: Brill Publishers.

Smith, R. A., & Fink, E. L. (2010). Compliance dynamics within a simulated friendship network I: The effects of agency, tactic, and node centrality. *Human Communication Research, 36*(2), 232–260.

Smith, R. A. & Baker, M. (2012). At the edge? HIV stigma and centrality in the community's network in Namibia. *AIDS & Behavior, 16*(3), 525–534. PMCID: PMC3337518 doi: 10.1007/s10461-012-0154-9

Snijders, T. A. B., &. Borgatti, S. P. (1999). Non-parametric standard errors and tests for network statistics. *Connections, 22*(2), 61–70.

Sudman, S. (1985). Experiments in the measurement of the size of social networks. *Social Networks*, 7(2), 127–151.

Valente, T. W. (2010). *Social networks and health: Models, methods, and applications.* New York, NY: Oxford University Press.

Wasserman, S., & Faust, K. (1994). *Social network analysis: Methods and applications.* New York, NY: Cambridge University Press.

CONTENT ANALYSIS OF HEALTH COMMUNICATION

Yan Tian and James D. Robinson

Health communication scholars frequently use content analysis in their research efforts. The topics of study are interestingly diverse, and even the most cursory examination of PubMed.gov yields thousands of studies employing content analysis on topics as varied as HIV and Kenyan newspapers (Muzyka, Thompson, Bombak, Driedger, & Lorway, 2012), online smoking cessation (van Mierlo, Voci, Lee, Fournier, & Selby, 2012), and Brazilian brochures about Hansen's disease (Santos, Ribeiro, & Monteiro, 2012). Content analysis is a method that allows researchers to analyze recorded communications, messages, or content. The content under analysis can come from traditional mass media channels such as TV programs, newspaper/magazine articles, books, or billboards. Content can also come from new Δ290media channels such as Twitter feeds, websites, or YouTube videos. In addition, the content can be public information presented to a mass audience (e.g., Facebook pages) or private information available only to a single individual (e.g., email messages). All types of recorded content can be analyzed using this method.

The term "analysis" refers to what the researcher does with the content. Typically, what the researcher does is count instances of something that occurs within the content. For example, an investigator could count the number of times characters eat snack foods during a program. This would allow for the description of TV portrayals of diet. The researcher might use this data to see how closely the diet of TV characters compares with the U.S. recommended daily allowances for dietary nutrients and vitamins, or the investigator might want to see if diets of audience members resemble the diets portrayed on TV.

Nature of Method

Description

Bernard Berelson is generally considered the modern father of content analysis. His book *Content Analysis in Communication Research* was published in 1952 and remains a seminal work. More recently, Holsti (1969), Krippendorff (2004), and Neuendorf (2002) have written books on content analysis that are invaluable and further explain its methodology. Like other research methods, content analysis has progressed a great deal over the past 50 years.

In its simplest form, content analysis is counting the frequency with which some event occurs. In many cases, it is about the presence or absence of some sign or symbol in communication texts (e.g., Daku, Gibbs, & Heymann, 2012; McCool, Cussen, & Ameratunga, 2011; Price & Grann, 2012). Before delving into the complexities of content analysis, a simple example of a research investigation employing content analysis should help provide some clarity and insight into the method.

Thompson, Robinson, Cusella, and Shellabarger (2000) used content analysis to determine which women's health issues were most commonly included within the storyline of daytime serial programming. Their rationale for the study was simple: (a) previous research suggests that people learn about health issues from TV programs; (b) soap opera viewers identify heavily with the characters, and typically watch the program several times in a given week and over a long period of time; (c) audience involvement with the TV character increases the likelihood of media portrayals impacting audience members; and (d) a desire to know how closely TV portrayals of health issues reflect actual health issues facing women.

Having clear research questions, Thompson et al. (2000) next developed a plan to gather the content for analysis. This step could have been done in at least two ways: (a) record all of the soap opera episodes, watch them, and code for instances of illness on the program; or (b) read the weekly synopses of daytime serials published in the Saturday edition of a local newspaper. They chose the latter method and ended up coding weekly synopses of the programs. As you can see, the term "content analysis" means exactly that—analyze content, and, in this case, it was those 754 weekly synopses of the daytime serials on air over this 14.5-year period. In each synopsis, they identified any and all of the health issues or problems facing a female character. Occasionally, the storyline would suggest that someone "almost drowned" or that someone thought they were pregnant (but ended up not being with child), and, in those cases, the health issue was excluded from the analysis.

Initially, each health problem was identified by the specific illness or health problem (e.g., a character fainted). Ultimately, the large number of specific illnesses were recoded into illness categories (e.g., somatic problems—which included fainting, collapsing, or passing out) so a less onerous and more reasonable number of statistical analyses could be conducted. At the end of the coding process, the researchers knew what types of illnesses occurred to female characters, and the researchers could then compare the occurrences of those illnesses to the health statistics of females in the America. Examples of health issues commonly found were: injuries due to violence, drug abuse, mental health issues (multiple personality and depression), automobile accidents, cancer, and accidents (e.g., falling down the stairs). This relatively simple study employing content analysis details the basic idea about the method.

Theoretical Assumptions

Berelson (1952) defined content analysis as "a research technique for the objective, systematic, and quantitative description of the manifest content of communication" (p. 18). While there are numerous definitions of content analysis (e.g., Krippendorff, 2004; Manganello & Blake, 2010), Neuendorf (2002) summarized the definition of content analysis with the following six parts: (a) scientific; (b) messages being the unit of analysis, data collection, or both; (c) quantitative; (d) summarizing; (e) applicable to all contexts; and (f) all message characteristics available to analysis (pp. 9–26).

Content analysis has traditionally been employed by communication scholars, but is gaining popularity among researchers in other disciplines, including health, psychology, sociology, political science, and gerontology (Manganello & Blake, 2010). There has been debate on whether it is valid or useful to make a difference between qualitative and quantitative content analysis, since "all reading of texts is qualitative" (Krippendorff, (2004), p. 16). On the other hand, Neuendorf (2002) argues that the term "content analysis" does not apply to all analyses of message content. Instead, content analysis is just one category of research techniques for analysis of message content, characterized by being systematic and measurable. Qualitative research techniques on message content, such as narrative analysis and rhetorical analysis, are not content analysis. In this chapter, we consider and detail content analysis as a quantitative research method, describing measurable characteristics of communication texts.

Since content analysis is quantitative, it relies on counting and assigning values to events or occurrences. For example, a researcher might be interested in what the most common types of exercises are that are portrayed in TV programs. This researcher may randomly select 1,000 TV shows from *TV Guide* and then divide each occurrence of exercise in each TV show into a category scheme. This category scheme should be made of categories that are mutually exclusive and exhaustive (Neuendorf, 2002). "Mutually exclusive" means that anything that is to be coded can only be coded into one category. For example, a content analytic scheme for coding TV portrayals of types of exercise might consist of two categories: aerobic exercises and anaerobic exercises. Unfortunately, the two categories are not mutually exclusive because many exercises are both aerobic and anaerobic (e.g., weight lifting/circuit training). A better system might be weight lifting and running or weight lifting, running, and swimming, since you can classify each exercise easily into these categories.

In addition to being mutually exclusive, a good content analytic scheme is also exhaustive. If we use the category system "weight training, running, and swimming," there would be no category for coding bike riding. This suggests you do not have enough categories to accurately code all types of exercise. A good content analysis scheme will allow you to classify each type of exercise into one category—and only one category. In addition, a good scheme will also contain enough categories to include all forms of exercise. Obviously, at times, you will need to employ a category called "other" for those unusual occurrences.

Many times, researchers using content analysis will employ an existing category scheme. For example, if a researcher (e.g., Haven, Burns, Britten, & Davis, 2006) wanted to look at TV portrayals of diet, the researcher could use the USDA food pyramid to categorize food people eat on TV (e.g., fruit, dairy, vegetables). Such an analysis would allow the researcher to compare the food eaten by characters with the food health professionals recommend. However, sometimes researchers might want to create their own category system, rather than use an existing system. For example, if researchers wanted to find out what kinds of messages healthcare professionals send in their emails, they might look at the emails to decide what is actually going on. In a study by Robinson, Turner, Levine, and Tian (2011), the coders coded five types of social support (e.g., emotional support and informational support) as well as a variety of other types of messages (e.g., self-disclosure and phatic messages) to see if patients receiving a particular type of message were more likely to improve their health. These categories emerged from the email messages and ended up being a combination of existing message types (social support) as well as other types of messages that were relatively unrelated to health.

At times you may read or hear that content analysis is problematic because it ignores context. While this issue is certainly true of some studies, it is not inherently a problem with content analysis. Many years ago, one of the authors of this chapter conducted a study looking at TV portrayals of sexual harassment (Skill, Robinson, & Kinsella, 1994). Part of our work in the investigation involved coding context, indicating, for example, if an unwanted sexual advance occurred within the workplace or a social setting; whether or not the unwanted sexual advance occurred with a laugh track; and even the type of character role (e.g., central character, peripheral character, guest character). In this way, an investigator can capture some of the most important elements of context as they code character behavior.

Applications

When researchers use content analysis, human subjects are not asked to participate in a study. Instead, they focus on describing and analyzing characteristics of recorded human verbal and visual communication. Content analysis can be used for a great variety of topics in health communication. Previous content analysis studies on health messages in traditional mass media have addressed topics such as violence, sex, tobacco, obesity/nutrition, alcohol, cancer, aging, body image/eating disorder, mental health, prescription drugs, illegal drugs, health providers/organizations, injury, death and disability, AIDS, women's health, and genetics (Manganello & Blake, 2010, p. 391). The Internet is proving to be a valuable resource for procuring content. A researcher could content analyze email communication between healthcare providers and their patients to evaluate the quality of provider–patient communication; code medical websites to rate the accuracy and/or credibility of online health information; or study transcripts of online support groups to identify supportive communication on the Internet. Content analysis can be used in a variety of ways—limited only by the imagination of the researcher.

Exemplars

Examples of health communication research employing content analysis abound. In many cases, the research resembles the study we introduced earlier to provide a general overview of a content analysis investigation. In this section, we will describe two additional lines of research that rely on content analysis. The first group of studies focuses on how the issue of organ donation is portrayed in traditional and new media outlets. These studies represent the examples of the most common usage of content analysis in health communication research: analyzing messages available to the public. The second study focuses on email messages sent by healthcare practitioners to their patients. This type of research, focusing on content produced by individuals and not publicly available, is less common within the literature.

Organ donation is an important topic in health communication. With the enormous gap between the number of people on the waiting list for an organ to be transplanted and the number of people who donate their organs, researchers use various research methods to investigate factors affecting people's attitudes toward organ donation. One of those factors is media content. Researchers have been using the method of content analysis to examine how media are presenting the issue of organ donation and the potential consequences of those presentations.

Feeley and Vincent (2007) conducted a content analysis on newspaper articles covering organ and tissue donation in the United States dated 2002 or 2003. The sample was 715 articles on organ and tissue donation from 20 high-circulation newspapers. Feeley and Vincent found that 57% of the articles were positive, 29% were neutral, and 14% were negative about organ donation. They also found that post-transplantation health and welfare, information on the shortage of organ donors, living donations, and information about the transplantation process were the most covered topics in the articles; in addition, the two most frequently covered organs were kidneys and hearts.

Similarly, Quick, Kim, and Meyer (2009) conducted a content analysis on TV news coverage of organ donation during a 15-year span. They coded 1,507 news broadcasts, and found that the majority of the news stories on organ donation were positive, but there was only modest coverage on the process of becoming a potential donor. When organ donation was mentioned in news stories, the majority of the excerpts had narratives of people waiting for an organ transplant, and some news broadcasts provided statistical evidence for organ shortage. Finally, this study found that the coverage on living and non-living donor donations was about equal.

Tian (2010) extended research on media presentation of organ donation from traditional media, such as newspaper and TV news, to the new media context. Specifically, she conducted a content analysis on organ donation videos on YouTube to investigate how YouTube users were presenting the issue of organ donation. Through analyzing 355 organ donation videos on YouTube, she found that more than 90% of those videos framed the issue of organ donation in a positive way, characterized by positive secondary frames including "donors are good people," "it is important to donate organs because of organ shortage," and "personal experience" (p. 242). Meanwhile, a content analysis on users' comments (N = 1,532) on those organ donation videos revealed a reciprocity relationship between media frames and audience frames.

Our research group has been studying patient–healthcare practitioner (HCP) interaction and the impact of that interaction on patient health. The first investigation (Levine, Turner, Robinson, Angelus, & Hu, 2009) coded email messages from HCP to patients using an extremely simple content analysis scheme. The patients were Native Americans with Type I or Type II diabetes. Simply, we coded each message as being sent by the patient or sent by the HCP. The messages sent by the HCP were then coded as either being patient specific or a system message. A patient-specific message was one that was sent by a HCP to a particular patient and to no one else. System messages were those messages sent to all of the patients and any HCP or administrator monitoring the research program. Our goal here was to see if patients receiving personal messages were more likely to upload their blood glucose scores (the way patients monitor their diabetes/health), and, indeed, the total number of personal messages received was related to blood glucose monitoring.

Our second investigation employed a more sophisticated content analytic scheme. In this investigation (Robinson et al., 2011), we analyzed all of the personal email messages sent by HCPs to their patients. These 924 messages were coded into 6,411 discrete message units, and then the message units were coded into 8 message types. The categories and the percentage of messages for each category type were phatic (32.2%), informational social support (21.1%), requests for health information (13%), social integration (9.0%), emotional social support (7.2%), esteem social support (6.7%), tangible social support (6.3%), and self-disclosure (< 1.0%). This study was one of the first large-scale studies designed to examine actual email messages from HCP to patients and, ultimately, predict patient involvement in their diabetes care.

Employing Content Analysis

Procedure

Conceptualization

Generally, research is guided by a theoretical rationale, and that means the research is actually a test of some component of the theory. So, the researcher reviews the theory and the extant literature and deduces hypotheses or research questions from that theory/literature. For example, in the telemedicine system study we mentioned earlier in this chapter, we started with the social support theory. We looked at the literature on different dimensions of social support and their relationship with health outcomes. Then, we were able to propose our research questions on what types of social support we could identify from the specific telemedicine system we were studying, and how those types of social support could be related to the system users' changes of specific health behaviors.

Sampling

Once the researchers formulate their research questions and/or hypotheses, they need to choose their sample—that is to say, the texts that they want to analyze. If the population is not too big, the researchers can analyze the entire population of documents, and this process is called a *census*. The study on how YouTube videos framed the issue of organ donation that we mentioned earlier in this chapter used the census approach. Because YouTube was relatively new when the study was conducted, the researcher located only 355 English videos relevant to organ donation. So, she analyzed all those 355 videos. In the perfect world, researchers would always analyze all of the texts.

Realistically, when researchers need to analyze large numbers of texts, they usually choose a sample that accurately reflects the entire population. This process of selecting or choosing which texts to analyze is called "sampling." There are a number of different sampling methods available to researchers, but they can best be understood as random sampling techniques or non-random sampling techniques. Researchers prefer to use random sampling, because, with random sampling, each text has an equal opportunity to be included or not included in the study, so the sample will be representative or similar to the entire population. Suppose a researcher finds 100,000 organ donation videos on YouTube. When researchers do not have enough resources to code all those 100,000 videos, they may decide to draw a random sample of 500 videos from all those 100,000 videos. To do that, researchers number those 100,000 videos first. Then, they use a computer program (e.g., Excel) to generate 500 random numbers between 1 and 100,000. After that, the researchers use those 500 random numbers to select 500 videos from the list of those 100,000 videos. By doing that, the 500 selected videos should be representative of all those 100,000 videos. This technique is called *simple random sampling*, and is perhaps the most commonly employed method of random sampling. Other methods of generating a random sample include *systematic* sampling, *stratified* sampling, and *cluster* sampling.

Most people understand the idea that a random or probability sample is preferred because it produces a sample that most closely resembles the population. Sometimes, the reasons for using non-random or non-probability samples are less clear. Generally, we use non-random samples in our research when it is too difficult, too expensive, or impossible to use a random sampling technique. For instance, let's say a researcher wants to interview heroin addicts to find out the problems they face in their daily lives. As you might guess, there is no giant list of heroin addicts so it would be impossible to use any of the random sampling techniques identified above. Instead, you might walk around until you identified a single heroin addict and then interview that addict. When you were done, you would ask the addict to identify another heroin addict and you would go find her or him to interview. This technique is called "snowball sampling" because the sample size increases, or the sample snowballs, by identifying one or more new potential participants. This would not produce a random sample, but it would produce a usable sample for better understanding heroin addicts.

As a second example of non-probability sampling, perhaps a researcher interested in content analyzing YouTube videos decides to select the 500 most relevant videos (as identified by YouTube) or the 500 most viewed videos (as determined by the audience). Neither of these techniques would produce a random sample, so the results of these investigations would not be generalizable to other YouTube videos about organ donation. But, without a doubt, it would provide insight into what audience members see about organ donation when they watch YouTube. That is, the sample is still meaningful, because the researchers want to focus on the most relevant or most viewed videos. That is what purposive sampling is designed to do.

Unit of Analysis

Once researchers have a theoretical rationale for their work and they have drawn a sample of content to study, they must begin to consider how they will analyze the data. The initial step in this process is defining the unit of analysis. A unit of analysis is the specific occurrence within the content that the researcher plans to study or code. In the research investigation examining provider–patient email messages discussed earlier (Robinson et al, 2011), you may recall that each email message was recorded. If the researcher examined each email message and treated each message as a single event, the unit of analysis would be the individual email message. However, in this investigation, the researchers chose to parse the email messages into individual sentences. Now the unit of analysis is each sentence found in an email message. The reason for this approach may be obvious—a single email message could contain a variety of different messages, and more precision is gained by examining each sentence in the email. However, that is not always the case. In the study by Levine et al. (2009), the researchers did use entire email messages as the unit of analysis. They simply coded each email message as "patient specific" or "messages sent to all patients." They used this approach to demonstrate it was the specific types of messages, and not simply receipt of the messages that motivated patients to monitor their blood glucose levels. Similarly, in the YouTube organ donation video study, the researcher used each video and each audience comment as unit of analysis. The decision about unit of analysis is made based on what the researchers believe about the nature of the content, the theory guiding their investigation, and the difficulty associated with coding the content. The more specific or finely grained the analysis, the more time consuming the process.

Coding

The best way to explain the coding process is to go through a simple content analysis project and explain each of the constituent parts within that process. The term "coding" refers to the process of transforming qualitative information in the texts into measurable values for further analysis. If the content analysis was coding portrayals of illness on daytime serial TV programming, coding would mean watching the program and identifying each time an illness is mentioned or depicted. At first, you might code every specific illness (e.g., flu or broken bone) or you might code categories of illnesses (e.g., mental illnesses). Before you can start coding, you must first develop a codebook, train individuals to code the content, and demonstrate that the coding process is both valid and reliable.

Codebook

You can think of the codebook as being like the blueprints of the investigation. The codebook identifies what will be coded and how each item to be coded is defined. These content category definitions must explain to everyone interested in the study what kinds of things get included within the category and what kinds of things get excluded. For example, if a researcher was coding incidents of drug abuse, the researcher would have to decide if smoking cigarettes or drinking alcohol should be included in the category "drug abuse." The point here is not to answer the question whether alcohol is a drug or not, but, rather, to ensure that all the coders are using the same rules for inclusion and/or exclusion during the coding process. Similarly, a researcher might be coding the race of characters on TV commercials in an effort to understand how food and nutrition are depicted on TV. The researcher could code race as being "Caucasians" and "non-Caucasians," or they could code race as being "Caucasian," "Asian," "Hispanic," "African American" and "Race other than Caucasian, Asian, Hispanic, or African American." This "other" category might include Native Americans. The researcher would decide based on their interests and what previous research suggests are best practices. You could code race using a 2-category system or a 22-category system, but, ultimately, you will find that commercials contain mostly Caucasians and very few Hispanics, Asians, or northern nomadic Inuit. Empty or nearly empty categories are not very useful beyond pointing out there are relatively few of something.

Think of a codebook like you would think about a definition. A good definition identifies what should be included and what should not be included. So does a good codebook. You might find out that, after you have created the codebook, you need to revise it. Common reasons for revision include missing categories (e.g., you forgot to include a particular race) and excessive categories (e.g., you find you are not using a particular category). There is nothing wrong with revising the codebook, but keep in mind you might have to recode all of the data you have already analyzed—depending on the changes to the codebook that you make. Similar to answers for multiple-choice questions in a survey questionnaire, the values or categories for a variable in a codebook should be exclusive to each other and exhaustive. This means your scheme should be able to account for all races that appear on the commercials and no individual appearing on a particular commercial should be coded into more than one category.

Coders

Once the researchers have a codebook established, they will need to train coders on how to use the codebook to code communication materials. Ideally, researchers would want to have two or more coders coding the materials. These coders should have no real idea about what the researcher is trying to do in the investigation (i.e., they don't know the research questions or hypotheses being tested by the researcher). This "blinding" of coders is done to ensure that the coders are not influenced by the goals of the study, and, instead, are coding based solely on the definitions included within the codebook. Using coders that do not know the purpose of the research helps ensure their coding efforts are not biased by their desire to "help the researcher," or by the assumptions they hold prior to beginning the process of coding. When researchers have limited resources, one or more of them may code the materials, but, ideally, at least one coder should be unaware of the research questions or hypotheses.

Having two or more coders coding the same communication texts makes it possible for researchers to test inter-coder agreement, or the reliability of the coding scheme. This is extremely important because inter-coder agreement is an indicator of the quality and reproducibility of the coding process. Without consensus or strong agreement on the coding process, there is little point to coding the material.

Normally, we expect the coders to agree at a rate of 70%. This means that, if there are two coders, in 70% of the cases, they would code some text identically. For example, both coders would agree that the flu is an illness or that a character on a TV show is Caucasian. The coders should be able to agree at a rate of 70%, or higher, or you cannot trust the data. If the coders do not agree 7 out of 10 times, you must modify/improve your codebook until they can reach that level of agreement.

Data Analysis

Since content analysis is a research method using measurement, its data analysis involves a variety of statistical techniques, ranging from simple descriptive statistics to more advanced techniques such as factor analysis and regression analysis. We will only cover the most frequently employed statistical techniques for content analysis in this chapter.

Descriptive statistics is probably the most important and most frequently used statistical technique for content analysis. Sometimes, researchers are just interested in the frequency of the occurrences of certain variables in certain communication texts. For example, a researcher is probably interested in which organ is covered most in newspaper articles (Feeley & Vincent, 2007) or YouTube videos (Tian, 2010) on organ donation. Then, the researcher simply needs to report the frequency of each organ (e.g., kidney, liver, lung) appearing in the sample (selected newspaper articles or YouTube videos). Statistics on frequencies typically go with statistics on percentages, as those numbers together indicate how prominent or important a value for a variable is in the communication texts being studied. So, a researcher may end up reporting something like "kidney was the most frequently covered organ in YouTube videos, mentioned in 136 (38.3%) videos; the second most frequently covered organ was liver, mentioned in 103 (29%) videos."

Descriptive statistics also includes mean and standard deviation. While mean is a measure of the average values for a group of scores, standard deviation indicates the variations of the values from the mean. Suppose a researcher is conducting a content analysis of anti-smoking public service announcements (PSAs) on TV.

One variable the researcher has is how many characters appear in each PSA, which could range from zero (no human character appearing in a PSA) to many (e.g., 100 individuals in one PSA). In that case, the researcher will need to report the mean and standard deviation of numbers of characters in all the anti-smoking PSAs being studied.

Researchers interested in the relationship between two or more variables often rely on the *chi*-square test for their analyses. Variables in content analysis are often nominal or categorical in nature (e.g., yes/no). Data measured at the ordinal level (e.g., low/medium/high) are also often analyzed using *chi*-square because the exact differences in the three categories are not known. You can think of ordinal measures as ranked categorical data. Let's assume a researcher is interested in determining if attitudes toward exercise differ across gender. The researcher would draw a sample of TV shows containing storylines on exercise. In the codebook, there is a gender variable, which has two values: male versus female. There is also the attitude variable, which has three values: positive, neutral, and negative. By coding TV shows with those two variables, the researcher will be able to calculate the crosstabs between gender and attitudes, and then to see if a significant difference exists. The researcher may report the final findings in a way such as "60% of females were positive about exercise, 30% of females were neutral about exercise, and 10% of females were negative about exercise. For the males, 50% were positive about exercise, 35% were neutral about exercise, and 15% were negative about exercise. The difference was not significant (X^2 (4) = 5.9, p = .21)."

T-test and analysis of variance (ANOVA) are used when the researchers are investigating differences of a ratio variable across different groups. Both *t*-test and ANOVA require a ratio variable (e.g., the length of newspaper articles on organ donations—how many words are in each organ donation article in newspapers) and a categorical variable (e.g., newspaper type—national versus regional newspapers). Then the researcher could use either *t*-test or ANOVA, with article length being the outcome variable and newspaper type being the group variable, to see if organ donation articles from national newspapers are significantly longer than organ donation articles from regional newspapers. When the categorical variable has three or more values (e.g., articles from newspapers in the United States, United Kingdom, Canada, and Australia), the researcher has to use ANOVA, with article length being the outcome variable and countries being the group variable.

Researchers could also use correlation analysis when they are interested in the relationship between two or more variables in a content analysis. The most commonly used correlation analysis is Pearson correlation analysis, which is used when both variables are ratio. Tian (2010), for example, was interested in the relationship among the frequency of viewing and rating of YouTube organ donation videos and the length of time a video had appeared on YouTube. Using Pearson correlation analysis, she found a positive relationship between the frequency of a video being viewed and the frequency of the video being rated (r = .94, p = .00). There was also a significant correlation between the length of time that a video had appeared on YouTube and frequency of viewing (r = .19, p = .00) and rating (r = .19, p = .00) of that video (Tian, 2010, p. 243).

Reliability and Validity

For a content analysis to make a substantial contribution to our understandings of a topic, the research measurement and procedure need to be reliable and valid. While reliability is about consistency and stability of a study, "validity" is about accuracy or truth. Similar to other social scientific research methods, such as survey (see Morgan & Carcioppolo, this volume) and experimental (see Morse, Quick, Volkman, & Whaley, this volume), content analysis should always aim for maximum reliability and validity. The concept of inter-coder reliability plays a central role in evaluating the reliability and validity of a content analysis.

Inter-coder Reliability

Inter-coder reliability is the most important indicator on the quality of content analysis data. Neuendorf (2002) suggests the goal of content analysis is to objectively identify and record characteristics of messages. Further, she argues that, without establishing the reliability of the coding scheme, the method is precariously close to useless. However, content analysis does rely on human coders. Researchers need to have two or more coders to code 10% to 20% of the sample texts independently, and then calculate inter-coder reliability with the codes they have.

Most studies published in communication journals reported statistics on inter-coder reliability (Manganello & Blake, 2010; Neuendorf, 2008). There are different ways to calculate inter-coder reliability. Intriguingly, Popping (1988) identified 39 "agreement indices," or ways to calculate inter-coder agreement for nominal variables. Fortunately, most of these methods are seldom used. Lombard, Snyder-Duch, and Bracken (2002) suggest the following indices are the most widely used in communication research: percent agreement, Holsti's method, Scott's pi (*p*), Cohen's kappa (*k*), and Krippendorff's alpha (*a*). We will introduce each of these indices briefly.

The simplest method for calculating inter-coder agreement is percentage of agreement. To calculate percentage of agreement, all you do is to add up the number of cases that were coded the same way by the two coders and divide that number (agreements) by the total number of cases. Table 10.1, below, is based on the coding of two independent coders watching the same newscast and identifying whether or not a story is a "health issue story" or "not a health issue story."

TABLE 10.1 Two Independent Coders Watching the Same Newscast

Story	*Coder 1*	*Coder 2*	*Agreement*
1. Cancer	Health Story	Health Story	Yes
2. School shootings	Health Story	Not a Health Story	No
3. Obesity	Health Story	Health Story	Yes
4. Health insurance	Not a Health Story	Health Story	No
5. Cyber bullying	Not a Health Story	Not a Health Story	Yes

As you can see, the two coders in this example did not agree on whether each story was an example of a health story. In this case, we employed 2 coders and each individual coded 5 stories. There was inter-coder agreement in 3 of the 5 stories, so we can see that the percentage of agreement was 60% (3 instances of agreement out of 5 total stories). Typically, we expect inter-coder agreement levels to exceed 70%, and are considered adequate, while 80% agreement is preferred.

Holsti (1969) suggested an alternative formula for calculating inter-coder agreement. Like percentage of agreement, Holsti's formula is commonly used and differs only in the way it is calculated. Holsti proposes the following formula for calculating inter-coder agreement:

> Inter-coder Agreement = $2M/(N_1 + N_2)$, where "M is the number of coding decisions on which the two judges are in agreement, and N_1 and N_2 refer to the number of coding decisions made by judges 1 and 2, respectively."
>
> *(p. 140)*

Using the same data from Table 10.1, Holsti's formula would produce the following mathematics and inter-coder reliability score: 2x3/10, or 60%. In this case, Holsti's formula produces the same inter-coder agreement percentage as the simple agreement method. But this is not always the case. Changing the number of coders (e.g., using 3 or more coders) or the number of categories (a scheme with 3 or more categories) changes the mathematics.

Cohen (1960) argues that percentage of agreement and Holsti's method artificially inflate agreement percentages. His argument is that some instances of inter-coder agreement happen by chance and those chance occurrences increase the percentage of agreement. He recommends using Cohen's kappa instead of simple agreement. Using SPSS software and the same data yields a kappa of .167, which indicates the level of agreement was significantly lower than Holsti's formula or simple percentage of agreement would suggest. The SPSS output can be seen below.

Not everyone agrees with Cohen's use of the kappa or the related statistic Scott's pi. Krippendorff (2004) and Hayes and Krippendorff (2007) discourage the use of Scott's pi and recommend using Krippendorff's alpha. All three of these

Coder1 * Coder 2 Crosstabulation

Count

		Coder 2		
		No	Yes	Total
Coder1	No	1	1	2
	Yes	1	2	3
Total		2	3	5

Symmetric Measures

		Value	Asymp. Std. Error[a]	Approx. T[b]	Approx. Sig.
Measure of Agreement	Kappa	.167	.446	.373	.709
N of Valid Cases		5			

a. Not assuming the null hypothesis.
b. Using the asymptotic standard error assuming the null hypothesis.

FIGURE 10.1 Coder 1–Coder 2 Crosstabulation

techniques are more conservative and generally considered superior to percentage of agreement or Holsti's formula. These three techniques differ primarily in the way they are calculated—which is beyond the scope of this chapter. Anyone interested in calculating reliability using Krippendorff's alpha should use the SPSS or SAS macros since the statistics are not natively available in either program. Fortunately, Hayes (2012) has made the macros readily available. More extensive discussions of reliability in content analysis are available (Krippendorff, 2004; Lombard, Snyder-Duch, & Bracken, 2002; 2004). In short, reliability refers to the reproducibility of research findings. A researcher should be able to give the content analysis scheme to another researcher and that researcher should find the same things within the data. This makes sense, since the point of content analysis is to identify and describe what occurs within a data set (e.g., group of documents, web pages, or television programs). If different researchers found different things within the same data set, the findings and the method would be worthless. Reproducibility is necessary, but not sufficient for researchers using content analysis. Researchers must also consider the issue of validity.

Validity

There are two types of validity for content analysis: *external validity* and *internal validity*. External validity in content analysis refers to the generalizability of the findings to other data sets. You may recall that, in an experiment, external validity refers to the findings of one experiment generalizing to the population. It is essentially the same here. External validity means the description of one sample of content should be similar to what you would find if you analyzed all of the content and not just a sample. Again, random sampling methods are used to ensure that a sample drawn from a population is representative of that population. As you would expect, the sample should be very similar to the population, so, if you have a reliable content analytic scheme, your findings should reflect the population.

Internal validity refers to the accuracy of your coding scheme. Internal validity is more difficult to demonstrate than external validity because there are four types of internal validity. They are: *face* validity, *content* validity, *criterion* validity, and *construct* validity. As you read more and more research employing content analysis, you will undoubtedly notice that, many times, researchers do not carefully address the issue of validity. However, they should, and this is a basic introduction to how it is done.

Pragmatically, a researcher simply looks at their coding scheme and declares that it has face validity. While this seems less than scientific, the rationale for simply declaring face validity is that, sometimes, things are so apparent or obvious that they do not need to be discussed. For example, a researcher looking at the variable "gender of characters in TV commercials" should code characters as being male or female. There is widespread agreement that there are only two genders and so the researcher can safely declare their coding scheme for gender has face validity. To the extent that others agree with you, your category system has face validity.

Next, content validity refers to the extent to which a content analytic scheme taps into the entire domain or universe of the thing being measured. For example, if a researcher was coding the credibility of public health officials testifying to congress, we would expect them to code the competence, character, and composure of the speakers. We would expect this because research into speaker credibility has indicated these three dimensions are primary or important. A scheme that omitted composure, for example, could be used, but would be missing part of what we believe to be included within the universe of the concept of credibility. If this is not clear, think of the things you would code if you were going to create a demographic profile of physicians on TV. If the coding scheme omitted gender or race, you would recognize that you had not tapped into the entire universe of character demographics and your scheme could be discredited for not having content validity.

The third type of internal validity discussed here is criterion validity. If a researcher used the food pyramid as the basis of their coding scheme, that would help establish the criterion validity of their measure. The term criterion refers to an accepted standard(s) used to make judgments. We are currently analyzing neurologist–stroke victim interactions that occur within emergency rooms employing telemedicine systems. One of the things we are trying to code is the effectiveness of telemedicine. To do that, we are coding the diagnostic process, so we are coding what the physician asks the patient to do (e.g., answer the question "Do you know what month it is?" or "Hold your head still and move your eyes and look at the wall on your left."). We can compare our coding of physician behavior with previous research on face-to-face diagnoses to establish the validity of our measure. In this way, we can demonstrate our coding scheme is accurate, in that our findings reflect the previous research.

The final type and "holy grail" of validity is construct validity. Typically, construct validity refers to demonstrating the relationship between a new measurement instrument and other constructs/measures that should be associated with the new measure. For example, everyone recognizes that the Stanford–Binet Intelligence Scales measure cognitive ability. If a researcher wanted to measure the intelligence of children who are so young that they could not read, such a test would not be possible to administer. So, a researcher might come up with an alternative method for measuring intelligence. That is exactly what the Goodenough–Harris Human Drawing Test purports to do. In a nutshell, a child aged 3 to 10 draws a picture of a person and the drawing is scored for the number and accuracy of the details included in the drawing. Since we know that the Stanford–Binet Intelligence Scales are valid, we could simply use the Goodenough–Harris Human Drawing Test on a group of children and then wait until they could take the Stanford–Binet test. We would expect the scores of the children to be highly correlated and that would help us demonstrate our new measure—the Goodenough-Harris Human Drawing Test—is a valid measure of IQ. We would also correlate "Goodenough" with other measures that should be associated with IQ (e.g., GPA at school) and problem solving. We would also correlate Goodenough with measures that should be unrelated to IQ, such as attention deficit measures, personality scales, or effort.

In terms of content analysis, you see little research focusing on construct validity. An example of such a study might look something like this. A researcher asks a group of people to keep a diary or journal. In that journal, the individuals keep track of how they spend their time. Then, the researcher analyzes those diaries to find out those individuals' perceptions of their own media use and interests. So, the diary is content analyzed and used as a measure of media usage. Now, the researcher asks those same individuals to wear a pager and to write down whatever they are doing whenever they get paged. The pager results and the diary results are then examined using simple correlations, and that would provide support for the construct validity of the diary/content analysis measure. Finally, the researcher could do the same type of correlational examination with both the pager and the diary reports and national averages. This would further bolster the researcher's claims that their measure (the content analysis of the diaries) is a valid measure of media usage.

Strengths and Limitations of Content Analysis

When researchers are interested in the quantitative nature of contents of communication texts themselves, content analysis is the method to use. Researchers conduct quantitative content analysis to get systematic understandings on the variables embedded in communication texts.

Strengths

One of the essential strengths of content analysis is that it is non-intrusive. As mentioned earlier in this chapter, researchers using content analysis do not have to invite human subjects to participate in the study. Researchers typically can get a good sample for content analysis; random sampling is seen more frequently in content analysis than in other methods, such as survey and experiment, with which researchers have to settle for convenient sample in many cases. Imagine you need to randomly select 100 TV shows that have storylines on STDs, and code those 100 TV shows with variables such as type of STDs and characters' attitudes toward each STD. Then imagine you need to randomly select 100 adults who have STDs and ask them to fill out your questionnaire on people's attitudes toward STDs. You probably would find that it is easier to reach those 100 TV shows than to reach those 100 randomly selected people.

Related to the non-intrusive nature of content analysis, this method also allows research process to be relatively free from the Hawthorne effect. Studies have found that, when research participants know they are being studied, they behave in ways different from how they really behave in their natural life (Roethlisberger & Dickson, 1939). This is similar to the social desirability concern we have on survey or interview research. When you ask people questions on certain health issues, a legitimate concern will be how many people are willing to answer the questions and how many will be honest with their answers. Those are challenges that reactive research methods face. With content analysis, since researchers can use existing communication texts, they do not need to worry about the Hawthorne effect or social desirability. For example, we could conduct a content analysis on how people communicate with one another on a health issue on some public discussion boards online. We would not have to worry about response rate, since the texts are already there, yet may still have to consider whether those individuals who post those messages are accurate or honest about what happens in reality or how they really think. However, at least we know the texts are from their anonymous communication with their peers who are interested in the same health issue, instead of the communication with researchers, and it is reasonable to expect that what they say on the anonymous discussion board would not be less accurate than what they say to a researcher.

Limitations

Despite the above strengths of content analysis, this method has limitations. Since content analysis does not involve human subjects, media effects or audience perceptions and interpretations of communication texts cannot be directly studied by analyzing content of traditional texts. Instead, methods such as survey and experiment are needed to measure audience response to communication texts or how those texts affect audience. For example, the studies of media presentation on organ donation in newspapers (Feeley & Vincent, 2007) could provide important understandings on how traditional media are framing the issue of organ donation; yet, we still need to employ interview, focus group, survey, or experiment to investigate how audience are responding to those frames, or how those frames affect audience members' willingness to donate an organ or not.

Using Content Analysis with Other Methods

Given content analysis's strengths and limitations, researchers can use it together with other research methods to better understand the content and effects of communication texts. As a matter of fact, two classical mass communicating theories—the agenda-setting theory (McCombs & Shaw, 1972) and cultivation theory (Gerbner, Gross, Morgan, & Signorielli, 1986)—both involve two research methods: content analysis and survey. For the agenda-setting theory, researchers employ content analysis to identify media agenda and survey to identify public agenda, and then they can test if the two types of agenda are consistent with each other. Similarly, for cultivation theory, researchers use content analysis to understand media profile and they use survey to understand viewer profile, and then they get to analyze if the relationship between TV-world portrayal and real-world perception is different between heavy and light TV viewers.

Niederdeppe, Fowler, Goldstein, and Pribble (2010), for example, used cultivation theory to investigate whether local TV news cultivates fatalistic beliefs about cancer prevention. Similarly to many cultivation studies, they conducted two studies using two research methods; one with content analysis and one with survey. In Study One, they content analyzed a national sample of local TV and newspaper coverage about cancer, and they found that local TV news stories about cancer were more likely to cover cancer causes and cancer research while less likely to provide follow-up information than newspaper stories. Then, in Study Two, they analyzed the 2005 Annenberg National Health Communication Survey (ANHCS) data, and found that local TV news viewing was positively associated with fatalistic beliefs about cancer prevention. The findings from both Study One and Study Two provide support for cultivation theory when communicating about cancer, with the content analysis indicating that the content of local TV news could potentially contribute to fatalistic beliefs about cancer prevention, and the survey data confirming the positive relationship between TV news consumption and fatalistic beliefs about cancer prevention.

Content analysis could also be used in experimental studies as a measurement method. In experimental studies, research participants are exposed to certain communication materials (e.g., health campaign messages). Sometimes, researchers would ask participants to write down their thoughts after they are exposed to the stimuli. Then, the researchers could employ coders to code those thoughts to understand participants' cognitive and/or emotional responses to the stimuli.

Challenges

One of the challenges in employing content analysis is using caution when interpreting findings. Keep in mind that what you are doing, ultimately, is counting the presence or absence of things within content. There is no way to move from knowing how often something appears on a newscast to suggesting social changes are due to TV portrayals. We can suggest there are negative models available in the media or that the media does not reflect reality particularly well, but we cannot know anything more—without additional research using alternative methods. Pay particular attention to this shortcoming in the discussion sections of research investigations. Researchers often wax poetic in the discussion section and overstate their findings using causal or quasi-causal language when they actually have correlational evidence, at best.

Without a doubt the biggest challenge to content analysis researchers is the fact that, if you count things, you will end up with numbers that can take on a life of their own. For example, if you find that a large number of stories in a newspaper focus on diet, you can argue that the focus on diet or obesity encourages eating disorders. If there are very few stories about diet in the newspaper, you can argue that public awareness about obesity needs to be raised. Thin models encourage eating disorders and fat models encourage obesity. Using this logic, thin models can also encourage lower levels of self-esteem. The point is that, if you count things, you will end up with a number, and there is a good chance that number will either be too low or too high. Further exacerbating this problem is the fact that all of the counts can be framed as if they are either positive or negative—depending on the underlying rationale. Believe it or not, people used to argue that, if violence were more realistic, audiences would not watch it. That argument is seldom foisted off on readers, and now we are more concerned that the realism is more impactful. Anyway, the point is that one thing to be concerned about when you use content analysis is that you use it to describe content, and not prescribe social change without additional audience research.

Recent Developments

New media presents new opportunities for content analysis (Freeman & Chapman, 2007; Keelan, Pavri-Garcia, Tomlinson, & Wilson, 2007; Quinn et al., 2012). With the highly interactive nature of new media, there are numerous user-generated contents on the Internet, and these contents help communication researchers conduct audience analysis through content analysis, which could have been very difficult for content analysis on traditional communication texts.

Studies on telemedicine systems (Robinson et al., 2010) and YouTube videos (Tian, 2010) mentioned earlier in this chapter are examples of employing content analysis for audience analysis in the new media context. Other new media channels (e.g., amazon.com or CNN.com) also provide a lot of user-generated content relevant to health products and issues. By analyzing these texts, researchers can investigate media effects in a non-intrusive way, relatively free from the Hawthorne effect or the social desirability issue that affects reactive research methods.

References

Berelson, B. (1952). *Content analysis in communication research*. New York, NY: Hafner Press.

Cohen, J. (1960). A coefficient of agreement for nominal scales. *Educational and Psychological Measurement*, *20*(1), 37–46.

Daku, M., Gibbs, A., & Heymann, J. (2012). Representations of MDR and XDR-TB in South African newspapers. *Social Science & Medicine*, *75*(2), 410–418.

Feeley, T. H., & Vincent, D. (2007). How organ donation is represented in newspaper articles in the United States. *Health Communication*, *21*(2), 125–131.

Freeman, B., & Chapman, S. (2007). Is "YouTube" telling or selling you something? Tobacco content on the YouTube video-sharing website. *Tobacco Control*, *16*(3), 207–210.

Gerbner, G., Gross, L., Morgan, M., & Signorielli, N. (1986). Living with television: The dynamics of the cultivation process. In J. Bryant & D. Zillmann (Eds.), *Perspectives on media effects* (pp. 17–40). Hillsdale, NJ: Lawrence Erlbaum Associates.

Haven, J., Burns, A., Britten, P., & Davis, C. (2006). Developing the consumer interface for the MyPyramid food guidance system. *Journal of Nutrition Education and Behavior*, *38*(6), S124–S135.

Hayes, A. F. (2012). Macros and code for SPSS and SAS [Software]. Available from: http://www.afhayes.com/spss-sas-and-mplus-macros-and-code.html

Hayes, A. F., & Krippendorff, K. (2007). Answering the call for a standard reliability measure for coding data. *Communication Methods and Measures*, *1*(1), 77–89.

Holsti, O. R. (1969). *Content analysis for the social sciences and humanities*. Reading, MA: Addison-Wesley.

Keelan, J., Pavri-Garcia, V., Tomlinson, G., & Wilson, K. (2007). YouTube as a source of information on immunization: A content analysis. *Journal of the American Medical Association*, *298*(21), 2482–2484.

Krippendorff, K. (2004). *Content analysis: An introduction to its methodology* (2nd ed.). Thousand Oaks, CA: Sage Publications.

Levine, B. A., Turner, J. W., Robinson, J. D., Angelus, P., & Hu, T. M.-J. (2009). Communication plays a critical role in web based monitoring. *Journal of Diabetes Science and Technology*, *3*(3), 461–467.

Lombard, M., Snyder-Duch, J., & Bracken, C. C. (2002). Content analysis in mass communication: Assessment and reporting of intercoder reliability. *Human Communication Research*, *28*(4), 587–604.

Lombard, M., Snyder-Duch, J., & Bracken, C. C. (2004). A call for standardization in content analysis reliability. *Human Communication Research*, *30*(3), 434–437.

McCombs, M. E., & Shaw, D. L. (1972). The agenda-setting function of mass media. *Public Opinion Quarterly, 36*(2), 176–187.

MacCool, J., Cussen, A., & Ameratunga, S. (2011). Media reporting of global health issues and events in New Zealand daily newspapers. *Health Promotion Journal of Australia, 22*(3), 228–230.

Manganello, J. A. & Blake N. (2010). A study of quantitative content analysis of health messages in U.S. media from 1985 to 2005. *Health Communication, 25*(5), 387–396.

Muzyka, C. N., Thompson, L. H., Bombak, A. E., Driedger, S., & Lorway, R. (2012). A Kenyan newspaper analysis of the limitations of voluntary medical male circumcision and the importance of sustained condom use. *BMC Public Health, 12*(1), 465. Available from: http://www.ncbi.nlm.nih.gov/pubmed/22720748

Neuendorf, K. A. (2002). *The content analysis guidebook.* Thousand Oaks, CA: Sage Publications.

Neuendorf, K. A. (2008). Reliability for content analysis. In A. B. Jordan, D. Kunkel, J. Manganello, & M. Fishbein (Eds.), *Media messages and public health: A decisions approach to content analysis* (pp. 67–87). New York, NY: Routledge.

Niederdeppe, J., Fowler, E. F., Goldstein, K., & Pribble, J. (2010). Does local television news coverage cultivate fatalistic beliefs about cancer prevention? *Journal of Communication, 60*(2), 230–253.

Popping, R. (1988). On agreement indices for nominal data. In W. E. Saris & I. N. Gallhofer (Eds.), *Sociometric research: Data collection and scaling* (Vol. 1) (pp. 90–105). New York, NY: St. Martin's Press.

Price, A., & Grann, V. R. (2012). Portrayal of complementary and alternative medicine for cancer by top online news sites. *Journal of Alternative and Complementary Medicine, 18*(5), 487–493.

Quick, B. L., Kim, D. K., & Meyer, K. (2009). A 15-year review of ABC, CBS, and NBC news coverage of organ donation: Implications for organ donation campaigns. *Health Communication, 24*(2), 137–145.

Quinn, E. M., Corrigan, M. A., McHugh, S. M., Murphy, D., O'Mullane, J., Hill, A. D., & Redmond, H. P. (2012). Who's talking about breast cancer? Analysis of daily breast cancer posts on the internet. *The Breast, 22*(1), 24–27. Available from: http://www.ncbi.nlm.nih.gov/pubmed/22683246

Robinson, J. D., Turner, J. W., Levine, B., & Tian, Y. (2011). Expanding the walls of the health care encounter: Support and outcomes for patients online. *Health Communication, 26*(2), 125–134.

Roethlisberger, F. J., & Dickson, W. J. (1939). *Management and the worker.* Cambridge, MA: Harvard University Press.

Santos, A. K., Ribeiro, A. P., & Monteiro, S. (2012). The production of social discourse on Hansen's disease and health education materials in Brazil: A skin patch as something harmless or a serious disease. *Leprosy Review, 83*(1), 24–33.

Skill, T., Robinson, J., & Kinsella, C. (1994). Sexual harassment in network television situation comedies: An empirical content analysis of fictional programming one year prior to the Clarence Thomas senate confirmation hearings for the U.S. Supreme Court. Paper presented at the Mass Communication Division of the Speech Communication Association national convention meeting, November 1994, New Orleans, Louisiana.

Thompson, T. L., Robinson, J. D., Cusella, L. P., & Shellabarger, S. (2000). Women's health problems in soap operas: A content analysis. *Women's Health Issues, 10*(4), 202–209.

Tian, Y. (2010). Organ donation on Web 2.0: Content and audience analysis of organ donation videos on YouTube. *Health Communication, 25*(3), 238–246.

van Mierlo, T., Voci, S., Lee, S., Fournier, R., & Selby, P. (2012). Superusers in social networks for smoking cessation: Analysis of demographic characteristics and posting behavior from the Canadian Cancer Society's smokers' helpline and stopsmokingcenter.net. *Journal of Medical Internet Research, 14*(3), e66. Available from: http://www.ncbi.nlm.nih.gov/pubmed/22732103

Causal Explication

ISSUES AND CHALLENGES IN CONDUCTING EXPERIMENTAL HEALTH COMMUNICATION RESEARCH

Christopher R. Morse, Brian L. Quick, Julie E. Volkman, and Bryan B. Whaley

The issue of health research is one that often transcends a single discipline. Researchers from a variety of fields and experiences can often find themselves working together to understand a specific aspect of health within the world at large. While the interdisciplinary nature of health research is both important and exciting, it also potentially brings with it some complications. Individuals with backgrounds in psychology, medicine, human development, public health, sociology, and communication not only have unique experience and knowledge that they can offer, but they also have different research training, terminology, and perspectives on how research should be conducted. To complicate matters even further, general trends within specific health-related fields can often focus on specific methodological techniques (e.g., design and analyses) at the exclusion of other research tools. To this end, the purpose of this chapter is to provide individuals interested in conducting health research (and, particularly, health communication research) with the prevailing practices, concerns, and terminology so they are equipped to conduct sound and beneficial investigations.

Specifically, this chapter addresses the issues and challenges that exist within research utilizing experimental designs. The authors focus on the issue of experimental research design as it applies to research in health—specifically, health communication—rather than a complete articulation of experimental design. This begins with a brief overview of sampling issues and techniques that may appear in health research. Following this discussion of sampling, a close look at different experimental designs researchers can employ when testing their hypotheses and searching for answers to their research questions is offered. In doing so, attention is given to the strengths and weaknesses of various true and quasi-experimental designs. Issues confronting health communication researchers, such as health literacy, message design, and induction checks, are also given consideration in this chapter. Finally, specific validity issues and challenges are addressed, such as attrition, testing sensitization, and timing of posttest measures, as well as how each factor relates to and impacts health communication research conducted within an experimental setting.

Sampling

Sampling, in the context of this chapter, is the process of selecting a fraction of the population of interest for participation in one's study. The assumption being that the results from the sample can be inferred to represent that of the population at large. However, researchers are often faced with two important questions during the sampling process: "Where is my sample going to come from?" and "How am I going to choose them?" Health communication researchers are often faced with the difficult task of attempting to recruit participants for their studies. While not always the case, many of the queries posed by health communication researchers cannot be examined utilizing the common "college-age" sample that is often used in communication research and related disciplines. While recruiting participants outside of the academic setting is potentially more difficult, it is critical for health communication researchers to do so. Many of the issues that can be researched regarding health fail to have a high incidence rate among the college population, or, in other cases, affect such a diverse population that college students represent only a fraction of the total. For instance, many cancer screening recommendations apply to men and women outside the 18–22 age range. Coronary heart disease (one of America's top health issues) has rates highest among adults in the age ranges of 45 to 64 years and 65 years and older (Centers for Disease Control and Prevention, 2011). Meanwhile, obesity is quickly becoming a health issue affecting individuals of every age. Given this, it is imperative that health communication researchers seek to work with others across the sciences, allied health, health services, and medical disciplines to reach populations that are truly influenced by the health issues of interest.

In response to this need, there is a growing trend now for academics in health communication to have joint appointments in other departments and agencies (e.g., medical school, public health, bio-behavioral health, health policy) for the sole purpose of working with colleagues from these areas. In addition, many of the funding agencies that provide grants for health research (e.g., National Institutes of Health, National Science Foundation, Centers for Disease Control and Prevention, Robert Wood Johnson Foundation, U.S. Department of Health and Human Services) recognize the importance of this issue and often look for research that is multi-/interdisciplinary in nature and draws from a wide variety of expertise and knowledge about a health issue.

Along with deciding "where" the sample is coming from, health communication researchers must also decide "how" they are going to select their participants. Within experimental research, there are two major types of sampling techniques—probability and non-probability—that can be used to select the potential participants from the population. Probability sampling is when each participant has a known non-zero probability of selection from the population. Random sampling concerns the assumption that every participant in the population has an equal chance of being selected as a member of the sample. In contrast, non-probability sampling involves techniques that violate these premises for various reasons, such as the purposeful selection of certain characteristics based on the research's purpose of inquiry (Cook & Campbell, 1979).

While both types of sampling are used in health communication research, those engaged in experimental designs are often encouraged to utilize probability (or random) samples. This preference is predicated on several key assumptions. First, true random samples are argued to be unbiased. Given that every participant in the population had an equal chance of being selected, then the factors that exist within the participants (known or unknown) is random. Second, random samples have a greater chance of being representative of the population from which the participants were recruited, compared to non-random samples. While there is no guarantee that a sample is truly representative of the population from which it is derived, random sampling techniques provide researchers with the highest probability of mirroring the characteristics of interest (based on the research) in the population. Finally, if the assumptions of being representative and unbiased hold true, then experimental designs that use a random sample have the greatest chance of possessing high external validity. That is, there is a greater chance that the results that are found based on the sample can be generalized to the population.

Random Sampling Techniques

Probability samples (those using random sampling) can be selected utilizing a variety of techniques. While each sampling technique is not without its own merits, selection is usually based upon cost (time, money, labor, etc.) to the researcher, as well as a function of the population under investigation. Within the area of health research, the following are a few of the more common techniques for sample recruitment.

Simple Random

In cases in which the population of interest is known, participants are selected by random (each participant having an equal chance of being chosen), often through the use of various sampling programs or tables—the basic understanding being that everyone in the population is attributed with some type or arbitrary marker (often a number) and then a specific number of those are randomly selected.

Stratified Random

In this technique, the population of interest is broken down into subgroups based on certain characteristics (e.g., age, sex, race, economic status, diagnosis). This is followed by an equal number of individuals being randomly selected from each group. This often requires more time and resources than simple random sampling, and relies heavily on the researcher clearly defining the subgroups.

Cluster

Often used when a population is known, but hard to get access to in entirety, cluster sampling techniques offer opportunities for health researchers to contact research participants. However, if the population can be clustered (in hospitals, departments, divisions, schools, geographic locations, for example), then these clusters can be randomly selected and so too can the individuals within them. Often called "multi-stage sampling," the idea is that one or more clusters are randomly selected from the whole, and, within these clusters, individuals are then randomly selected.

Non-Random Sampling Techniques

It is important to note, however, that, while the assumptions of experimental design research are often better served by probability samples, they are not always practical. Some situations can (and often do) occur in health research that may make random sampling techniques more problematic, or, in other cases, less preferred to non-probability samples. Researchers in the health field often face various constraints, such as time, financial considerations, access to participants, occurrence of variable of interest, and ethical considerations, that often prevent them from being able to engage in the ideal of random sampling. Thus, several non-random sampling techniques are often employed by researchers in this field. While a more in-depth description of these techniques (and others) can be found in classic research methods texts, the following are brief descriptions of some of the more common non-random sampling techniques used in the health field.

Convenience

Participants are selected due to the ease of accessibility to the researcher. Often, research using this sampling technique is comprised of people who are already associated with the researcher in some form or another (e.g., work for, live near, attend a similar institution, are admitted in the hospital or clinic that the researcher works for). This type of sampling technique can result in fairly large samples. Researchers are cautioned to access within-group representativeness of participant sample.

Purposive (Judgmental)

Participants are purposefully selected by the researcher due to the fact that they have some characteristic that the researcher believes will make them more likely to engage in the research, or they will be more likely to benefit from the research and findings. Obviously, in this scenario, the researcher's bias (albeit potentially altruistic) is now present in the study.

Snowball

Often utilized in hard-to-find (or hard-to-reach) samples, this technique involves participants in the active recruiting of "like qualified" others. Researchers identify a small number of individuals that possess the characteristics needed to be part of the sample, and then ask those participants to utilize their connections (friends, family members, support groups, etc.) to recruit other participants who also share those same characteristics.

Again, there is a growing trend for interdisciplinary collaborations within health research not only to increase knowledge but also gain access to samples. Often, these collaborations will lead to specific sampling techniques based on the variables of interest, or the location (clinical, medical, or health services setting). For instance, provider–patient communication research would require collaborating with or studying physicians, clinicians, nurses, patients, and the like. As providers often operate within a general practice, clinic, or office, it poses an interesting decision for health communication researchers to consider how best to recruit and sample patients or providers. For some, a clustering sampling method (see above), where they randomize at the practice level, may be considered advantageous and economical (Bowling, 2009). Depending on the health issue, researchers may also want to use the stratified random sampling technique (Bowling, 2009).

Certain health issues may influence one segment of the population versus another. For instance, researchers may oversample in an area where a specific population dominantly lives for use in later analyses or to have a full representation of those affected by the health issue (Bowling, 2009). In either case, sample size to satisfy statistical power is always a concern. When it comes to experimental research, *who* is participating in your research and how many are participating is just as important as *how* you are doing your research.

Experimental Designs

Two common research designs within the communication field are typically labeled as *true* experimental designs and *quasi*-experimental designs. To be classified as such, the research design must have two or more differently treated groups (often designated as experimental groups and control groups). In the case of true experimental designs, the participants must also be randomly assigned into one of the treatment groups. While researchers in the communication field (as well as certain social sciences) tend to use these terms (true experimental or quasi-experimental) when referring to these types of research designs, others in health research (clinical) generally refer to them as *randomized controlled clinical trials* (RCT) and *non-randomized controlled clinical trials* (NRCT). Regardless of the nomenclature, the philosophy behind true experimental design/RCT is that research conducted this way minimizes the impact of confounding variables, allows for control over the independent/predictor variable, and theoretically allows for the presence of causal relationships. Furthermore, in instances where a pretest–posttest is included (common but not required in these types of research designs), researchers are able to control for time-related validity concerns as well as measure change in the dependent variable.

True Experimental Designs/RCTs

Randomization

As posited, one of the criteria for this design type is the random assignment of participants. More specifically, randomization can be defined as "the assignment to experimental treatments of members of a universe in a way such that, for any given assignment to a treatment, every member of the universe has an equal probability of being chosen for that assignment" (Kerlinger & Lee, 2000, p. 170). Randomization can often be a difficult concept, both in definition and application. This circumstance is often compounded in health settings, where it is often hard to explain the justifications for a particular research design to participants with regard to their placement in specific conditions (Krieger, Parrott, & Nussbaum, 2011). Regardless, it is an important element in experimental methods, and one that should not be overlooked. Perhaps the best example regarding the need for randomization is to look at one in a clinical health research setting. Imagine that medical researchers are interested in testing a new drug and using the process of RCT. In clinical trials, a subset of the population is studied, and patients in the trial are either given the new drug or the standard drug (or usual care). Researchers use randomization as a part of the design to ensure that participants in the trial have an equal chance of being given the new drug or the standard drug. The research (and, thereby, the results) are considered to be less biased because everyone has an equal chance of being put in any condition (new drug vs. standard drug)—no favoritism is given to participants. It is important that the experimental research be as fair and balanced as possible to help give validity to the study outcomes.

Another key need for randomization is that it helps balance any unique differences between participants that may influence the outcomes of the study.

In other words, it attempts to reduce the impact of potentially confounding variables that might be unforeseen by the researchers. Investigators cannot identify every potential confounding variable within a study, especially when conducting experimental research in non-controlled laboratory settings. For this reason, randomization helps to balance the odds of participants with distinctive characteristics consistently being placed in the same condition (or, as in the example mentioned previously, being given the new drug compared to the standard drug).

Design Types

In conducting research within the health context, four of the more common true experimental designs/RCTs include: (a) Solomon four-group design, (b) pretest–posttest control group design, (c) posttest-only control group design, and (d) complete factorial design. In discussing each, it is important for readers to know that *R* stands for random assignment, *X* represents the treatment stimuli, and *O* equals the observation.

Solomon Four-Group Design

The classic and idealized design for true experiments/RCTs is the Solomon four-group design (Solomon, 1949). If a researcher possessed unlimited resources, arguably there is no design more advantageous. The Solomon four-group design is diagrammed below:

$$
\begin{array}{llll}
R & O_1 & X & O_2 \\
R & O_3 & & O_4 \\
R & & X & O_5 \\
R & & & O_6
\end{array}
$$

As the name implies, four groups comprise the Solomon four-group design, which combines several designs and, as a result, presents the most robust defense against threats to internal and external validity (discussion to follow). That is, this design reduces threats to validity such as history, maturation, testing sensitization, pretest sensitization, and instrumentation. The major purpose of this design is to assess the effect of a pretest on the outcomes of an intervention. For example, Aschen (1997) utilized the Solomon four-group design to determine that schizophrenic and depressive patients receiving assertion training therapy experienced less anxiety and greater responsiveness following training compared to patients receiving no training. The greatest strength of this design is the myriad testing opportunities for researchers. First, researchers can test for differences between groups 1 and 2 prior to the intervention (O_1 and O_3) and then after exposure to the treatment (O_2 and O_4). Additionally, researchers can test for within-subject differences between group 1 (O_1 and O_2) and 2 (O_3 and O_4). In testing for the interaction between the pretest and the intervention, the Solomon four-group design enables researchers to examine pretest influence on subsequent observations (O_2 and O_5). With four groups, a variation of tests can be utilized to examine the effectiveness of the intervention utilizing one within-subject test (O_1 and O_2) as well as several between-subject tests, including (O_2 and O_4), (O_2 and O_6), (O_5 and O_6), (O_5 and O_4), (O_5 and O_3), and (O_5 and O_1).

Clearly, as evidenced above, the strength of this design rests in the various number of tests offered to researchers. However, it should be noted that, while ideal, this design is often impractical due to the financial costs and time constraints required to conduct it effectively. Thus, its use within health research is often limited. In contrast, the remaining three designs that follow are more often represented within health research in this area.

Pretest–Posttest Control Group Design

The pretest–posttest control group design consists of at least two groups: the treatment group and the control group. The design can be diagrammed as follows:

$$\begin{array}{llll} R & O_1 & X & O_2 \\ R & O_3 & & O_4 \end{array}$$

This particular design is strengthened because researchers can examine the effectiveness of the treatment via three important comparisons. First, a researcher can assess differences between the treatment and control groups prior to the treatment group's exposure to the intervention (O_1 and O_3). Second, researchers utilizing this design can examine differences between the treatment and control group following exposure to the intervention (O_2 and O_4). Third, researchers can determine if the difference between the pre- and post-intervention scores differed significantly between the treatment and control group by taking the difference between the pre- and post-intervention assessment (O_1/O_2 and O_3/O_4). Smith, Egbert, Dellman-Jenkins, Nanna, and Palmieri (2012) employed this experimental design to assess the effectiveness of a web-based intervention delivered to male stroke survivors and their caregivers in hopes of reducing depression. Despite the advantages offered through each of the abovementioned analyses, many researchers elect to use this particular design because it controls for several threats to internal validity, such as history, maturation, testing sensitization, and instrumentation, equally for individuals exposed to the intervention and those randomly assigned to the control group. Finally, an advantage of the pretest–posttest control group design is the gain of enhanced statistical power through within-group analysis. Despite all of these strengths, the major shortcoming associated with this design rests in pretest sensitization. That is, participants are likely aware of the purpose of the research project following their participation in the pretest, which could affect their processing of the treatment and their responses at the follow-up observation. To overcome this limitation, health researchers should employ this pretest well in advance of the intervention to mitigate this threat to validity.

Posttest-Only Control Group Design

In some cases, researchers may not be able to administer a pretest due to patient health, lack of time, or fear of biasing the participant. In cases such as this, the posttest-only control group design offers a comparable true experimental design for researchers to employ when gauging the effectiveness of an intervention. The posttest-only control group design is diagrammed below:

$$\begin{array}{lll} R & X & O_1 \\ R & & O_2 \end{array}$$

Unlike other designs, the posttest-only control group design limits researchers to one comparison (O_1 and O_2; Campbell & Stanley, 1967). This design is boosted by the fact that it controls for threats to internal validity in much the same way as the previous designs; however, the external and internal validity of this design is strengthened because pretest sensitization concerns are no longer problematic. Roberto, Meyer, Johnson, and Atkin (2000) utilized this design in their gun safety intervention aimed at participants enrolled in a hunter safety course. Their results demonstrated that participants exposed to the intervention listed significantly more recommended gun safety practices, greater susceptibility to gun injuries, and perceived gun injuries as more serious than individuals in the control group. With only a posttest administered, another advantage of this design compared to the previous design rests in its affordability, both in terms of cost and time. However, critics of this design rightfully recognize the discomfort of not knowing with certainty if the two groups were similar prior to the treatment group's exposure to the intervention. For this reason, researchers are reluctant to use this design when randomization is questionable or in situations with a limited sample size. However, as the sample size grows, concerns over group differences prior to the intervention are often abated.

Complete Factorial Design

Similar to the designs above, complete factorial designs incorporate an intervention as well as experimental and control groups. However, what distinguishes this design type from others is the presence of more than one experimental or control group. One example is below:

$$\begin{array}{llll} R & O_1 & X_1 & O_2 \\ R & O_3 & X_2 & O_4 \\ R & O_5 & & O_6 \end{array}$$

While researchers within the communication field will often categorize this design type as either a type of pretest–posttest control group design or a posttest-only control group design, it is important to note that researchers in other areas of health (clinical/public health) will often make a distinction. The strength of this design type (in the example of multiple experimental conditions) is the ability to introduce either multiple intervention types or multiple levels of the same intervention. For example, using the design above, a researcher may want to examine the impact of various health behaviors (X) on patients' blood pressure (O). In this case, the researchers may have a control group that is not given any health behavior regimen, one experimental group that is required to exercise (X_1), and another experimental group that is required to engage in a low sodium diet (X_2). Here, the researchers are comparing multiple intervention types (exercise vs. diet) with regard to their impact on patients' blood pressure levels. In contrast, researchers may choose to compare levels of a single intervention instead of multiple intervention types. Using the same example, researchers may compare one experimental group that is required to exercise for 1 hour twice a week (X_1), a second experimental group that is required to exercise for 2 hours twice a week (X_2), and the control group (which receives no exercise regimen) with regard to patients' blood pressure.

Similarly, researchers using this design can also introduce multiple control conditions rather than experimental ones. Often, this is seen in instances where a standard procedure or treatment is already in existence (control$_1$) and the researcher wants to compare a "new" treatment (experimental) to it as well as a placebo condition (control$_2$; Bowling, 2009).

In either case, this design offers benefits similar to the pretest–posttest control group design or a posttest-only control group design mentioned previously. In addition, it also provides the researcher with the ability to simultaneously compare multiple types of interventions or intervention levels.

Quasi-Experimental Designs/NRCTs

While true experimental designs/RCTs are often touted as the preferred design choice, based on the advantages mentioned previously, they are not always feasible or, for that matter, permissible. Within a health context, there are often instances in which random assignment is not feasible (e.g., the intervention is a message or program that already exists in the population and cannot be removed or modified) or unethical (e.g., when withholding an intervention with potential health benefits from a segment of the population is prohibited by law or organizational policy). In situations such as these, where true experimental designs cannot be employed, health researchers often rely on quasi-experimental designs or NRCTs. The following are two designs that are often employed.

Pretest–Posttest Design

The most commonly employed quasi-experimental design is the pretest–posttest design. The pretest–posttest design is diagrammed below:

$$\begin{array}{ccc} O_1 & X & O_2 \\ O_3 & & O_4 \end{array}$$

Similar to the pretest–posttest group design, the pretest–posttest design allows for four different tests. Specifically, researchers can assess between group differences prior to (O_1 and O_3) and after the intervention (O_2 and O_4). Additionally, researchers can assess within-subject differences for individuals exposed to the treatment (O_1 and O_2) as well as differences for individuals not exposed to the intervention (O_3 and O_4). An example of this research design is a mass mediated intervention designed to elicit positive attitudes and intentions toward living kidney donation among Arizona Hispanics (Alvaro, Siegel, Crano, & Dominick, 2010). The major shortcoming of this particular design is that participants are not randomly assigned to a group. Because participants have been assigned to either the treatment or control group prior to the intervention, they likely differ prior to the launch of the intervention or the experimental stimulus. With this limitation in mind, researchers employing this design must utilize a variety of measures at the pretest to better understand the similarities and differences between groups prior to the treatment. Despite this limitation, the pretest–posttest design controls reasonably well for internal validity threats such as testing sensitization and history even though the control group is nonequivalent with the treatment group.

Posttest-Only Design

This design is similar to the pretest–posttest design without the pretest. The posttest-only design is diagrammed below:

$$\begin{array}{cc} X & O_1 \\ & O_2 \end{array}$$

For this design, a researcher can test for differences between both groups (O_1 and O_2) following the implementation of the stimulus (X). The strength with this particular design is that pretest sensitization is not an issue. However, the downside of not administering a pretest is that it is impossible to measure the equivalence of the treatment and control groups prior to the experimental stimulus. For this reason, attributing differences to the stimuli between individuals exposed to the treatment and those not exposed to the treatment can be an arduous task.

We should remind readers that, while quasi-experimental designs are sometimes argued as not ideal, this should not be taken as indication that they should be avoided. While they do have weaknesses derived from the lack of randomization, these can often be addressed and these design types certainly have a place at the table in health communication research. More importantly, these designs are often the only options available to researchers.

Issues with Experimental Designs in Health Contexts

In any form of research, issues with methodology (both in components and implementation) have the potential to threaten the reliability and validity of the results, the generalizations that can be made, and even the possibility that the research can be conducted. Research within health contexts is no exception. While many of the concerns faced by health researchers are similar to those found in other areas, there are several issues to which health communication researchers should pay particular attention. The importance of these issues are predicated on either the frequency with which they appear in health research, the unique situations that manifest in health research, or the deviation from common trends in other areas of communication research.

Message Effects and Generalizing about Health Messages

An essential methodological issue of health communication research concerns generalizability of findings of message effects. Jackson (1992) and colleagues have detailed the theoretical, experimental design, and statistical underpinnings of enhancing this confidence (see Jackson, 1992; Jackson & Jacobs, 1983; Jackson, O'Keefe, & Brashers, 1994; Jackson, O'Keefe, & Jacobs, 1988; Jackson, O'Keefe, Jacobs, & Brashers, 1989). These researchers posit three premises critical to enhancing confidence of generalizability of findings: (a) inclusion of multiple message instantiations (i.e., examples) of treatment, (b) acknowledging that these multiple examples of the same message type is a source of random variation in the valuation of treatment effects, and (c) that researchers do their best to have instantiations be naturally occurring examples of the message type under investigation (Brashers & Jackson, 1999; Jackson & Jacobs, 1983). Several additional recommendations regarding message effects research also exist (see Jackson et al., 1994).

Taking Jackson and colleagues' suggestions into consideration when investigating the effects of rebuttal analogy, Whaley and associates (Whaley &

Wagner, 2000; Whaley, Wagner, Cook, & Jeha, 2002) used a 2 (rebuttal analogy, no analogy) × 4 (message topic) factorial design, and utilized four different naturally occurring messages and respective analogies that varied across topics and context. They found only main effects for rebuttal analogy on the dependent measures, and no interactions. Because of the adherence to Jackson and colleague's suggestions (i.e., experimental design; using multiple, naturally occurring instantiations; statistically treating instantiations as random sources of variation), investigators can be most confident of the generalizability of the effects of rebuttal analogy demonstrated in this study.

Similarly, Whaley, Stone, Brady, and Whaley (2014) investigated explanatory analogies, which are frequently used linguistic devices for explaining illness. Using the same core message explaining diabetes (i.e., control condition) to create two message conditions employing two naturally occurring analogies to aid in diabetes explanation ("key/lock" analogy, "driveway" analogy) embedded in the core message, Whaley et al. found significant differences in the effects of explanatory analogy. Specifically, they found differences not only between the two analogies on several dependent measures, but that the control message (i.e., core message without analogy) was rated better on several key dependent measures than either or both analogy messages. Again, considering the design issues posited by Jackson et al., there appears to be little to no generalizability concerning within-message category effects of these explanatory analogies.

Induction Checks

Research in health communication often involves the induction of some type of message component designed to impact a dependent variable in some way (e.g., the use of fear appeals in health campaigns). Before any conclusions can be made on the results, one must first make sure that the participants perceived the message in the intended way. Referring back to the example of fear appeals in health campaigns, before one determines the impact that fear might have on a health behavior, one must make sure that the participants actually perceived the fear appeal as fearful. An induction check, by definition, examines the degree to which the experimental stimulus is perceived as the researcher intended. In his thought-provoking essay on the role of induction checks in persuasion research, O'Keefe (2003) presented three classes of claims that interest message effect researchers. The first class of claims involves the relationship between a psychological state (e.g., beliefs, emotions) and an outcome variable of interest (e.g., message persuasiveness). The second type of claim examines the association between a message induction (e.g., message length, explicitness) and the outcome variable of interest. The final type of claim investigates the relationship between the message induction and psychological state as well as the relationship between psychological state and the outcome variable of interest.

In short, for researchers defining their message manipulations in terms of effect-based variations, manipulation checks will be necessary. However, as O'Keefe (2003) persuasively argued, such claims are limited in that they do not inform health communication researchers about the specific message properties necessary to bring about the desired psychological state. Rather than relying on effect-based message variables, it is more advantageous for researchers to define variables based on their intrinsic message properties. It is important to note that we are not dismissing the importance of measuring psychological state. As shown in the third class of research claims, psychological state can serve as a useful mediator connecting the intrinsic message properties and the outcome variables of interest.

General Validity Issues

While the issues mentioned above can impact a research study on multiple levels, there are also several specific validity threats that health communication scholars should be aware of when conducting research. Validity refers to the veracity of a research claim—the likelihood that the researcher successfully tested the issues of interest. Common threats to validity within health research include: (a) history, (b) testing sensitization, (c) instrumentation, (d) timing of posttest measures, (e) attrition, and (f) social desirability bias.

"History" refers to events that occur between data-collection time points. The concern here is that events in a participant's life, events completely isolated from the experiment, may influence posttest reactions, thereby introducing confounding variables. For example, following a pretest regarding the dangers of drinking and driving, an individual learns of a friend who was killed by a drunk driver. A traumatic event such as this could impact the participant, likely resulting in an increased desire to not drink and drive measured in the second data collection. This participant's levels on the measures of interest could be above that accounted for by the intervention admonishing against the dangers of drinking and driving.

As mentioned earlier, several research designs available to health researchers involve the use of a pretest. While there are numerous benefits to this, it also presents one with a potential validity threat. *Testing sensitization* occurs when the administration of a pretest enhances issue salience. As a result, a participant's measurement on the posttest may be attributed to familiarity from the pretest and not the intervention. In another scenario, the pretest may influence the participant's perceptions about a message or issue. Thus, change in the posttest could be a reflection of this and not the intervention.

Whereas testing sensitization refers to changes in the participants over time, *instrumentation* refers to changes in the measures employed to observe the outcomes of interest following exposure to the experimental treatment (Kazdin, 2003). While having the potential to appear in any type of health research, instrumentation issues are more common in clinical settings; for example, when medical personnel witness progress in a patient's health. With an improving patient, clinicians often adjust their scoring criteria to gauge the effectiveness of the treatment intervention. In other words, sometimes changes in the dependent variable are a result of the scoring criteria rather than the behavior observed.

The "timing of posttest measures" often plays an important role in health research. In all of the design types discussed in this chapter, a stimulus/intervention is introduced at some point in the study, and the impact of its presence (or absence) is measured at a later point in time. Often, the effect of a stimulus/intervention in health research is not instantaneous; it takes time for a drug, behavior modification, or attitude shift, among others, to take affect and thus produce measureable change. The question for health researchers then becomes "How long do I wait?" before administering the posttest. If it is conducted too early, a posttest runs the risk of measuring participants before the stimulus/intervention can produce change. If one waits too long, the chance of measureable data important to the study being lost is increased. Given the nature of stimulus/interventions commonly used in health research, one must give careful consideration to their nature and plan the implementation of the posttest accordingly.

"Attrition" occurs when participants drop out of a study for any number of reasons, causing the current or final sample size to be different from the initial one. Within health contexts, several factors, such as worsening of health condition, requirements of participating conflicting with care, and even death, can cause an individual's participation in a study to stop. Furthermore, the nature of the patient's condition (such as studies involving stress, depression, anxiety, etc.) may cause them to be less likely to maintain participation. Either way, researchers run the risk of having a final sample that is too small (issues of statistical power) or unrepresentative (only healthy individuals remain).

Finally, "social desirability bias" also presents a legitimate threat to validity. Within the context of health research, many of the issues examined can involve illegal (e.g., illicit substance use), altruistic (e.g., organ donation), or identity-threatening (e.g., sexual behavior, alcohol consumption) activities. The mere fact that participants are aware that they are being observed as they participate in an experiment produces a potential risk. Often, participants may seek to please the researcher with a socially desirable response, or avoid responding in ways that would present themselves in an unfavorable light. This potential often reduces the validity and generalizability of a study's findings.

In conclusion, messages are used to get much of our daily tasks accomplished, and this is especially indicative of the health context. Here, like other contexts, messages are employed to achieve a variety of effects or goals—expressions of pain, delivering bad news, comforting, instructions, medical adherence, illness explanations, and the like. Ultimately, health communication researchers are concerned with effects of the messages. Being aware of and attuned to the aforementioned experimental design options and issues related to the multitude of messages created and exchanged in the health context, health communication researchers can conduct studies that enhance and propel our understanding of the effects of health messages—with unwavering confidence in the generalizability of the findings.

References

Alvaro, E. M., Siegel, J. T., Crano, W. D., & Dominick, A. (2010). A mass mediated intervention on Hispanic organ donation. *Journal of Health Communication, 15*(4), 374–387.

Aschen, S. R. (1997). Assertion training therapy in psychiatric milieus. *Archives of Psychiatric Nursing, 11*(1), 46–51.

Bowling, A. (2009). *Research methods in health: Investigating health and health services* (3rd ed.). Maidenhead, Berkshire, England: McGraw-Hill/Open University Press.

Brashers, D. E., & Jackson, S. (1999). Changing conceptions of "message effects": A 24-year overview. *Human Communication Research, 25*(4), 457–477.

Campbell, D. T., & Stanley, J. C. (1967). *Experimental and quasi-experimental designs for research.* Chicago, IL: Rand McNally.

Centers for Disease Control and Prevention. (2011). Prevalence of coronary heart disease—United States, 2006–2010. *Morbidity and Mortality Weekly Report, 60*(40), 1377–1381.

Cook, T. D., & Campbell, D. T. (1979). *Quasi-experimentation: Design and analysis for field settings.* Chicago, IL: Rand McNally.

Jackson, S. (1992). *Message effects research: Principles of design and analysis.* New York, NY: Guilford Press.

Jackson, S., & Jacobs, S. (1983). Generalizing about messages: Suggestions for design and analysis of experiments. *Human Communication Research, 9*(2), 169–181.

Jackson, S., O'Keefe, D. J., & Jacobs, S. (1988). The search for reliable generalizations about messages: A comparison of research strategies. *Human Communication Research, 15*(1), 127–141.

Jackson, S., O'Keefe, D. J., & Brashers, D. E. (1994). The messages replication factor: Methods tailored to messages as objects of study. *Journalism Quarterly, 71*(4), 984–996.

Jackson, S., O'Keefe, D. J., Jacobs, S., & Brashers, D. E. (1989). Messages as replications: Toward a message-centered design strategy. *Communication Monographs, 56*(4), 364–384.

Kazdin, A. E. (2003). *Research design in clinical psychology* (4th ed.). Needham Heights, MA: Allyn & Bacon.

Kerlinger, F. N., & Lee, H. B., (2000). *Foundations of behavioral research* (4th ed.). Fort Worth, TX: Harcourt College Publishers.

Krieger, J. L., Parrott, R. L., & Nussbaum, J. F. (2011). Metaphor use and health literacy: A pilot study of strategies to explain randomization in cancer clinical trials. *Journal of Health Communication, 16*(1), 3–16.

O'Keefe, D. J. (2003). Message properties, mediating states, and manipulation checks: Claims, evidence, and data analysis in experimental persuasive message effects research. *Communication Theory, 13*(3), 251–274.

Roberto, A. J., Meyer, G., Johnson, A. J., & Atkin, C. K. (2000). Using the parallel process model to prevent firearm injury and death: field experiment results of a video-based intervention. *Journal of Communication, 50*(4), 157–175.

Smith, G. C., Egbert, N., Dellman-Jenkins, M., Nanna, K., & Palmieri, P. A. (2012). Reducing depression in stroke survivors and their informal caregivers: A randomized clinical trial of a web-based intervention. *Rehabilitation Psychology*, *57*(3), 196–206.

Whaley, B. B., & Wagner, L. S. (2000). Rebuttal analogy in persuasive messages: Communicator likability and cognitive responses. *Journal of Language and Social Psychology*, *19*(1), 66–84.

Whaley, B. B., Wagner, L. S., Cook, K. E., & Jeha, N. (2002). Individual differences and rebuttal analogy in persuasive messages: Effect of need for cognition. *Communication & Cognition*, *35*(3/4), 193–209.

Whaley, B. B., Stone, A. M., Brady, S. A., & Whaley, R. C. (2014). Explaining diabetes: Studying the effects of using analogies to talk about illness. *Journal of Diabetes Nursing*, *18*(2), 72–76.

BUILDING CUMULATIVE KNOWLEDGE IN HEALTH COMMUNICATION

The Application of Meta-Analytic Methods

Seth M. Noar and Leslie B. Snyder

Traditionally, cumulative knowledge in the social sciences has been built through research synthesis articles known as *narrative* or *integrative research* reviews of the literature (Cooper & Hedges, 2009; Johnson & Eagly, 2000). In fact, the "review article" is something of a staple in the social and behavioral sciences, so much so that specialized publications are often devoted to such endeavors (e.g., *Communication Yearbook*, *Annual Review of Public Health*). Review articles often aim to integrate existing studies in a line of inquiry in order to (a) create generalizations from the literature; (b) focus on applicable theories and critically analyze studies; (c) attempt to resolve conflicts in the literature; and, finally, (d) identify gaps in the literature and point to directions for future research (Cooper, 1988; Cooper & Hedges, 2009).

Although this review method has been used for decades, and will likely continue to be used, critics of the strategy point to a number of deficiencies with the method. For instance, Rosenthal (1991) suggested that narrative review articles often yield little new information, and do not solve and perhaps contribute to the problem of *poor cumulation of research findings* and thus slow research progress within the social sciences (also see Schmidt, 1992). A number of scholars have also criticized the informal nature of narrative reviews, and the lack of systematic and thorough literature searching that often goes into such reviews (Cooper & Rosenthal, 1980; Johnson & Eagly, 2000). Indeed, many narrative reviewers begin their review projects with differing goals and methods in mind—with some not gathering all of the relevant literature on a given topic (Cooper & Hedges, 2009).

Moreover, when there are contradictory research findings in a given area, narrative reviewers often have difficulty making sense of the literature, which can lead different reviewers to come to conflicting conclusions regarding the same set of studies (Cook & Leviton, 1980; Schmidt, 1992). For example, while observers have come to both positive (Rogers, 1996) and negative (Wallack & Dorfman, 2001) conclusions about the effects of health communication campaigns, meta-analyses (Derzon & Lipsey, 2002; Snyder et al., 2004) have brought a measure of objectivity and precision to this discussion. In addition, empirical studies directly comparing the narrative reviewing strategy to meta-analysis have suggested that meta-analysis is a superior research synthesis technique (Bearman, 1991; Bushman & Wells, 2001; Cooper & Rosenthal, 1980).

In addition to the above criticisms, perhaps the most central criticism of the narrative review method is its over-reliance on statistical significance as the primary criterion for judging the results of empirical studies (Cohen, 1994; Hunter & Schmidt, 2004; Rosenthal, 1991). Many narrative reviews use "vote counting" procedures, in which they compare the number of statistically significant ($p < .05$) to non-significant studies in a given area and make conclusions based on this comparison. There are many problems with such an approach, including: (a) studies that were statistically underpowered, for instance because of small sample sizes, may be counted as having *no effects* when effects may have existed; (b) studies with very large sample sizes may be counted as having *meaningful effects* when such effects are minimal or perhaps even nonexistent; and (c) this dichotomous decision making ignores the magnitude of effect within given studies (i.e., effect size). Central criticisms of narrative reviewing directly lead to central criticisms of null hypothesis significance testing (NHST) as it is currently practiced in the literature (Cohen, 1994; Meehl, 1978; Schmidt, 1992). Though many have called for increased reporting of effect sizes, in part to allay concerns about NHST procedures (APA Publications and Communications Board Working Group on Journal Article Reporting Standards, 2008), such reporting is still varied and inconsistent.

Meta-Analysis: An Alternative Method for Integrating Research Findings

Meta-analysis is a systematic approach to research synthesis that is focused on the quantitative integration of research findings. It is a technique that applies only to quantitative empirical studies, and typically focuses on the *magnitude* of study effects (effect size) rather than on the statistical significance of those effects. Effect size is viewed as superior to statistical significance for a number of reasons, including that such estimates are more precise as well as the fact that, unlike statistical significance tests, such estimates are independent of sample size (see Table 12.1 for a comparison of traditional narrative reviews and meta-analysis).

Meta-analytic techniques were initially developed in the 1970s, largely out of frustration with the status quo narrative review method (Rosenthal, 1991). Many point to Smith and Glass's (1977) work on outcomes of psychotherapy as the

TABLE 12.1 Comparison of Traditional Narrative Reviews and Meta-Analysis

	Narrative Review	*Meta-Analysis*
Applicable to ...	Virtually any type of research	Studies must be quantitative, and effect sizes must be able to be retrieved and/or calculated from study reports
Ease of conducting synthesis	Any researcher with knowledge of the area and access to the studies should be able to conduct such a review	Requires knowledge of the literature, access to the studies, and specialized skills in meta-analysis
Literature review	Varies in different reviews—many narrative reviews are not explicit about literature boundaries or comprehensive in the search	Comprehensive review must be conducted, based upon explicit inclusion criteria indicating boundaries of the literature
Key criterion for evaluating study effects	Varies. The researcher may use significance tests, typically $p < .05$, or may apply other criteria.	Effect size
Integration of research findings	Varies. May be the researcher's judgment and logic. Sometimes a "vote count" of significant versus non-significant studies.	Quantitative integration—weighted average of effect sizes; relies more on interpretation of effect size
Ability to handle large numbers of studies	When number of studies becomes large (e.g., > 50), review may become unwieldy	Able to handle large numbers of studies with relative ease
Replicability	Typically not possible. Different researchers conduct unique searches, use their own criteria to integrate the studies, and may reach different conclusions.	Possible when all procedures are specified in the methods section.
Ability to explain contradictory findings in the literature	Difficult to sort out given the many factors that vary across studies	Easier to discover, as moderator tests can empirically examine factors associated with larger or smaller effect sizes
Conclusions of the synthesis based on ...	Researcher's judgment about the overall literature, and sometimes a "vote count" of significant studies. Lack of clear guidelines for the narrative review method may open the door to biased conclusions.	Quantitative results are examined, and researcher interprets results of the meta-analysis as if interpreting the results from a primary study.

"first" meta-analysis, although other researchers were concurrently and independently developing what later become known as meta-analytic procedures (Rosenthal & Rubin, 1978; Schmidt & Hunter, 1977). In addition, meta-analytic methods can be viewed in terms of three sets of approaches, including those of Hedges and Olkin (1985), Hunter and Schmidt (2004), and Rosenthal (1991). All three approaches are conceptually quite similar and have essentially identical aims. The differences emerge in the methodological details of how effect sizes are calculated, corrected (or not) for potential sources of bias, and analyzed. In addition, all of the approaches are commonly used in the literature, and, although there are proponents of each approach, at the moment, there does not appear to be evidence of the clear superiority of any one approach over the others (Johnson, Mullen, & Salas, 1995). Also, in practice, some researchers use a mixture of the approaches; for example, using Hedges and Olkin's (1985) methods for weighting and Hunter and Schmidt's (2004) methods for correcting for bias in effect sizes (these are discussed more below).

There are numerous examples of meta-analyses in health communication (Noar, 2006), and the application of meta-analysis to health communication appears to be growing over time (Snyder & LaCroix, 2013). In the message design area alone, there have been several recent meta-analyses on message framing (Gallagher & Updegraff, 2012; O'Keefe & Jensen, 2007) and tailored messaging (Lustria, Noar, Cortese, Van Stee, & Glueckauf, 2013; Noar, Benac, & Harris, 2007). The field is accumulating more meta-analyses of campaign (Derzon & Lipsey, 2002; Snyder et al., 2004) and intervention (Snyder & LaCroix, 2013) effectiveness, too. It is also possible to use meta-analyses to address questions about methods, as in which evaluation methods have led to greater effect sizes in the literature (Snyder, Hamilton, & Huedo-Medina, 2009). All of these studies have helped to provide a "report card" to the field on where a particular literature is and what future directions may be fruitful to pursue. As one example of their impact on the field, a Google Scholar search (conducted on April 15, 2014), indicated that O'Keefe and Jensen's (2007) framing meta-analysis had been cited 170 times, Snyder et al.'s (2004) campaigns meta-analysis had been cited 210 times, and Noar et al.'s (2007) tailoring meta-analysis had been cited 389 times.

Rationale for Method

Meta-analysis corrects for the deficiencies in the narrative review method in many ways. First, meta-analysis corrects for the lack of a thorough literature search by mandating a comprehensive and systematic review of the literature. While narrative reviews often do not include comprehensive literature searches and may also have "fuzzy" criteria in terms of the boundaries of the literature that were searched, meta-analysis is quite explicit about the search methods and the inclusion and exclusion criteria that were applied to each study. In fact, the level of detail in specifying which literature to include is similar to a content analysis, and reporting guidelines instruct meta-analysts to report all inclusion criteria as well as the "flow" of how many studies were excluded, and for what reasons (APA Publications and Communications Board Working Group on Journal Article Reporting Standards, 2008; Moher, Liberati, Tetzlaff, Altman, & the PRISMA Group, 2009).

Next, meta-analysis corrects for the problem of potential bias in narrative reviews by implementing strict coding procedures. Again, similar to content analysis, meta-analysts develop a coding form and pretest it for accuracy and comprehensiveness. Multiple coders code study characteristics, and inter-coder reliability is tracked, computed, and reported. This provides a "checks and balances" element to the review, giving readers more confidence that the literature is accurately described in the review. It also provides transparency as to what was coded and how it was coded that is not found in most narrative reviews.

Third, by their very nature, meta-analysis corrects for the problem of poor synthesis of research findings in narrative reviews, as meta-analysts convert study findings into a common effect size metric and analyze those data using sophisticated statistical methods. Weighted mean effect sizes are calculated, heterogeneity is examined, and moderator analyses (which attempt to explain the variability across studies) are conducted. While the statistical significance of effect sizes is examined, the focus is on the magnitude of those effect sizes as well as how they vary across studies, more so than whether or not such effect sizes are statistically significant. The focus on effect sizes and variability aids in testing the hypotheses under study in an unbiased manner and in planning future research (e.g., use in power analyses and setting evaluation goals; see Snyder et al., 2004).

Finally, there is an overall transparency to a meta-analysis that is exceedingly valuable to science. Just as in other quantitative studies, replication is possible because the procedures are clearly stated. Readers are informed about the search procedure, inclusion criteria, operationalization of key terms, and statistical approach. In addition, many studies present the "raw data" used in the analysis—the coded effect sizes for each study. When narrative reviews arrive at differing conclusions, it is often hard to reconcile their differences. In contrast, it is much easier to compare meta-analyses on similar topics. For example, the level of detail reported in multiple meta-analyses of computer and web interventions on alcohol made it possible to use the results from the relevant studies and arrive at an average effect size across all of the studies (Snyder & LaCroix, 2013).

Applications of Meta-Analysis

The purpose of conducting any meta-analysis is to answer two key questions. First, what is the magnitude of effect of a particular phenomenon? In its most basic form, this is an average of the effects of all of the studies. However, in meta-analysis, effect sizes are typically weighted before they are combined into a mean effect size, such that larger studies (which are presumed to have more accurate effect estimates) are given more weight in the mean effect size than smaller studies (which are presumed to have less accurate effect estimates; Borenstein, Hedges, Higgins, & Rothstein, 2009; Lipsey & Wilson, 2001). Next, what are the moderators of the effect? This second question is concerned with understanding which study features are associated with stronger study outcomes (i.e., larger effect sizes). These analyses are often conducted on simple descriptive characteristics, conceptual characteristics emanating from relevant theoretical perspectives, and/or methodological characteristics that may influence study outcomes (Hall & Rosenthal, 1991). While many meta-analyses conduct analyses examining one moderator at a time, meta-regression (in which many potential moderators are examined together in a multivariate analysis) is becoming an increasingly popular technique (Borenstein et al., 2009).

In communication and the social sciences in general, meta-analyses typically fall into two categories. The first is meta-analyses examining an association between variables, and these are often meta-analyses of correlations. For example, what is the association between sensation seeking and risky sexual behavior (Hoyle, Fejfar, & Miller, 2000), or what is the association between cancer patient characteristics (e.g., gender, age, education level, and stage of diagnosis) and their information needs (Ankem, 2006)? Such meta-analyses involve synthesizing correlations across many studies, which first involves recording correlations reported in the studies themselves as well as converting other statistics reported in the studies into correlations, where necessary. The second category is meta-analyses examining the impact of interventions, and these are typically syntheses of mean differences. For example, what is the impact of computer-delivered interventions on health-related behaviors (Portnoy, Scott-Sheldon, Johnson, & Carey, 2008), or what is the impact of fear appeal messages on attitude and behavior change (Witte & Allen, 2000)? Such meta-analyses involve computing standardized mean effect sizes from intervention studies, which conceptually is the intervention group mean minus the control group mean divided by a pooled standard deviation. Thus, most meta-analyses in health communication are likely to be either syntheses of correlations or syntheses of mean differences.

Meta-Analytic Exemplars

We recently undertook a large meta-analytic project that was the first to synthesize the growing literature on computer technology-based interventions in HIV prevention, and will use this project as a detailed example here. The goal of the project was to understand whether technology-based HIV prevention health communication interventions are capable of impacting (a) theoretical mediators of safer sex and (b) key safer sex behaviors, such as condom use. Given the fact that these two outcomes were largely mutually exclusive (most studies fell into either category (a) or category (b)), a decision was made to carry out and publish these projects as two separate meta-analyses. Each is now described in turn.

The first meta-analysis was undertaken to examine the potential efficacy of computer technology-based interventions in changing theoretical mediators of safer sex, such as knowledge, attitudes, self-efficacy, and so forth (Noar, Pierce, & Black, 2010). Both the published and unpublished literatures were searched for studies that evaluated the ability of a computer technology-based intervention (relative to a comparison condition) to change theoretical mediators of safer sex. A total of k = 20 studies met criteria and were included in the meta-analysis.

Populations studied in this literature included men who have sex with men (15%), heterosexually active adolescents (55%), and young adults/adults (30%). The most common intervention type was a group targeted intervention (65%). This was followed by individually tailored interventions (15%), virtual decision-making interventions (10%), and multiple type interventions (10%). Most interventions were delivered via the Internet (55%) or on-screen using a computer located on site (40%). One intervention (Scholes et al., 2003) was delivered via a computer-generated magazine (5%). Just over half of the interventions (55%) were theory based, and just under half of the studies were conducted outside the United States (45%).

Analyses were conducted on all theoretically-oriented outcome variables measured in the studies, one at a time. The results indicated that computer-based interventions significantly improved the three outcome variables most often reported in studies, including HIV/AIDS knowledge ($d = .276, p < .001$), sexual/condom attitudes ($d = .161, p < .001$), and condom self-efficacy ($d = .186, p < .001$). Interventions also significantly improved perceived susceptibility ($d = .131, p < .01$), condom communication ($d = .119, p < .01$), and condom intentions ($d = .110, p < .05$). No significant effects were found on refusal self-efficacy ($d = .056, p = .31$).

Many of the mean effect sizes listed above were found to be heterogeneous, suggesting the presence of moderator variables that impacted study outcomes. Analysis of moderator variables revealed some significant differences. For example, interventions were significantly ($p <.05$) more likely to have improved sexual or condom attitudes if they (a) targeted men who have sex with men (versus heterosexuals), (b) were delivered online, or (c) utilized individualized tailoring.

A second meta-analysis was undertaken to examine the ability of computer technology-based interventions to impact safer sexual behavior (Noar, Black, & Pierce, 2009). Again, both the published and unpublished literatures were searched for studies that evaluated the ability of a computer technology-based intervention (relative to a comparison condition) to change safer sexual behaviors. A total of k = 12 studies met criteria and were included in the meta-analysis.

Populations studied included men who have sex with men (17%) as well as heterosexually active adolescents (33%) and young adults/adults (50%). The most common intervention type was an individually tailored intervention (50%), followed by group targeted (25%), virtual decision making (17%), and mixed type interventions (8%). Most interventions were delivered on-screen using a computer located on site (67%), while the remainder was delivered over the Internet (25%) or via a computer-generated magazine (8%). Most of the interventions (83%) were theory based, with a stages of change model being the most popular theoretical perspective applied (50% of the theory-based interventions). Virtually all of the studies (92%) were conducted in the United States, with the exception of one study conducted in the Netherlands.

Results of the meta-analysis indicated that computer-based interventions had a statistically significant effect on condom use, $d = .259$, $p < .001$. While fewer studies measured other behavioral outcomes, the existing data suggested that interventions reduced numbers of sexual partners ($d = .422$, $p < .01$), frequency of sexual activity ($d = .427$, $p < .001$), and incident STDs ($d = .140$, $p < .01$). Given that the effect size for condom use was heterogeneous, moderator analyses were conducted to examine this variability in relation to key study characteristics. Interventions were found to be significantly more efficacious when they (a) were targeted to a single gender ($p < .01$), (b) applied individualized tailoring ($p < .001$), (c) used a stages of change model ($p < .001$), and (d) had a "high" intervention dose (3+ contacts; $p < .05$).

The above meta-analyses were the first to demonstrate that computer technology-based interventions are efficacious in changing theoretical mediators of safer sex and safer sexual behaviors. They also point to features—in particular, the use of message targeting and tailoring—that may enhance the efficacy of such interventions. In both projects, publication bias analyses were conducted, and, in both cases, suggested that it is unlikely that the observed effect sizes were inflated by publication bias. Moreover, both projects compared observed effect sizes to effect sizes from meta-analyses of human-delivered behavioral interventions, and, in both cases, effect sizes were (remarkably) found to be similar (Noar, et al., 2009; Noar, et al., 2010).

Employing Meta-Analysis

Conducting a meta-analysis is a step-by-step process. Several authors have offered lists of such steps (Cooper & Hedges, 2009). The basic steps of the process are: (a) defining the research question, (b) setting boundaries for the literature and developing inclusion criteria, (c) locating all relevant literature, (d) developing a coding sheet and coding studies, (e) calculating the magnitude of effect (effect size) for each study, (f) analyzing the meta-analytic database, and (g) presenting results and drawing conclusions (Table 12.2). *The Handbook of Research Synthesis*

TABLE 12.2 Steps in Conducting a Meta-Analysis

Step 1: Define the research question
Step 2: Set boundaries for the literature (i.e., inclusion criteria)
Step 3: Locate all relevant literature
Step 4: Develop a coding form and code study characteristics
Step 5: Calculate the magnitude of effect in each study
Step 6: Analyze the meta-analytic database
Step 7: Present results and draw conclusions

(Cooper & Hedges, 1994), recently updated as *The Handbook of Research Synthesis and Meta-Analysis* (Cooper, Hedges, & Valentine, 2009), is generally considered the most complete treatment of meta-analysis, and readers interested in learning in depth about particular aspects of meta-analysis are referred to this comprehensive source. A resource specific to communication research is available from Johnson, Scott-Sheldon, Snyder, Noar, and Huedo-Medina (2008). In the next section, we describe each of these steps in more detail.

Meta-Analytic Procedures

The first step in a meta-analysis is to define the research question to be examined. For example, in our meta-analysis discussed above (Noar, et al., 2009), we asked the question of whether computer technology-based HIV prevention interventions were efficacious in changing behavior. As in primary research, reviewers give a justification for a given meta-analysis. In the above case, there had been several studies in this area, but no meta-analysis conducted to date. Also, while several human-delivered interventions had previously shown efficacy in meta-analysis (Albarracin et al., 2005; Noar, 2008), dissemination challenges with some of those interventions were moving the HIV prevention field toward using more technology for delivery of interventions.

The next step (Step 2) involves setting boundaries for the literature to be reviewed, as well as developing explicit inclusion criteria for the review. It is critical that the studies chosen have *conceptual comparability*, meaning that the primary studies are similar enough that synthesizing them will result in a meaningful outcome (Lipsey & Wilson, 2001). This helps one to avoid the "apples and oranges" criticism—or the idea that one is averaging qualitatively different types of studies together, resulting in an effect size that has no real meaning (Sharpe, 1997).

A variety of factors are typically considered and ultimately used in inclusion criteria, including type of publication (and years published), study population, type of research design used, treatment/intervention applied, and outcome measure(s). For example, the Noar et al. (2009) meta-analysis included all published and unpublished studies available through March of 2008, if they met the following criteria: (a) tested the efficacy of an HIV prevention behavioral intervention focused on changing sexual risk behavior among individuals of HIV-negative or unknown serostatus; (b) measured condom use or unprotected sex as a dependent variable; (c) used computer technology to deliver the intervention, including computers, the Internet, and mobile devices; and (d) utilized an experimental design in which individuals were randomized to conditions. These inclusion criteria make it very clear how the boundaries of this particular literature were defined in this review, and, specifically, which studies were to be included and excluded.

The next step (Step 3) in the process is to locate all relevant literature for the meta-analysis. This can (and should) be undertaken using a variety of literature search methods. Widely used search methods include database searches (e.g., Communication and Mass Media Complete, Medline, PsycINFO), citation searches (i.e., examining reference lists in review articles or key primary studies and/or examining all articles that have cited a particular seminal article in the field), and journal searches (i.e., searching contents of relevant journals). Other methods (particularly to find unpublished works) include personal communications via email and relevant listservs and searching conference proceedings. Since each search method may lead the reviewer to different studies, it is critical that meta-analyses apply multiple search strategies (Lipsey & Wilson, 2001).

In our 2009 meta-analysis, we conducted searches of the Medline and PsycINFO electronic databases, using numerous relevant keyword combinations. We also conducted forward citation searches on all articles located in our database searches, using Social Science Citation Index. Further, we examined reference lists of review articles in the area. In addition, we searched the reference lists of the final set of articles to look for any possible additional studies. Finally, in order to potentially include unpublished work, we sent out an email message that went to a large number of researchers working in this area, soliciting unpublished studies for inclusion in the meta-analysis.

Step 4 involves developing a coding sheet and coding studies' key characteristics, which may include descriptive, conceptual, and/or methodological characteristics. In meta-analysis, coding is conducted for two reasons. First, it allows one to describe the set of studies, both individually and as a collective whole. And, second, it allows one to conduct analyses testing whether a given variable moderates the effect of a treatment or intervention. For example, in our meta-analysis, we coded population type (heterosexual or men who have sex with men) to both describe the set of studies on this characteristic as well as to analyze whether interventions targeted to differing populations had differing effects.

Coding in meta-analysis is a challenging process. This is the case because (a) authors of studies often report demographic and other characteristics in different forms; (b) reliability is critical, and this can only be achieved with a clear and well thought-out coding sheet and trained coders; and (c) since we cannot know everything that will be encountered at the start of the coding process, it is sometimes an iterative process where a coding form is revised at different points in the process. The literature makes several important suggestions for successful coding in meta-analysis (Lipsey & Wilson, 2001; Wilson, 2009). Those who are familiar with content analytic procedures can apply many of those recommendations as well (Krippendorff, 2004).

Step 5 focuses on estimating the magnitude of effect for each study, and this step begins by deciding on a common effect size (such as *r* or *d*) that is appropriate for a particular group of studies, and then converting all study outcomes into that metric. Many treatments of meta-analysis detail how to make such effect size conversions (Cooper et al., 2009; Lipsey & Wilson, 2001; Rosenthal, 1991). These writings point out that the three most common effect size indicators used in meta-analysis are (a) the correlation coefficient (Pearson's *r*), used to characterize associations between continuous variables; (b) the standardized mean difference (*d*), which is applied in cases with a categorical independent variable and a continuous dependent variable; and (c) the odds ratio (*OR*), which is applied in cases with a dichotomous independent and dependent variable. The goal of the meta-analyst is to choose the effect size that is most appropriate to the type of data reported in the majority of studies being reviewed (Johnson et al., 2008). The analyst can also take into account which statistics are most understood by likely readers of the article. As indicated above, in the social sciences, most meta-analyses employ *r* or *d*, which can be easily converted between the two statistics. However, since health communication inquiry often crosses disciplines, particularly into medicine and public health, meta-analyses using odds ratios are likely to be evident in the health communication literature (see Table 12.3) (though note that conversions between odds ratios and *r* or *d* are more controversial).

As an example, we (Noar et al., 2009) converted all study findings into the standardized mean difference statistic, or *d*. We chose this statistic because many (if not most) studies reported outcomes in terms of means. Also, in our meta-analysis, several outcomes were of interest, and data on each available outcome (condom use, frequency of sexual behavior, number of sex partners, and incident STDs) from each study was extracted and converted to a *d* statistic. This resulted in four meta-analytic databases, one for each outcome.

In Step 6, the meta-analytic database(s) containing the coding and effect sizes for each study is analyzed. Effect sizes are weighted such that larger studies, which contain more precise effect size estimates, are weighted more heavily in the aggregation of the mean effect size than are smaller studies. Some approaches to meta-analysis also advocate making additional statistical corrections (for methodological factors) to each individual effect size before aggregation (Hunter & Schmidt, 2004). The weighted mean effect size is calculated along with its 95% confidence interval, and the statistical significance of the effect size is examined (Lipsey & Wilson, 2001). Whether the mean effect size is homogeneous or heterogeneous is also examined statistically. For example, do study effect sizes vary

TABLE 12.3 Some Common Statistics Used in Meta-Analysis

Statistic	*Symbol*	*Description*	*Notes*
Effect Size			
Correlation coefficient	r	Measure of association between two continuous variables. Varies from −1 to 1.	Mainstream meta-analytic approach implements a Fisher's r-to-z transform before conducting analyses due to non-normal distribution of r. Results are then transformed back to r for presentation and interpretation (Lipsey & Wilson, 2001, pp. 63–64)
Standardized mean difference	d	Mean difference statistic. Typically falls in the −1 to 1 range.	Hedges' small sample size correction is typically applied to this statistic (Lipsey & Wilson, 2001, pp. 48–49)
Odds ratio	OR	Measure of association between two dichotomous variables. Falls between 0–1 or above 1 (a 1 indicates no association)	Analyses are conducted on the natural log of the odds ratio, due to the unusual distribution of the odds ratio statistic (Lipsey & Wilson, 2001, p. 53)
Heterogeneity			
Q statistic	Q	Test of the homogeneity (versus heterogeneity) of a distribution of effect sizes. Distributed as a chi-square with k-1 degrees of freedom, where k is the number of effect sizes	A statistically significant Q statistic results in the rejection of the null hypothesis of homogeneity (Lipsey & Wilson, 2001, p. 116)
I-squared statistic	I^2	A homogeneity index that is a ratio of excess to total variability. Ranges from 0 to 100%.	Rather than a dichotomous significance test, I^2 provides a variability ratio: 25% low, 50% moderate, 75%+ high heterogeneity (Borenstein et al., 2009; Higgins & Thompson, 2002)

(*Continued*)

TABLE 12.3 (*Continued*)

Statistic	*Symbol*	*Description*	*Notes*
Moderator Analysis			
Q^B statistic	Q^B	Index of the variability between group means. If mean effect sizes vary across categories by more than sampling error alone, this statistic will be statistically significant	This statistic is analogous to analysis of variance (ANOVA) in primary research (Lipsey & Wilson, 2001, pp. 135–137)

Note: For additional details on these statistics, see text as well as the sources referred to in this table.

more than would be expected based upon sampling error alone (i.e., does significant heterogeneity exist?)? Heterogeneity is commonly examined by testing the statistical significance of the Q statistic as well as examining the size of the *I*-squared statistic. If the distribution of effect sizes is homogenous, then it is likely that studies only vary with regard to sampling error and there are no meaningful between study differences. However, in cases where significant heterogeneity among study effect sizes is found, moderator analyses are then conducted in attempts to explain the variability in effect sizes according to moderator variables specified a priori. In those cases, more emphasis should be put on the findings of such analyses and less emphasis on the weighted mean effect size itself.

In many cases, moderator analyses examine and compare effect sizes that are stratified by particular variables. For example, in our 2009 meta-analysis, we grouped studies into group targeted (d = .113), virtual decision making (d = .240), and individually tailored (d = .361) interventions. A comparison of the effect sizes for these different intervention types found that they were statistically different, (Q_B = 15.73, df = 2, p <.001), suggesting that type of intervention may act as a moderator of intervention efficacy. While we did not calculate a meta-regression where several potential moderators are examined in a multivariate model, this is another technique that can be used to examine the possible influence of moderator variables. Meta-regression is similar to multiple regression except that several statistics—including standard errors of the regression coefficients, *t*-test values, and the significance of the *t*-tests—are adjusted to yield appropriate values for meta-analysis (Lipsey & Wilson, 2001). Thus, several independent (moderator) variables are entered into the equation to predict the dependent variable (effect size), and the meta-analyst can examine what variables remain significant in the presence of other moderator variables.

A brief diversion is necessary at this point. The procedures just described above represent a "fixed effects" statistical approach to meta-analysis. A fixed effects approach makes the assumption that there is a *single* population-level effect size, and thus studies may vary from effect size only because of sampling error as well as other "fixed" moderator variables. If a meta-analyst takes this view, then a fixed effects analysis approach may be fine. However, it may be the case that a meta-analyst does not believe that these assumptions are true for a given set of studies. For example, he or she may believe that there are other, *random* sources of variability across studies due to variations in study procedures or settings. In that case, studies may be viewed as being drawn from a larger population of studies that do *not* share a single population-level effect size. If one takes this latter view, and one's set of studies are heterogeneous, then a random effects analysis model is most appropriate (Lipsey & Wilson, 2001). Such a model would include not only the *subject-level* sampling error component but also a *study-level* sampling error component, and, functionally, this would involve using a different inverse variance weights in one's analyses. Thus, weighted mean effect sizes and confidence intervals are likely to be different when employing a fixed versus random effects approach.

Further, there is one final option here: a *mixed effects* model. As the name implies, this approach mixes the assumptions of the fixed effects with random effects models. In this case, the assumption is made that there are three sources of variability: subject-level sampling, study-level sampling error, and systematic "fixed" factors. This model would allow one to pursue moderator analyses, operating under the assumption that, although there are other random sources of variability, fixed factors still represent a systematic variability component that can be meaningfully analyzed (for more details on these models, see Borenstein et al., 2009; Lipsey & Wilson, 2001).

Meta-analysts also recommend publication bias analyses to guard against what Rosenthal coined the "file drawer problem" (Rosenthal, 1992). The problem here is that researchers are more likely to submit for publication (and journal editors are more likely to accept for publication) studies with statistically significant findings. Thus, a meta-analysis may overestimate the true effect size based only on meta-analyzing studies with significant results. What is a meta-analyst to do? First, one can solicit and include unpublished studies in one's meta-analysis, which may help guard against the problem. Second, one can calculate a *Fail Safe N*, which answers the question of how many null studies would need to exist to reduce the observed weighted mean effect size to one of trivial magnitude (Lipsey & Wilson, 2001; Rosenthal, 1992). In our 2009 meta-analysis, such an analysis revealed that 51 non-significant studies would need to exist in order to reduce the observed effect size to one of trivial magnitude, which seems quite unlikely given the relatively small number of researchers working in that particular area.

It is important to note that, while meta-analysts tend to agree on much of the general analysis approach just described above, several details of how analyses are undertaken may differ when applying different statistical approaches to meta-analysis (Cooper et al., 2009; Johnson et al., 1995). For example, rather than examining the significance of the Q statistic and examination of I^2 for heterogeneity, Hunter and Schmidt (2004) instead recommend use of a "75%" variance rule. Those who wish to use a particular set of meta-analytic methods should thus refer to sources specific to that method.

Finally, with regard to actually undertaking analyses, software that has been designed specifically for meta-analysis is often used, including Comprehensive Meta-Analysis, DSTAT, and RevMan. Some treatments of meta-analysis also discuss how to use more standard software packages, such as Statistical Analysis Software (SAS) and the Statistical Package for the Social Sciences (SPSS), for meta-analysis (Lipsey & Wilson, 2001). David Wilson (2010) has a website with downloads to help with analysis, including meta-analysis macros for SAS, SPSS, and Stata.

In Step 7, meta-analysts present their results and draw conclusions. Given that meta-analysis converts each study's findings into a common metric, allowing for head-to-head comparisons of studies, it is common to present effect sizes not only in tabular form but also in visual form. A variety of figure types are available for this purpose, including forest plots, box and whisker plots, and stem and leaf plots (Cooper et al., 2009; Lipsey & Wilson, 2001; Rosenthal, 1991). Such figures give the reader a useful visual means with which to interpret the pattern of findings across studies. In our meta-analysis, we presented a forest plot displaying the effect sizes for condom use. As depicted in Figure 12.1, this plot displays the effect size

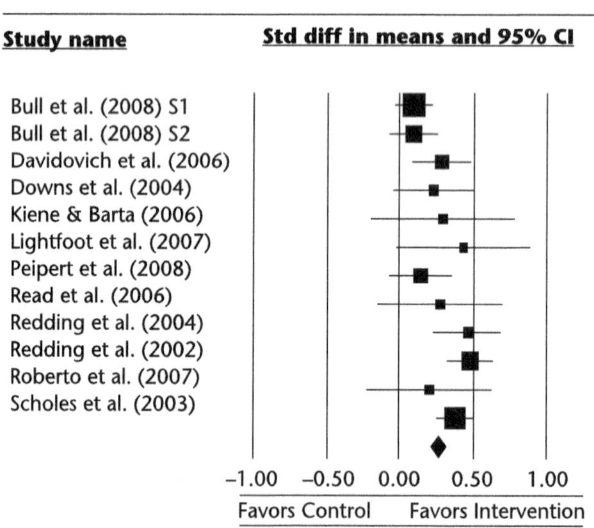

FIGURE 12.1 Forest Plot Displaying Effect Sizes and 95% Confidence Intervals From a Meta-Analysis of the Effects of Computer Technology-Based Interventions on Condom Use (Noar et al., 2009)

for each study (square), the weight of the effect size in our analysis (size of square), the 95% confidence interval representing the precision of the estimate (line through square), and the overall weighted mean effect size (diamond at bottom of plot).

Finally, researchers draw conclusions from meta-analysis, may discuss limitations of the project or potential alternative explanations for findings, and discuss gaps in the literature and implications for future research. This section of a meta-analysis is quite important, as it is an opportunity to reflect on the entire literature to date and point toward fruitful directions for future scholarship. In our meta-analysis, we concluded that computer technology-based HIV prevention interventions are efficacious, and we also emphasized several factors that appear to moderate the efficacy of such interventions. We concluded that additional investment in this area would be wise and that additional research is needed to further advance this area.

Ensuring Reliability and Validity of Meta-Analysis

Any meta-analysis requires numerous decisions and careful implementation, as well as a very detailed write up of the report for reasons of transparency and replicability. To encourage the highest quality in both the conduct and reporting of meta-analyses, several efforts have been undertaken. Early efforts included the Quality of Reporting of Meta-Analysis of Randomized Controlled Trials (QUOROM) statement (Moher et al., 1999) and the *Handbook of Research Synthesis* (Cooper & Hedges, 1994). More recent efforts include an updated set of standards (to replace QUOROM) that applies to both systematic reviews and meta-analyses, referred to as the Preferred Reporting Items for Systematic Reviews and Meta-Analyses (PRISMA) statement (Moher et al., 2009); an updated *Handbook of Research Synthesis and Meta-Analysis* (Cooper et al., 2009); and new guidelines from the American Psychological Association (APA) on the reporting of meta-analysis, referred to as Meta-Analysis Reporting Standards (APA Publications and Communications Board Working Group on Journal Article Reporting Standards, 2008). While the *Handbook* is a lengthy and extremely in-depth treatment of meta-analysis, covering all aspects of the technique, the PRISMA and APA efforts are aimed in particular at the quality of meta-analytic reports. These efforts may also ultimately affect the *conduct* of systematic reviews and meta-analyses, however, as more complete and transparent reporting will likely encourage researchers to perform more methodologically rigorous reviews.

Both the APA and PRISMA statements include tables that describe recommended sections of meta-analytic reports as well as the information that should be reported in each of those sections. For example, perhaps the simplest recommendation is to include the term "meta-analysis" in the title of the report. Such a simple action can have an important pragmatic benefit, however, in that it instantly clarifies the type of review conducted and makes it easier to locate the review in a database search. The PRISMA statement also includes a flow diagram illustrating the flow of studies through the search process, including how many studies were excluded during different phases of the search process and for what reasons.

Completeness of reporting is particularly important in meta-analyses, because they are such large and complex projects, and because they have a unique potential to greatly influence a particular field of study. Numerous decisions must be made in the course of a systematic review for meta-analysis that will be unknown to the reader of that review if the information is not reported. Thus, many meta-analyses have lengthy methods sections (and, increasingly, an online methods appendix) containing details about search procedures, screening of studies, the coding process, and effect size conversion and analysis. Indeed, one should be suspicious of any meta-analysis with a short methods section that lacks sufficient detail.

Strengths and Limitations of Meta-Analysis

The strengths of the meta-analytic technique should be apparent by now, and include the comprehensiveness of the literature search (and implications for external validity of findings), the objectivity of the coding process, and the focus on precise effect sizes of study findings. Most limitations of meta-analysis are seen when the technique is not properly applied. For example, when a search is incomplete (e.g., the review searched too few sources for articles, ignored the unpublished or "gray" literature, or used poor search terms), the external validity of a meta-analysis is greatly threatened. Also, if a coding form is not carefully developed with thoughtful coding categories, and coding is not carefully conducted and tracked, this limits the contribution and robustness of a meta-analysis. Finally, when the methods used in a meta-analysis are not adequately described, it gives the impression that careful thought was not given to the finest details in the project itself.

One limitation of meta-analysis is really more a limitation of a particular literature. A meta-analysis cannot make up for a lack of studies on a topic, nor can it make up for poorly conceptualized or poorly conducted studies. That is, a meta-analysis is only as good as the set of studies that are being synthesized, and thus one should avoid the temptation of synthesizing studies that may be interesting and important but that are not methodologically rigorous.

Also, we should be careful not to generalize our findings beyond the range of variables, outcomes, and populations included in a given meta-analysis. In fact, one little-discussed limitation of many literatures is the excessive use of college student convenience samples. If most of one's samples are college students, then many of our meta-analytic findings may be biased. If there are enough studies in one's meta-analytic database, one can treat the population as a moderating variable to examine whether associations are similar or different across different types of samples or populations.

Finally, a limitation that applies to most meta-analyses (even those that are well conducted) has to do with analyses of possible moderating variables. Analyses of moderators essentially stratify one group of studies on a particular variable and compare them to another group of studies. In many ways, moderator analyses have the potential to greatly advance a field, as they attempt to get at study mechanisms through empirical testing of a priori hypotheses. The key limitations of these analyses, however, are (a) moderator variables are often missing from some of the coded studies, perhaps in a biased way, and (b) some moderator variables may be confounded with others. Thus, there is a danger of making conclusions from moderating analyses that are the result of spurious associations (Lipsey, 2003). While meta-regression may help with the problem of confounded moderators (Borenstein et al., 2009), there is no obvious solution with the exception of interpreting the results of such analyses with some caution.

How to Get Started

If a researcher wishes to begin a meta-analytic project, he or she may wonder how to get started. There are several steps that can be recommended. First, there is no substitute for knowing the literature in a particular area extremely well. Because a researcher knows how to conduct meta-analysis does *not* mean that they are expert in meta-analyzing any research literature. Rather, being familiar with the particular literature to be examined is crucial in undertaking a number of tasks. For instance, developing inclusion criteria for the study involves thinking about how broad or narrow the project should be as well as what kinds of studies can and cannot be usefully synthesized together. Developing a coding sheet, coding articles and subsequently analyzing the data all involve a deep understanding of the substantive research questions at hand in a particular literature. Careful training of all coders is critical, too. Finally, the meta-analyst must carefully interpret the results and make conclusions and recommendations for the field based on a large and sophisticated dataset, and this is no small task. Thus, in order to perform all of these important tasks, one should either be knowledgeable about the literature or bring on a collaborator who is knowledgeable.

We also recommend a *feasibility stage* as the first step in any project. That is, because one wants to conduct a particular meta-analysis does not mean that a particular meta-analysis is capable of being conducted. In fact, there are many potential (and common) barriers to conducting a meta-analysis. For instance, in some cases, there are simply not enough studies to conduct a meaningful meta-analysis. Although, theoretically, the technique can be applied to just two studies, it is more fruitfully applied to situations when a dozen or more studies exist. In addition, in some cases, effect sizes cannot be extracted or calculated. For example, if one is conducting a meta-analysis of correlations, one must be sure that bivariate correlations (or other statistics that can be converted to correlations) are actually reported in the studies. Unfortunately, multivariate statistics from multiple regression and structural equation modeling generally *cannot* be meta-analyzed (Lipsey & Wilson, 2001). Also, meta-analyses of mean differences can be problematic if corresponding standard deviations are not reported in the articles, a situation more common that one may think (though contacting authors can result in recovering those data). Finally, in some cases, one cannot code the features of the studies that the meta-analyst had planned to code, which can result in few if any moderator variables to analyze. This tends to occur where there is little consensus on moderator variables in an area of inquiry. In addition, a related problem is that the features that one planned to code are not reported in enough detail to make coding feasible.

To allay the potential problems above, one can begin with a feasibility stage in which numerous articles are collected and examined for relevance. Initial inclusion criteria are developed, effect sizes are calculated, and some preliminary coding is done. At a certain point in this process, it will either become clear that the project is feasible, in which case, the meta-analyst can now spend the time necessary to locate all of the relevant articles and begin the meta-analysis in earnest, or it will become clear that the project is *not* feasible and should be abandoned. Of course, sometimes it turns out that the project *is* feasible but not in the form in which it was originally conceived. If that occurs, changes can be made to the conceptualization of the project *before* large amounts of time are devoted to it.

Conclusion

Meta-analyses have greatly advanced the science of cumulative knowledge-building in health communication and many related fields. Meta-analyses have advanced our understanding of fear-arousing communications, health communication campaigns, computer-tailored interventions, and behavioral interventions, among many other areas (for recent reviews of meta-analyses, see Johnson, Scott-Sheldon, & Carey, 2010; Noar, 2008; Snyder & LaCroix, 2013). This technique gives health communication researchers a method to accurately summarize research literatures where previously no real method existed. Thus, while poor cumulation was, in the past, a serious impediment to scientific progress (Rosenthal, 1991), we now have tools that allow us to summarize what is known more accurately, as well as to test which mechanisms may account for particular effects. Indeed, the strengths of meta-analysis rest on the basic tenets of science: no one study is perfect, and replication is necessary. Only when we see consistent effects across a body of research can we have great confidence in a particular effect. Additional meta-analyses in health communication will continue to help advance the science of this rapidly growing field.

References

Albarracin, D., Gillette, J. C., Earl, A. N., Glasman, L. R., Durantini, M. R., & Ho, M.-H. (2005). A test of major assumptions about behavior change: A comprehensive look at the effects of passive and active HIV-prevention interventions since the beginning of the epidemic. *Psychological Bulletin, 131*(6), 856–897.

Ankem, K. (2006). Factors influencing information needs among cancer patients: A meta-analysis. *Library & Information Science Research, 28*(1), 7–23.

APA Publications and Communications Board Working Group on Journal Article Reporting Standards. (2008). Reporting standards for research in psychology: Why do we need them? What might they be? *American Psychologist, 63*(9), 839–851.

Bearman, A. L. (1991). An empirical comparison of meta-analytic and traditional reviews. *Personality and Social Psychology Bulletin, 17*(3), 252–257.

Borenstein, M., Hedges, L.V., Higgins, J. P. T., & Rothstein, H. R. (2009). *Introduction to meta-analysis*. Chichester, West Sussex, England: John Wiley & Sons.

Bushman, B. J., & Wells, G. L. (2001). Narrative impressions of literature: The availability bias and the corrective properties of meta-analytic approaches. *Personality and Social Psychology Bulletin, 27*(9), 1123–1130.

Cohen, J. (1994). The earth is round (p<.05). *American Psychologist, 49*(12), 997–1003.

Cook, T. D., & Leviton, L. C. (1980). Reviewing the literature: A comparison of traditional methods with meta-analysis. *Journal of Personality, 48*(4), 449–472.

Cooper, H. M. (1988). Organizing knowledge syntheses: A taxonomy of literature reviews. *Knowledge in Society, 1*(1), 104–126.

Cooper, H. M., & Hedges, L. V. (1994). *The handbook of research synthesis*. New York, NY: Russell Sage Foundation.

Cooper, H. M., & Rosenthal, R. (1980). Statistical versus traditional procedures for summarizing research findings. *Psychological Bulletin, 87*(3), 442–449.

Cooper, H. M., & Hedges, L. V. (2009). Research synthesis as a scientific process. In H. M. Cooper, L.V. Hedges, & J. C. Valentine (Eds.), *The handbook of research synthesis and meta-analysis* (2nd ed.) (pp. 3–16). New York, NY: Russell Sage Foundation.

Cooper, H. M., Hedges, L. V., & Valentine, J. C. (2009). *The handbook of research synthesis and meta-analysis* (2nd ed.). New York, NY: Russell Sage Foundation.

Derzon, J. H., & Lipsey, M. W. (2002). A meta-analysis of the effectiveness of mass-communication for changing substance-use knowledge, attitudes, and behavior. In W. D. Crano & M. Burgoon (Eds.), *Mass media and drug prevention: Classic and contemporary theories and research* (pp. 231–258). Mahwah, N.J.: Lawrence Erlbaum Associates.

Gallagher, K. M., & Updegraff, J. A. (2012). Health message framing effects on attitudes, intentions, and behavior: A meta-analytic review. *Annals of Behavioral Medicine, 43*(1), 101–116.

Hall, J. A., & Rosenthal, R. (1991). Testing for moderator variables in meta-analysis: Issues and methods. *Communication Monographs, 58*(4), 437–448.

Hedges, L. V., & Olkin, I. (1985). *Statistical methods for meta-analysis*. Orlando, FL: Academic Press.

Higgins, J. P. T., & Thompson, S. G. (2002). Quantifying heterogeneity in a meta-analysis. *Statistics in Medicine, 21*(11), 1539–1558.

Hoyle, R. H., Fejfar, M. C., & Miller, J. D. (2000). Personality and sexual risk taking: A quantitative review. *Journal of Personality, 68*(6), 1203–1231.

Hunter, J. E., & Schmidt, F. L. (2004). *Methods of meta-analysis: Correcting error and bias in research findings* (2nd ed.). Thousand Oaks, CA: Sage.

Johnson, B. T., & Eagly, A. H. (2000). Quantitative synthesis of social psychological research. In H. T. Reis & C. M. Judd (Eds.), *Handbook of research methods in social and personality psychology* (pp. 496–528). New York, NY: Cambridge University Press.

Johnson, B. T., Mullen, B., & Salas, E. (1995). Comparison of three major meta-analytic approaches. *Journal of Applied Psychology, 80*(1), 94–106.

Johnson, B. T., Scott-Sheldon, L. A. J., & Carey, M. P. (2010). Meta-synthesis of health behavior change meta-analyses. *American Journal of Public Health, 100*(11), 2193.

Johnson, B. T., Scott-Sheldon, L. A. J., Snyder, L. B., Noar, S. M., & Huedo-Medina, T. B. (2008). Contemporary approaches to meta-analysis in communication research. In A. F. Hayes, M. D. Slater, & L. B. Snyder (Eds.), *The Sage sourcebook of advanced data analysis methods for communication research* (pp. 311–347). Thousand Oaks, CA: Sage Publications.

Krippendorff, K. (2004). *Content analysis: An introduction to its methodology* (2nd ed.). Thousand Oaks, CA: Sage Publications.

Lipsey, M. W. (2003). Those confounded moderators in meta-analysis: Good, bad, and ugly. *Annals of the American Academy of Political and Social Science, 587*(1), 69–81.

Lipsey, M. W., & Wilson, D. B. (2001). *Practical meta-analysis*. Thousand Oaks, CA: Sage Publications.

Lustria, M. L., Noar, S. M., Cortese, J., Van Stee, S. K., & Glueckauf, R. L. (2013). A meta-analysis of web-delivered, tailored health behavior change interventions. *Journal of Health Communication, 18*(9), 1039–1069.

Meehl, P. E. (1978). Theoretical risks and tabular asterisks: Sir Karl, Sir Ronald, and the slow progress of soft psychology. *Journal of Consulting and Clinical Psychology, 46*(4), 806–834.

Moher, D., Liberati, A., Tetzlaff, J., Altman, D. G., & the PRISMA Group. (2009). Preferred reporting items for systematic reviews and meta-analyses: The PRISMA statement. *PLoS Medicine, 6*(7), e1000097.

Moher, D., Cook, D. J., Eastwood, S., Olkin, I., Rennie, D., & Stroup, D. F. (1999). Improving the quality of reports of meta-analyses of randomised controlled trials: the QUOROM statement. *Lancet, 354*(9193), 1896–1900.

Noar, S. M. (2006). In pursuit of cumulative knowledge in health communication: The role of meta-analysis. *Health Communication, 20*(2), 169–175.

Noar, S. M. (2008). Behavioral interventions to reduce HIV-related sexual risk behavior: Review and synthesis of meta-analytic evidence. *AIDS and Behavior, 12*(3), 335–353.

Noar, S. M., Benac, C. N., & Harris, M. S. (2007). Does tailoring matter? Meta-analytic review of tailored print health behavior change interventions. *Psychological Bulletin, 133*(4), 673–693.

Noar, S. M., Black, H. G., & Pierce, L. B. (2009). Efficacy of computer technology-based HIV prevention interventions: A meta-analysis. *AIDS, 23*(1), 107–115.

Noar, S. M., Pierce, L. B., & Black, H. G. (2010). Can computer-mediated interventions change theoretical mediators of safer sex? A meta-analysis. *Human Communication Research, 36*(3), 261–297.

O'Keefe, D. J., & Jensen, J. D. (2007). The relative persuasiveness of gain-framed and loss-framed messages for encouraging disease prevention behaviors: A meta-analytic review. *Journal of Health Communication, 12*(7), 623–644.

Portnoy, D. B., Scott-Sheldon, L. A. J., Johnson, B. T., & Carey, M. P. (2008). Computer-delivered interventions for health promotion and behavioral risk reduction: A meta-analysis of 75 randomized controlled trials, 1988–2007. *Preventive Medicine, 47*(1), 3–16.

Rogers, E. M. (1996). The field of health communication today: An up-to-date report. *Journal of Health Communication, 1*(1), 15–23.

Rosenthal, R. (1991). *Meta-analytic procedures for social research* (rev. ed.). Thousand Oaks, CA: Sage Publications.

Rosenthal, R. (1992). Effect size estimation, significance testing, and the file-drawer problem. *Journal of Parapsychology, 56*(1), 57–58.

Rosenthal, R., & Rubin, D. B. (1978). Interpersonal expectancy effects: The first 345 studies. *Behavioral and Brain Sciences, 1*(3), 377–415.

Schmidt, F. L. (1992). What do data really mean? Research findings, meta-analysis, and cumulative knowledge in psychology. *American Psychologist, 47*(10), 1173.

Schmidt, F. L., & Hunter, J. E. (1977). Development of a general solution to the problem of validity generalization. *Journal of Applied Psychology, 62*(5), 529–540.

Scholes, D., McBride, C. M., Grothaus, L., Civic, D., Ichikawa, L. E., Fish, L. J., & Yarnall, K. S. (2003). A tailored minimal self-help intervention to promote condom use in young women: Results from a randomized trial. *AIDS (London, England), 17*(10), 1547–1556.

Sharpe, D. (1997). Of apples and oranges, file drawers and garbage: Why validity issues in meta-analysis will not go away. *Clinical Psychology Review, 17*(8), 881–901.

Smith, M. L., & Glass, G. V. (1977). Meta-analysis of psychotherapy outcome studies. *The American Psychologist, 32*(9), 752–760.

Snyder, L. B., & LaCroix, J. M. (2013). How effective are mediated health campaigns? A synthesis of meta-analyses. In R. E. Rice & C. K. Atkin (Eds.), *Public communication campaigns* (4th ed.) (pp. 113–129). Thousand Oaks, CA: Sage Publications.

Snyder, L. B., Hamilton, M. A., & Huedo-Medina, T. B. (2009). Does evaluation design impact communication campaign effect size? A meta-analysis. *Communication Methods and Measures,* 3(1–2), 84–104.

Snyder, L. B., Hamilton, M. A., Mitchell, E. W., Kiwanuka-Tondo, J., Fleming-Milici, F., & Proctor, D. (2004). A meta-analysis of the effect of mediated health communication campaigns on behavior change in the United States. *Journal of Health Communication, 9*(Suppl. 1), 71–96.

Wallack, L., & Dorfman, L. (2001). Putting policy into health communication: The role of media advocacy. In R. E. Rice & C. K. Atkin (Eds.), *Public communication campaigns* (3rd ed.) (pp. 389–401). Thousand Oaks, CA: Sage Publications.

Wilson, D. B. (2009). Systematic coding. In H. M. Cooper, L. V. Hedges & J. C. Valentine (Eds.), *The handbook of research synthesis and meta-analysis* (2nd ed.) (pp. 159–176). New York, NY: Russell Sage Foundation.

Wilson, D. B. (2010). Meta-analysis macros for SAS, SPSS, and Stata. Retrieved from http://mason.gmu.edu/~dwilsonb/ma.html

Witte, K., & Allen, M. (2000). A meta-analysis of fear appeals: Implications for effective public health campaigns. *Health Education & Behavior, 27*(5), 591–615.

META-SYNTHESIS

The Utility of Synthesizing Qualitative Health Communication Research

Anne M. Stone and Aaron T. Seaman

Scholars across disciplines (e.g., communication, nursing, medicine) are working to advance knowledge by synthesizing research findings through a variety of innovative methodologies (Cook, Mulrow, & Haynes, 1997; Estabrooks, 1999; Estabrooks, Field, & Morse, 1994; Harrison, 1996). Researchers have started using methodologies that organize, make sense of, and further develop existing bodies of data and theory in an effort to reduce "information anxiety" (Harrison, 1996, quoted in Sandelowski & Barroso 2007). Meta-analysis (Noar & Snyder, this volume) and meta-synthesis—the subject of this chapter—are two such methodologies that are commonly applied.

Glass (1977) described the importance of meta-analysis centering on the growth of research. Although Glass' concern was with burgeoning research in the field of education, we see a similar need for meta-study, and particularly meta-synthesis, in health communication. For example, a simple search in the database Communication and Mass Media Complete yields more than 6,000 articles that have been published on the topic of HIV or AIDS. Lack of proper synthesis of findings from existing literature may have deleterious effects on researchers aimed at designing and implementing interventions. Different types of qualitative meta-study have been developed and implemented, including meta-ethnography (Noblit & Hare, 1988) and meta-synthesis (Jensen & Allen, 1996; Sandelowski & Barroso, 2007).[1]

Indeed, inasmuch as meta-studies are useful for furthering knowledge in the academy, Sandelowski (1997) highlighted that scholars' "heightened accountability to the public" carries a responsibility for scholars to be aware that research findings have important implications for practitioners designing interventions (Goldsmith & Brashers, 2008). This may be particularly important for health communication researchers, as they are uniquely positioned to develop interdisciplinary scholarship that answers important questions about the role of communication in improving health experiences and outcomes for healthcare providers, patients, and families (Parrott, 2004; Rimal & Lapinski, 2009).

The Nature of Meta-Synthesis

More than 20 years ago, Stern and Harris (1985) used grounded theory techniques (Glaser & Strauss, 1967; Glaser, 1978; Stern, 1980; Stern, Allen, & Moxley, 1982) to conduct a "qualitative meta-analysis" of women's self-care practice. Walsh and Downe (2005) noted that Stern and Harris (1985) "were the first to coin the phrase 'qualitative meta-synthesis' with reference to the amalgamation of a group of qualitative studies" (Walsh & Downe, 2005, p. 204). Unlike secondary analysis, where a researcher reanalyzes data from a single study using different techniques (Glass, 1977; Thorne, 1994), meta-studies, which include meta-analysis and meta-synthesis, work across studies to evaluate their data and findings in the context of a larger body of research. Although some scholars have distinguished between "analysis" and "synthesis" to argue that the use of the term "meta-study" is more appropriate because it combines the two (Paterson et al., 2001), others commonly use the terms "meta-analysis" and "meta-synthesis" to distinguish between meta-studies of quantitative work (i.e., meta-analysis) and qualitative work (i.e., meta-synthesis). Paterson et al. (2001) described meta-synthesis research as being able to offer "a critical, historical, and theoretical analytic approach to making sense of qualitatively derived knowledge" (p. 2).

One of the major differences between meta-analysis and meta-synthesis, as Walsh and Downe (2005) noted, stems from the assumptions made by researchers about knowledge influenced by different paradigms. Although the approaches seem to share a common goal, the outcome of the meta-study is different largely because of the approach taken. A meta-analysis aims to develop larger sample sizes from an aggregate of published research to describe relationships between variables with increased certainty than smaller sample and effect sizes allow. Meta-synthesis, on the other hand, seeks to explain and understand phenomena by pulling together findings from qualitative research.

Description

Meta-synthesis as a method of conducting research refers to the systematic study and integration of qualitative research findings. Qualitative research syntheses often draw from a variety of specific qualitative approaches, including ethnography, phenomenology, thematic analysis, and grounded theory (Sandelowski & Barroso, 2007), with data collected via focus group interviews, individual interviews, observations, and texts (Sandelowski & Barroso, 2002). Sandelowski and Barroso (2007) outlined five characteristics of qualitative meta-synthesis: "(a) systematic and comprehensive retrieval of all relevant reports of completed qualitative studies in a target domain of empirical inquiry, (b) systematic use of qualitative and quantitative methods to analyze these reports, (c) analytic and interpretive emphasis on the findings in these reports, (d) systematic and appropriately eclectic use of qualitative methods to integrate the findings in these reports, and (e) the use of reflexive accounting practices to optimize the validity of study procedures and outcomes" (p. 22). Together, these characteristics highlight the comprehensive, systematic nature of the meta-synthetic method. They also point to several challenges of conducting meta-syntheses, including ensuring complete retrieval of extant studies, comparing across a diverse set of research projects, and maintaining transparency of the research process to increase consistency and validity.

The increasing popularity of qualitative research and meta-synthesis as a useful method of inquiry (Morse, 1994), especially in health-related fields, makes this chapter and research that describes this method particularly important for training health communication scholars. Scholars who undertake a meta-synthesis project must first articulate the purpose for the synthesis. Sandelowski and Barroso (2007) identified three major reasons to write a meta-synthesis. First, meta-synthesis is a useful way to "sum up the knowledge generated in an area in order to draw conclusions directly relevant to practice or chart directions for future research" (p. 23). Next, meta-synthesis techniques give researchers an opportunity to identify research discrepancies in a subject area and work to "resolve these discrepancies" (p. 23). Finally, meta-syntheses are useful for "clarifying or modeling the relationships among research variables, defining the conditions under which a phenomenon appears, explaining or providing a context for the findings of primary quantitative research or research syntheses, or mapping knowledge fields" (p. 23). In our review of recent studies that have used meta-synthesis techniques, scholars across disciplines engaged topics related to the hope experience of family caregivers of persons with chronic illness (Duggleby et al., 2010), caring within nursing education (Beck, 2001), and models of chronic illness (Paterson, 2001) to name just a few. This chapter draws on a meta-synthesis we conducted to synthesize literature on deception in the context of dementia and Alzheimer's disease to highlight the utility of qualitative meta-synthesis for health communication researchers.

Theoretical Assumptions and Challenges of Meta-Synthesis Projects

Van Maanen (1983) described qualitative methods as "an umbrella term covering an array of interpretive techniques which seek to describe, decode, translate, and otherwise come to terms with the meaning, not the frequency, of certain more or less naturally occurring phenomena in the social world" (p. 9). Qualitative methodologies elucidate the complexities of an issue by allowing the researcher to explore topics without restraint (Babbie, 2004). Additionally, qualitative methods focus on participants' words and meanings, highlighting the communicative nature of the process and discerning how those involved in this important speech act make sense of what they are doing. Interpretive research aims to collect descriptive data through qualitative methods including participant observation, focus groups, and individual interviews (Taylor & Bogdan, 1998). Meta-synthesis techniques are a type of qualitative method developed out of an interpretive perspective on research design. A meta-synthesis allows the opportunity to articulate the themes that are evident across studies while keeping in tension the differences that arise between studies' findings (Thorne et al., 2004).

Alongside efforts to develop meta-synthesis techniques, scholars have also identified challenges that face qualitative researchers. First, as we describe in the following sections, there are different ways of applying the methodologies described in the literature (Bondas & Hall, 2007). Sandelowski and Barroso (2007) also noted that there is a debate over the similarities and differences between qualitative research synthesis (i.e., meta-synthesis) and quantitative research synthesis (i.e., meta-analysis). The major concern surrounding this debate is how to maintain the theoretical assumptions of qualitative research through synthesis, and if a streamlined approach to the method of synthesis is appropriate, given the importance of achieving understanding in interpretive research.

Exemplars

Meta-synthesis as a method for integrating qualitative research findings has become increasingly popular, with several notable studies published. Duggleby and colleagues (2010) synthesized qualitative research reports on the hope experience of family caregivers of persons with chronic illness. They included 14 studies in their meta-synthesis that described the role of hope in coping with caregiving. The authors followed the procedures outlined by Sandelowski and Barroso (2007) and developed a conceptual model of hope based on four major themes from the research reports, including: (a) transitional refocusing from a difficult present to a positive future, (b) dynamic possibilities within uncertainty, (c) pathways of hope, and (d) hope outcomes. This meta-synthesis described clear implications for practice, and noted that the model presented highlights the different factors that influence a caregiver's experience of hope, which can be a focal point for hope interventions.

A second exemplar is Metcalfe, Coad, Plumridge, Gill, and Farndon's (2008) meta-synthesis of family communication between children and their parents about inherited genetic conditions. Metcalfe et al. (2008) reviewed research from major health and medical research databases and identified relevant research from 1980 to 2007. After identifying 17 articles relevant to their research question, the authors used a meta-ethnographic approach (Noblit & Hare, 1988) to analyze key themes. Metcalfe et al. (2008) argued that providing information, checking understanding, and explaining and managing the emotional feelings that arise as part of the conversation were essential components in supporting children's coping with genetic risk information.

Beck (2001) sought to uncover what generalizations could be derived from qualitative research studies on the importance of caring within nursing education. Fourteen studies met the inclusion criteria for this meta-synthesis, based on Noblit and Hare's (1988) criteria. Beck's (2001) analysis yielded five metaphors that were associated with caring in nursing education, including the reciprocal connection between presencing, sharing, supporting, competence, and the positive impact of caring. Beck (2001) concluded her meta-synthesis with clear implications for how the findings from her meta-synthesis can be used by nursing educators.

It is clear, from the brief descriptions of the exemplar studies that we chose, that there are different ways of designing a qualitative meta-synthesis. In the sections that follow, we outline how health communication scholars can employ the method of meta-synthesis in their research program by first describing the procedures and then highlighting some further considerations related to strengthening the validity of the project and its relative strengths and weaknesses.

Employing Meta-Synthesis: A Study of Deception and Dementia

In this section, we use a case study example to demonstrate the logistics of conducting a meta-synthesis. The example is a meta-synthesis we undertook to examine the research on deception in the context of dementia.[2] As discussed below, when beginning our research on deception, it quickly became clear that a meta-synthesis was the ideal methodology for our aims. In the following, we detail the procedures for undertaking a meta-synthesis. Despite the theoretical instability accompanying this nascent methodology, the procedural form is fairly standard and includes the following steps: (a) determining topical focus/research aims and appropriateness of methodology, (b) designing and conducting the search, (c) analyzing research findings, and (d) synthesizing and presenting research findings (see Table 13.1).

Determining Topical Focus and Appropriateness of Methodology

The choice to conduct a meta-synthesis, or to use meta-synthetic techniques to investigate a particular topic, is one that should be guided by the topical focus and the current body of literature, which dictate the appropriateness of the methodology. As scholars have described, researchers spend considerable time determining what might be an appropriate topic for a meta-synthesis (Finfgeld, 2003; Sandelowski, Docherty, & Emden, 1997; Schreiber, Crooks, & Stern, 1997). And, while beginning researchers might see a meta-study as a means to bypass the time-consuming, challenge-laden process of data collection, these same scholars

TABLE 13.1 Meta-Synthesis Procedures

Stage 1:	**Determining topical focus/research aims and appropriateness of methodology** Determine the purpose of the synthesis Decide on the topic/phenomenon of interest
Stage 2:	**Designing and conducting the search** Decide which online databases to search for qualitative research reports Choose key terms to search online databases Decide on the inclusion criteria for qualitative research reports Create a spreadsheet to keep track of relevant research articles
Stage 3:	**Analyzing research findings** Work with members of your team to code a subset of the articles from the spreadsheet for themes Discuss themes from individual articles noting relevant examples to illustrate categories
Stage 4:	**Synthesizing and presenting research findings** Organize recurrent themes into explanatory categories Develop your argument to clarify how the findings were synthesized

are quick to point out that to do so would be a mistake as a meta-study requires the same interpretive rigor as primary data-collection procedures (Bondas & Hall, 2007, p. 114).

Health communication scholars have many options for choosing a topical focus, including a specific disease, a particular aspect of the disease experience, a health-related event, a specific intervention, an organization (e.g., hospital), or a communicative relationship (Sandelowski & Barroso, 2007). The choice for methodological approach is just as varied (as, among others, this volume duly demonstrates). While ideally, perhaps, methodological choice would be solely guided by the questions that spring from the empirical world, unconstrained by individual histories of scholarly growth, the reality is that the question of which comes first, a topical focus or a research methodology, is often a chicken-and-egg affair of co-development. Researchers' approach to topics and discovery of new research questions often is guided by the methodologies in which they have been trained, while their use of different methodologies just as frequently is influenced by the kinds of questions they ask and answers they seek. This simultaneous development certainly has been evidenced in our own process.

Before we decided on a methodology (and, before this project became the example for this chapter), we had determined that we had questions about the role of deception in the context of dementia. These stemmed, in part, from broader topical interests that have guided previous research that we have conducted with dementia patients and their caregivers (Seaman, 2010; Stone & Jones, 2009) and with professional caregivers of persons with Alzheimer's disease (Stone, 2013), including a concern with relationships of care, questions about communication and cognitive capacity, and interests in knowledge production in medical and bioethical contexts. These larger interests condense quite concretely in discussions surrounding the use of deception with people diagnosed with dementia, a commonly employed yet ethically controversial communication-based means for others to control the information that person receives and their behavior.

Alongside this, our methodological training and inclinations also shaped the project. Reading the extant literature on deception in the context of dementia, we quickly realized that we had questions, such as the following, that would not be answered in the course of conducting a traditional literature review:

- When is a communicative interaction called "deception," and when is it something else (e.g., "non-disclosure," "concealment")? Are these categories that research participants—or researchers—use?
- Who can deceive? Who cannot?
- Are the ethical standards surrounding deception different for different interactions?
- What is the historical trajectory of deception research, given the changes in what it means to be a "person with dementia" as people are diagnosed increasingly earlier and with more cognitive capacity?

Especially given our concerns with research design and the assumptions about deception as a construct, a meta-study seemed most appropriate. The question became "meta-analysis or meta-synthesis?" By training, one of us (Stone) is a health communication scholar, and the other (Seaman) a medical anthropologist. At the most general level, this leads us to seek answers (and, thus, ask questions) in particularity, "to seize upon the interpretations people place on existence and to systematize them so they are more readily available to us" (Carey, 1975, p. 190). Based on our search, the body of literature on deception and dementia produced from quantitative studies also appears quite substantive (see Pinner & Bouman, 2002, for a review), so a meta-analysis might well have been appropriate. Yet, a meta-synthesis allows us to describe the complexities of how deception is communicated in the context of dementia.

After determining that a meta-synthesis was appropriate, given our questions, we next considered which approach to synthesis best fit with our question of interest. In her analysis of meta-syntheses published since 1994 related to health issues, Finfgeld (2003) outlined three types of meta-synthesis research: theory building, theory explication, and descriptive. Theory building approaches, she argues, include grounded formal theory (e.g., see Kearney, 2001) and meta-study (e.g., see Paterson, 2001). Given the data upon which they draw, theory building meta-syntheses ideally are able to offer a complexity that extends what is possible in any single study, resulting in new theoretical contributions. Theory explication, in contrast, works within existing theoretical and conceptual terrain, reconceptualizing it in light of cross-study data. Such work allows for themes to be reimagined to more clearly explicate a concept (Finfgeld, 2003;

Schreiber et al., 1997). Finfgeld (1999) took this approach when she synthesized literature on the concept of courage for people with chronic illness. Both the theory building and theory explication approaches call for a deconstruction of the data itself, whereby the data is stripped from the researchers' findings and reworked into, ultimately, new thematic and theoretical findings. Our project was slightly different in nature: We found ourselves concerned with exactly the links that researchers were building between their data and their eventual findings. Therefore, we used the third type of meta-synthesis research that Finfgeld discussed: the descriptive approach. This approach "involves the synthesis of qualitative findings and results in a comprehensive analysis of phenomena" (Finfgeld, 2003, p. 897). Instead of deconstructing findings as we would have from a theory building or theory explication approach, we engage with the data as the original researchers did, analyzing the actual text from their results and findings in our own analysis and synthesis (Finfgeld, 2003; Schreiber et al., 1997).

Designing and Conducting the Search

After deciding on the initial topical focus of deception in the context of dementia, and determining that our research questions would be suited to a meta-synthetic analysis, we began to develop the parameters that would guide our search of the extant literature. Conducting a thorough review of qualitative studies relevant to your project is essential for a successful meta-synthesis. Sandelowski and Barroso (2007) described recall and precision as "the most commonly used performance measures in information retrieval" (p. 35). Where "recall" refers to "the percent of relevant documents in the database that have been retrieved," "precision" refers to "the percent of documents that have been retrieved that are relevant" (p. 35). Because one goal of a meta-synthesis is to be exhaustive, it is important for scholars to stress recall over precision. Emphasizing precision may lead to the exclusion of relevant work.

In order to be as complete as possible, we conducted a two-stage search. For the first stage, we chose seven databases that, together, provided comprehensive coverage of the fields where qualitative work on deception was likely to have been published. PubMed, PsycInfo, Medline, and CINAHL were included for their focus on medical, psychological, and nursing literature; Communication Abstracts and Sociological Abstracts for academic discussions of deception; and JSTOR for its comprehensive general collection. All databases were searched for the entirety of their available date range.[3] We used search terms designed to capture as broad a range of articles as possible (*Alzheimer's disease* and *dementia*, each combined with deception, lying, lie, redirection, validation, reality, covert, honesty, truth, trust, fals*, mislead*, dece*, and pretend*), searching each database with these 28 permutations. After deleting all duplicate articles, this process resulted in 8,158 unique articles.

The second stage of our search comprised two parallel processes. To determine its relevance to the meta-synthesis, we reviewed each article using the four inclusion criteria below.[4] When formulating our inclusion criteria, we attempted to maintain a balance between, on one hand, keeping the criteria as broad as possible, while, on the other hand, drawing the line between those articles germane to our topical focus and those outside the purview of our interests (Jensen & Allen, 1996).

Is the Article Published Research? And Does it Appear in a Peer-Reviewed Publication?

Within discussions about meta-synthesis, there is debate about whether to include unpublished or non-peer-reviewed works (Beck, 2002; Bondas & Hall, 2007). Dissertations, theses, and conference presentations often include the most recent (and, frequently, most innovative) research, and can provide valuable data that have not yet reached publication (or may never do so; Finfgeld, 2003). And publications such as book chapters and specially edited journal issues arguably have gone through some review process. Yet, the credibility and trustworthiness of published, peer-reviewed data is still considered the gold standard (Barroso & Powell-Cope, 2000). Therefore, for the purposes of this meta-synthesis, we opted to only include published, peer-reviewed work.

Does the Study Use Qualitative or Mixed Methodologies?

Given the nature of meta-synthesis, this is an obvious criterion, yet what counts as "qualitative" might not be self-evident. In some cases, the study will not explicitly state the methodology used. In others, the methodology might be unusual; one of the pleasures of qualitative research is its amenability to creative methodological approaches, yet some of the more boundary-pushing approaches might not be appropriate to include. This is especially true when doing health-related research, where the standards of acceptably valid and rigorous research can be conservative.

Generally, the purpose of qualitative research is to gain a deep understanding of a phenomenon as it occurs in a natural setting and describe the meaning constructed by the participants (Denzin & Lincoln, 1994; Patton, 2002). Qualitative health-related studies can employ a range of methodologies, including ethnography, grounded theory, phenomenology, thematic analysis, and narrative analysis. The studies we included in the meta-synthesis used grounded theory (Day, James, Meyer, & Lee, 2011; Derksen, Vernooij-Dassen, Gillissen, Olde-Rikkert, & Scheltens, 2005; Keightley & Mitchell, 2004), phenomenology (Karnieli-Miller, Werner, Aharon-Peretz, & Eidelman, 2007; Langdon, Eagle, & Warner, 2007), narrative analysis (MacQuarrie, 2005), and ethnography (Blum, 1994; Hertogh, The, Miesen, & Eefsting, 2004; Tuckett, 2007, 2012). In addition, seven of the articles stated only that the studies were conducted using "qualitative methods" (Aminzadeh, Byszewski, Molnar, & Eisner, 2007; Byszewski et al., 2007; Hayes, Zimmerman, & Boylstein, 2010; Hughes, Hope, Reader, & Rice, 2002; James, Wood-Mitchell, Waterworth, Mackenzie, & Cunningham, 2006; Kaduszkiewicz, Bachmann, & van den Bussche, 2008; Smith & Beattie, 2001). We excluded prescriptive articles based in personal experience and observation, articles that grew from workshop sessions, discussion articles based on vignettes or case studies, review articles, and letters to the editor.

Mixed methodologies also are increasingly popular (Morgan, 1998). For studies that included both quantitative and qualitative findings, we examined the qualitative findings apart from the quantitative analysis to determine if the project would contribute to our synthesis. If the qualitative portion was robust enough (i.e., the study actually involved a qualitative sub-study, rather than, for example, the analysis of anecdotal observations collected unsystematically during administration of a survey), we included that article in the meta-synthesis (James et al., 2006; Kaduszkiewicz et al., 2008).

Does the Article Discuss Deception and/or Lying?

At some point in the process, you will decide upon a criterion that draws the line between those articles you include, and those you do not. This criterion was ours, and, ultimately, it proved incredibly difficult to settle upon.[5] Over the course of the meta-synthesis project, we vacillated between two wordings that had implications for the articles that we included in the study. The first you see above; the second read: "Does the article specifically mention deception and/or lying?" While the distinction might seem small, it had sizable consequences for the argument we were able to make.

Designing and Conducting the Search

As we worked through the articles that were gathered in our search, we found that there were two types of articles that seemed to be discussing deception. One group of articles explicitly said they were studying deception or lying. The second group, while discussing interactions that seemed deceptive, never explicitly stated that deception was their specific object of study. Instead, these articles—which we refer to as "gray area" articles—talked about the issues surrounding "disclosure" of diagnosis, or when families or people with dementia "conceal" or "cover up" symptoms, or "keeping" information. As we began conducting our thematic analysis (see below, *Synthesizing and Presenting Research Findings*), this distinction became increasingly meaningful, for, as we discuss elsewhere, whether researchers choose to label an interaction as deceptive reflects the agency they are granting actors within that interaction. Importantly, researchers never called acts by people with dementia acts of deception—a choice, we argue, that ripples outward, effecting larger implications for research design and interpretation of findings. We finally settled on the more broadly worded criterion to reflect our interest in including both groups of articles, which allowed us to discuss the important differences between them.

Is the Article Published in English?

Returning to Sandelowski and Barroso's (2007) advice to maximize your search recall, you should search as broadly as possible. Research published in other languages may not ever be translated into multiple languages, and the data presented may be relevant to your study. However, this, of course, will be limited by your language proficiency.

While engaged in the first process of checking the original list of 8,158 articles against the above four criteria, we simultaneously conducted a hand search through the bibliographies of relevant articles from that same list to see whether they contained references we had missed in our original search. Although online database tools are expansive in their reach, they are not always perfect, and occasionally articles do slip through their electronic fingers (e.g., Duggleby et al., 2010).[6] Meta-synthesis techniques generally favor depth of analysis over sample size, and Sandelowski et al. (1997) caution researchers from including more than 10 studies in a meta-synthesis because "overly large sample sizes tend to impede deep analysis and, therefore, threaten the interpretive validity of findings" (p. 368). Although, in many cases, fewer studies would allow for more in-depth analysis, in this case, we felt that the inclusion criteria that we had selected would lead to a complex analysis of the topic rather than the more cursory analysis that fewer articles would have given us.

Analyzing the Data

Once we had the set of articles in hand, our next step was to analyze the data. Broadly, we followed qualitative analysis procedures outlined by Lincoln and Guba (1985) and Strauss and Corbin (1990), a collaborative and iterative process of coding the data and developing themes. First, each author independently coded a subset of the articles for themes that were present within individual studies. Given that we were conducting what Finfgeld (2003) typologized as a descriptive meta-synthesis, throughout this process, we were careful to approach the data as the article authors presented it. To facilitate this, we started with a table of all the articles, detailing four areas of information as outlined below.

Basic Information About the Articles (Author(s), Title, Publication Year, Discipline)

Basic article information is important not only for the obvious reason of tracking the article under examination, but also because it allows you to note historical and disciplinary trends in publication. Is the bulk of research being done in health communication? Public health? Nursing? These differences can affect the kinds of disciplinary conversations the authors are entering and the interventions they are seeking to make, which will shape the way they present data. For our purposes, the historical trends were key, as what it means to be a "person with dementia" has changed significantly in the past 30 years, in light of increased awareness, earlier diagnostic technologies, and, to a much lesser extent, minimal treatment of symptoms. In addition, the care philosophy toward people with dementia has changed as a person-centered care model has become more popular. Therefore, the very milieu in which interactions of deception take place is markedly different between the earliest article (Blum, 1994) and the most recent (Day et al., 2011), which affects the meta-synthetic comparisons drawn across them.

Method (Data Collection Method, Sample Size and Demographics, Data Analysis Method)

Tracking methods of data collection and analysis allows for comparisons across these (Bondas & Hall, 2007, Paterson et al., 2001). This can be especially important if radically different methods of collection are used, if sample sizes are drastically different, and if the means of data analysis is not explicitly stated (Finfgeld, 2003).

Results or Findings

The results or findings will form the basis of much of what Bondas and Hall (2007), based on a system articulated by Paterson et al. (2001), call "meta-data analysis": "an analysis of 'processed data' from selected qualitative research studies in light of data and findings from other studies" (Bondas & Hall, 2007, p. 115). As we tracked the results or findings at this early stage, we were particularly careful to maintain the authors' language. This helped to ensure that our subsequent analysis maintained verisimilitude with the original authors' analysis.

Material from the Discussion

Finally, we tracked the interpretations of findings and recommendations for practice and future research that authors presented in the articles' discussion sections separately. Doing so separately from results and findings allowed us to see the ways in which authors extrapolated from those findings to make broader claims, evaluating the argumentative connections between data and claim, as well as questioning why some claims were articulated while others remained unvoiced.

From the population of this table, we then moved slowly outward from those isolated article "nodes" to coding and thematic development across the articles. This was deeply iterative, as we worked between the table, growing lists of possible themes, and the articles themselves. As we worked through the articles, we met at regular intervals to compare and discuss our developing coding schemes. From there, we examined the findings as a whole, noting the clarity of each example in illustrating the theme. Finally, we engaged in a collaborative process, which resulted in the synthesis that we have described in this paper (Seaman & Stone, 2012).

Synthesizing and Presenting Research Findings

The final stage in the process—synthesizing and presenting research findings—involves organizing and writing up the meta-synthesis. During this stage, we believe it is important to remember—perhaps especially when employing the meta-synthetic method—that arguments are developed through the writing of them. This point may seem elementary, but, too often, this synthesizing stage can be viewed as "simply" writing up, a plodding through that must be endured to communicate the important material—the data (if you doubt this, think about the last time you sat down to read an article, skipped the introduction, pored over the results, and skimmed the discussion). Yet, one of the strengths of qualitative literature is the understanding that the presentation of an argument is also an (ideally complementary) argument, and that coming to both actually involves the engagement of writing (Denzin & Lincoln, 2000). This attention to the writing itself as integral is the process we recognize and employ here, and, in the case of the meta-synthesis on deception, it became critical in helping determine our final organization and arguments.

As we approached a point of completion in analyzing the data, we found ourselves with a matrix of different data elements, including forms of deceptive interaction, rationales for deception, contexts where deception occurred, and people involved in these deceptive interactions. As writing—and particularly writing for print media (certain forms of electronic media allow you to disrupt this somewhat)—is a linear form of communication, the presentation of these elements is necessarily nested and hierarchical, even if explicit attempts are made to disrupt the effects of this linearity. Thus, to organize the presentation in a certain order highlights some arguments and obscures others. For example, organizing by forms of deceptive interaction would allow us to foreground certain arguments about the various verbal and nonverbal communicative elements that can be involved in deception, while an organization focusing on contexts where deception occurred would most readily lead to a discussion on the ways that certain types of deceptive interactions occur most frequently in certain contexts—non-disclosure of diagnosis in the clinic, covert medicine administration in long-term care facilities, or white lies to coax a parent to their adult day program from home.

Throughout our discussions of coding, we had realized that we both were most interested in the relationships between people involved in deceptive interactions and, as sketched above, the ways in which context seemed to constrain the kinds of deception that occurred. We tried writing in both ways and ended up appreciating the flexibility that organizing by the people involved (physicians, nurses and other healthcare providers, familial caregivers, and persons with dementia) allowed us. As we wrote, one primary argument that emerged was that people moved fluidly across these spaces, yet the extant literature did not treat them as such, instead treating them as though they were "siloed," only existing statically in particular contexts (e.g., physicians only deceive at moments of diagnosis in the clinic). Organizing by context makes this argument more challenging to present, while, organizing by people, it emerges "naturally" over the course of the presentation of the data, such that, when the reader reaches the point in the discussion where we state it explicitly, it is almost obvious.

It is important to note here that this does not mean that other points about rationales or forms of deceptive interaction disappeared, only that they were not the organizing principle. Indeed, as we wrote up the meta-synthesis, we discovered a model of deception, implicit across the studies, comprising motives, modes, and outcomes of deception. This ended up being a central part of the contribution made by the meta-synthesis.

Evaluating Meta-Synthesis

Reliability and Validity

As with all research, it is essential to optimize the reliability and validity of the project in order to demonstrate the quality of the research (Patton, 2002). Stenbacka (2001) argued that "the concept of reliability is even misleading in qualitative research. If a qualitative study is discussed with reliability as a criterion, the consequence is rather that the study is no good" (p. 552). Not all qualitative researchers, though, make this argument. Healy and Perry (2000), for example, argued that quantitative and qualitative projects should be evaluated using criteria relevant to the paradigms from which each method was developed. Because qualitative research is guided by principles of the interpretive paradigm (Lindlof & Taylor, 2002), standards for judging reliability and validity have been developed apart from quantitative research (Golafshani, 2003; Lincoln & Guba, 1985; Patton, 2002). For qualitative research generally (Angen, 2000; Golafshani, 2003) and meta-synthesis in particular, there are several ways to enhance the reliability and validity of a study (Sandelowski & Barroso, 2007).

Instead of using the term "reliability," qualitative researchers are concerned with dependability (Lincoln & Guba, 1985) or consistency (Clonts, 1992; Seale, 1999). Campbell (1996) suggested that achieving consistency (i.e., reliability) occurs when the data collection and analysis procedures are verified through the data audit process, which often involves reviewing the data as well as memos detailing the process. We worked to establish consistency in our meta-synthesis in a number of ways. First, we documented the literature search process using an Excel spreadsheet. This allowed us to track the number of articles that each search yielded with each combination of terms. Second, we kept records of the analysis procedures through memo writing and notes from meetings where we discussed the parameters of our search criteria within the overall aims of the project.

The terms "quality" and "trustworthiness" are commonly used to describe the validity of a qualitative study (Lincoln & Guba, 1985; Mishler, 2000). Trustworthiness of findings suggests that the researcher describes the data collection and analysis procedures in detail so that the researcher and other readers are confident in the findings (Johnson, 1997; Lincoln & Guba, 1985). First, a team approach is one way of enhancing validity. This approach involved consulting with a research librarian. This is an important part of this process, as librarians are highly skilled in conducting this type of information search. In addition to consulting with a reference librarian, researchers can increase the validity of a project if at least two members of the research team are trained to conduct the searches. This will decrease the likelihood of missing a relevant article across all stages of the search process. Weekly meetings with the research team and keeping detailed memos of the search process will aid in discussions of search strategies. Additionally, peer review by other researchers who are experts in qualitative methods and in the subject area you are examining further enhance the validity of the project (Sandelowski & Barroso, 2007). In addition to the team approach, researchers can enhance validity by carefully tracking their collection and analysis procedures. As Sandelowski and Barroso (2007) suggested, we used a bibliographic citation management software program to track search outcomes.[7] Tracking search outcomes in this way was helpful because it allowed us to keep track of notes on each of the articles, and to search for key terms we were interested in describing in our analysis. An iterative approach to searching for literature also will increase the descriptive validity of the study, or "the factual accuracy of the account as reported by the qualitative researcher" (Johnson, 1997, p. 284), if all major databases and search engines are used. Finally, as with other forms of qualitative research (e.g., grounded theory studies), keeping close track of search procedures and analysis through an audit trail further enhances the validity of the qualitative meta-synthesis (Sandelowski & Barroso, 2007).

Strengths and Limitations of Method

There are several strengths and limitations that should be noted about the meta-synthetic method. A major strength of this approach is that the meta-synthesis allows researchers to track a body of knowledge to draw conclusions across studies that scholars may not benefit from without such an exhaustive review. Instead of a literature review, a qualitative meta-synthesis pushes scholars to go beyond summary to create models of communication processes that may be useful for future research designed to implement various changes related to important health outcomes.

One clear weakness that scholars have long acknowledged is related to the generalizability of qualitative research generally and meta-synthesis projects specifically (Sandelowski & Barroso, 2007, p. 2). Because qualitative research reports are designed in the tradition of interpretive research, scholars acknowledge that the interpretation of the findings is based on social constructions that may be analyzed from multiple perspectives. Although this may also be considered a strength of qualitative research generally, with the push to more generalizable findings useful for interventions and having policy implications, the lack of generalizable qualitative research is a limitation to be noted. Paterson and colleagues (2001) highlighted two additional limitations that researchers should consider. First, they suggested that decontextualizing the data, or "removing them from the emotional and physical context within which they were originally constructed," is a limitation of meta-synthesis projects because qualitative research aims to provide context and detailed explanations of phenomena in the words of the participants. Second, Paterson et al. (2001) argued that "the quality of the meta-study is to a large degree dependent on the primary researcher's ability to articulate the research design and research findings in such a way that the meta-study researcher can follow the primary researcher's decisions" (p. 15). Finfgeld (2003) suggested that one way to have better access to the primary data is to include dissertations in meta-synthesis work because of the level of detail provided to discuss key findings.

Conclusion

For these last paragraphs, we want to turn briefly to Babrow and Mattson's (2003) discussion of theorizing in health communication. In that piece, they are clear to assert the "interpenetrating" link between theory and practice (p. 38). Beginning from the stance that "health communication theory is meaningless if it does not influence practices related to health and illness" (p. 37), they elegantly illustrate that theory and practice are, in effect, two sides of the same intellectual project coin.

Into that conversation, we would like to interject two related points. First, preceding both theory and practice is a third concern—that of this volume: methodology. Unfortunately, in the discussions of theory and practice, methodology, and the actual work of research, is rarely mentioned. Yet, without a well-grounded, well-structured, and well-implemented methodology, neither of the subsequent two, theory or practice, can be meaningfully developed. Therefore, we argue that methodology is not only the third leg of some research stool, it is the sole root, from which well-constructed research, theory, and practice spring.

Second, we suggest that meta-synthesis, in particular, has much to offer health communication, as well as the other way around. Returning to Babrow and Mattson (2003), early on, they offer a definition of theory as a "consciously elaborated, justified, and uncertain understanding" (p. 36). The motivation to articulate such an understanding is fueled, in part, by a desire to deepen our knowledge of four key tensions that they posit drive health communication: between "body and communication," "science and humanism," "idiosyncrasy and commonality," and "(un)certainties and values, expectations, and desires" (Babrow & Mattson, 2003, pp. 39–45). As with all methodologies, researchers use meta-synthesis in an effort to elaborate and justify their theoretical understandings. Yet, meta-studies have the benefit of working across multiple studies, drawing into a single frame the data collection, analysis, and theorizing of a host of researchers. This allows for improved understanding of phenomenon (Jensen & Allen, 1996). In addition, the meta-synthetic method is uniquely situated to address the uncertainties inherent in both the theory-building and intervention-oriented projects of health communication. In their work on meta-ethnography, Noblit and Hare (1988) wrote of the distinction between reciprocal and refutational findings—findings across studies that are, as Finfgeld (2003) described them, "comparable" or "in opposition" (p. 901). In particular, both note the importance of refutational findings: "[I]t is these types of analyses and discussions that are useful for preserving and emphasizing the uniqueness of individual studies while building a comprehensive whole around reciprocal relationships and parallel lines of argument" (Finfgeld, 2003, p. 901). Meta-synthesis is an ideal methodology to explicate the gaps, discrepancies, and misunderstandings that run through not only the contexts we, as health communication scholars, study, but also the studies we conduct. As we, the authors, found in our meta-synthesis, misunderstandings in the power of labeling something as "deception" and a siloing of particular people in particular contexts had led to a thin, partial portrait of deception in the context of dementia, a fact that has had deep implications for theories of deception, understandings of dementia, and the treatment of people with dementia, as well as those who provide them care.

Although meta-synthesis has been described as "a relative 'newcomer'" (Zimmer, 2006, p. 311) to qualitative research, Sandelowski and Barroso (2007) highlighted the increasing popularity of meta-synthesis research, saying "reports of qualitative research now appear regularly, not only in exclusively qualitative research publication venues, but also in venues that once rejected qualitative studies as unscientific" (p. 2; see also Britten, 2011). Researchers must avoid doing work that does not build on the knowledge we have by drawing from previous studies to better inform our research questions. Instead of creating "little islands of knowledge," as Glaser and Strauss (1971, p. 181) feared we might, qualitative meta-synthesis gives us the important opportunity to integrate research findings and further push the questions, theories, and interventions that drive our discipline. In return, working within the field of health communication can help to deepen and solidify understandings of the methodology. In these ways, both the meta-synthetic method and the discipline of health communication have much to gain from each other.

Notes

1. For an excellent discussion of the types of meta-study written by the authors of the approaches themselves, please see Thorne, Jensen, Kearney, Noblit, & Sandelowski (2004).
2. Dementia is a clinical diagnosis of symptom presentation defined as "the development of multiple cognitive deficits that include memory impairment and at least one of the following cognitive disturbances: aphasia, apraxia, agnosia, or a disturbance in executive functioning. The cognitive deficits must be sufficiently severe to cause impairment in occupational or social functioning and must represent a decline from a previously higher level of functioning" (American Psychiatric Association, 2000, p. 148). "Dementia" has several etiologic possibilities, of which Alzheimer's disease is one. Alzheimer's disease, while its coherence as a disease entity is contested (George, Whitehouse, & Ballenger, 2011; Richards & Brayne, 2010), is based in the characteristic pathology of neurological tangles and amyloid plaque buildups (American Psychiatric Association, 2000). For the purposes of this paper, we will be using the term "dementia" to describe the condition, except where the studies themselves refer to "Alzheimer's disease" and are quoted directly.
3. Available date ranges for individual databases were as follows: PubMed, 1965–2012; PsycInfo, 1889–2012; Communication Abstracts, 1915–2012; Sociological Abstracts, 1962–2012; Medline, 1965–2012; JSTOR, 1840–2012; and CINHAL, 1982–2012.
4. We began by reviewing the title, keywords, and abstracts. However, if the article's relevance was not clear at that point, we delved into the body text as necessary.
5. This is, of course, in service of a full archaeological disclosure of our application of the meta-synthetic method. Indeed, what is the purpose of this volume, if not the exposing of just such method-in-practice challenges? Too often, we find, the toil that goes on behind the closed doors of offices and research labs is neatly written over, smoothed out, and left on the cutting room floor, in such a way that those seeking to learn a method find themselves frustrated at the amount of angst that can accompany the project. We hope to hold no such illusions here, and, instead, seek to present the process of meta-synthesis in all its occasionally maddening, but, ultimately, rewarding glory.
6. We used a bibliographic citation manager to help us organize the articles into a searchable database. This also allowed us to create a duplicate database so that we could retain one file with the complete 8,158 articles and a second file with narrowed list of 17 articles that met our inclusion criteria.
7. There are several options for bibliographic citation manager software, many of which are accessible through a university library or are available free online.

References

American Psychiatric Association. (2000). *Diagnostic and statistical manual of mental disorders: DSM-IV-TR*. Washington, D.C.: American Psychiatric Association.

Aminzadeh, F., Byszewski, A., Molnar, F. J., & Eisner, M. (2007). Emotional impact of dementia diagnosis: Exploring persons with dementia and caregivers' perspectives. *Aging and Mental Health, 11*(3), 281–290.*

Angen, M. J. (2000). Evaluating interpretive inquiry: Reviewing the validity debate and opening the dialogue. *Qualitative Health Research, 10*(3), 378–395.

Babbie, E. (2004). *The practice of social research.* Belmont, CA: Wadsworth Publishing Company.

Babrow, A. S., & Mattson, M. (2003). Theorizing about health communication. In T. L. Thompson, A. Dorsey, K. Miller, & R. Parrott (Eds.), *Handbook of health communication* (pp. 35–61). Mahwah, NJ: Lawrence Erlbaum Associates.

Barroso, J., & Powell-Cope, G. M. (2000). Metasynthesis of qualitative research on living with HIV infection. *Qualitative Health Research, 10*(3), 340–353.

Beck, C. T. (2001). Caring within nursing education: A metasynthesis. *The Journal of Nursing Education, 40*(3), 101–109.

Beck, C. T. (2002). Postpartum depression: A metasynthesis. *Qualitative Health Research, 12*(4), 453–472.

Blum, N. S. (1994). Deceptive practices in managing a family member with Alzheimer's disease. *Symbolic Interaction, 17*(1), 21–36.*

Bondas, T., & Hall, E. O. C. (2007). Challenges in approaching metasynthesis research. *Qualitative Health Research, 17*(1), 113–121.

Britten, N. (2011). Qualitative research on health communication: What can it contribute? *Patient Education and Counseling, 82*(3), 384–388.

Byszewski, A. M., Molnar, F., Aminzadeh, F. Eisner, M., Gardezi, F., & Bassett, R. (2007). Dementia diagnosis disclosure: A study of patient and caregiver perspectives. *Alzheimer's Disease and Associated Disorders, 21*(2), 107–114.*

Campbell, T. (1996). Technology, multimedia, and qualitative research in education. *Journal of Research on Computing Education, 30*(2), 122–133.

Carey, J. (1975). Review essay: Communication and culture. *Communication Research, 2*(2), 173–191.

Clonts, J. G. (1992). The concept of reliability as it pertains to data from qualitative studies. Paper presented at the Annual Meeting of the Southwest Educational Research Association, January 31–February 2, 1992, Houston, Texas.

Cook, D. J., Mulrow, C. D., & Haynes, R. B. (1997). Systematic reviews: Synthesis of best evidence for clinical decisions. *Annals of Internal Medicine, 126*(5), 376–380.

Day, A. M., James, I. A., Meyer, T. D., & Lee, D. R. (2011). Do people with dementia find lies and deception in dementia care acceptable? *Aging and Mental Health, 15*(7), 822–829.*

Denzin, N. K., & Lincoln, Y. S. (2000). *The Sage handbook of qualitative research.* Thousand Oaks, CA: Sage Publications.

Derksen, E., Vernooij-Dassen, M., Gillissen, F., Olde-Rikkert, M., & Scheltens, P. (2005). The impact of diagnostic disclosure in dementia: A qualitative case analysis. *International Psychogeriatrics, 17*(2), 319–326.*

Duggleby, W., Holtslander, L., Kylma, J., Duncan, V., Hammond, C., & Williams, A. (2010). Metasynthesis of the hope experience of family caregivers of persons with chronic illness. *Qualitative Health Research, 20*(2), 148–158.

Estabrooks, C. A. (1999). Will evidence-based nursing practice make practice perfect? *Canadian Journal of Nursing Research, 30*(4), 273–294.

Estabrooks, C. A., Field, P. A., & Morse, J. M. (1994). Aggregating qualitative findings: An approach to theory development. *Qualitative Health Research, 4*(4), 503–511.

Finfgeld, D. L. (1999). Courage as a process of pushing beyond the struggle. *Qualitative Health Research, 9*(6), 803–814.

Finfgeld, D. L. (2003). Metasynthesis: The state of the art—so far. *Qualitative Health Research, 13*(7), 893–904.

Glaser, B. (1978). *Theoretical sensitivity*. Mill Valley, CA: Sociology Press.

Glaser, B. G., & Strauss, A. L. (1967). *The discovery of grounded theory: Strategies for qualitative research*. New York, NY: Aldine Publishing Company.

Glaser, B. G., & Strauss, A. L. (1971). *Status passage*. Chicago, IL: Aldine Publishing Company.

Glass, G. V. (1977). Integrating findings: The meta-analysis of research. *Review of Research in Education, 5*(1), 351–379.

George, D. R., Whitehouse, P. J., & Ballenger J. F. (2011). The evolving classification of dementia: Placing the DSM-V in a meaningful historical and cultural context and pondering the future of "Alzheimer's". *Culture, Medicine, & Psychiatry, 35*(3), 417–435.

Golafshani, N. (2003). Understanding reliability and validity in qualitative research. *The Qualitative Report, 8*(4), 597–607.

Goldsmith, D. J., & Brashers, D. E. (2008). Communication matters: Developing and testing social support interventions. *Communication Monographs, 75*, 320–330.

Harrison, L. L. (1996). Pulling it all together: The importance of integrative research reviews and meta-analyses in nursing (Editorial). *Journal of Advanced Nursing, 24*(2), 224–225.

Hayes, J., Zimmerman, M. K., & Boylstein, C. (2010). Responding to symptoms of Alzheimer's disease: Husbands, wives, and the gendered dynamics of recognition and disclosure. *Qualitative Health Research, 20*(8), 1101–1115.*

Healy, M., & Perry, C. (2000). Comprehensive criteria to judge validity and reliability of qualitative research within the realism paradigm. *Qualitative Market Research, 3*(3), 118–126.

Hertogh, C. M., The, B. A., Miesen, B. M., & Eefsting, J. A. (2004). Truth telling and truthfulness in the care for patients with advanced dementia: An ethnographic study in Dutch nursing homes. *Social Science and Medicine, 59*(8), 1685–1693.*

Hughes, J. C., Hope, T., Reader, S., & Rice, D. (2002). Dementia and ethics: The view of informal carers. *Journal of the Royal Society of Medicine, 95*(5), 242–246.*

James, I. A., Wood-Mitchell, A. J., Waterworth, A. M., Mackenzie, L. E., & Cunningham, J. (2006). Lying to people with dementia: Developing ethical guidelines for care settings. *International Journal of Geriatric Psychiatry, 21*(8), 800–801.*

Jensen, L. A., & Allen, M. N. (1996). Meta-synthesis of qualitative findings. *Qualitative Health Research, 6*(4), 553–560.

Johnson, R. B. (1997). Examining the validity structure of qualitative research. *Education, 118*(2), 282–292.

Kaduszkiewicz, H., Bachmann, C., & van den Bussche, H. (2008). Telling "the truth" in dementia—Do attitude and approach of general practitioners and specialists differ? *Patient Education and Counseling, 70*(2), 220–226.*

Karnieli-Miller, O., Werner, P., Aharon-Peretz, J., & Eidelman, S. (2007). Dilemmas in the (un)veiling of the diagnosis of Alzheimer's disease: Walking an ethical and professional tightrope. *Patient Education and Counseling, 67*(3), 307–314.*

Kearney, M. H. (2001). Enduring love: A grounded formal theory of women's experience of domestic violence. *Research in Nursing and Health, 24*(4), 270–282.

Keightley, J., & Mitchell, A. (2004). What factors influence mental health professionals when deciding whether or not to share a diagnosis of dementia with the person? *Aging and Mental Health, 8*(1), 13–20.*

Langdon, S., Eagle, A., & Warner, J. (2007). Making sense of dementia in the social world: A qualitative study. *Social Science and Medicine, 64*(4), 989–1000.*

Lincoln, Y. S., & Guba, E. G. (1985). *Naturalistic inquiry*. Newbury Park, CA: Sage Publications.

Lindlof, T. R., & Taylor, B. C. (2002). *Qualitative communication research methods* (2nd ed.). Thousand Oaks, CA: Sage Publications.

MacQuarrie, C. R. (2005). Experiences in early stage Alzheimer's disease: Understanding the paradox of acceptance and denial. *Aging and Mental Health, 9*(5), 430–441.*

Metcalfe, A., Coad, J., Plumridge, G. M., Gill, P., & Farndon, P. (2008). Family communication between children and their parents about inherited genetic conditions: a meta-synthesis of the research. *European Journal of Human Genetics, 16*(10), 1193–1200.

Mishler, E. G. (2000). Validation in inquiry-guided research: The role of exemplars in narrative studies. In B. M. Brizuela, J. P. Stewart, R. G., Carrillo, & J. G., Berger (Eds.), *Acts of inquiry in qualitative research* (pp. 119–146). Cambridge, MA: Harvard Educational Review.

Morgan, D. L. (1998). Practical strategies for combining qualitative and quantitative methods: Applications to health research. *Qualitative Health Research, 8*(3), 362–376.

Morse, J. M. (1994). On the crest of a wave? (Editorial). *Qualitative Health Research, 4*(2), 139–141.

Noblit, G. W., & Hare, R. D. (1988). *Meta-ethnography: Synthesizing qualitative studies*. Newbury Park, CA: Sage Publications.

Parrott, R. (2004). Emphasizing "communication" in health communication. *'Journal of Communication, 54*(4), 751–787.

Paterson, B. L. (2001). The shifting perspectives model of chronic illness. *Journal of Nursing Scholarship, 33*(1), 21–26. doi: 10.1111/j.1547-5069.2001.00021.x

Paterson, B. L., Thorne, S. E., Canam, C., & Jillings, C. (2001) *Meta-study of qualitative health research: A practical guide to meta-analysis and meta-synthesis*. Thousand Oaks, CA: Sage Publications.

Patton, M. Q. (2002). *Qualitative research and evaluation methods*. Thousand Oaks, CA: Sage Publications.

Pinner, G., & Bouman, W. P. (2002). To tell or not to tell: On disclosing the diagnosis of dementia. *International Psychogeriatrics, 14*(2), 127–137.

Richards, M., & Brayne, C. (2010). What do we mean by Alzheimer's disease? *British Medical Journal, 341*(7778), 865–867.

Rimal, R. N., & Lapinski, M. K. (2009). Why health communication is important in public health. *Bulletin of the World Health Organization, 87*(4), 247.

Sandelowski, M., & Barroso, J. (2002). Reading qualitative studies. *International Journal of Qualitative Methods, 1*(1), 74–108.

Sandelowski, M., & Barroso, J. (2007). *Handbook for synthesizing qualitative research*. New York, NY: Springer.

Sandelowski, M., Docherty, S., & Emden, C. (1997). Qualitative metasynthesis: Issues and techniques. *Research in Nursing & Health, 20*(4), 365–371.

Schreiber, R., Crooks, D., & Stern, P. N. (1997). Qualitative meta-analysis. In J. M. Morse (Ed.), *Completing a qualitative project: Details and dialogue* (pp. 311–326). Thousand Oaks, CA: Sage Publications.

Seale, C. (1999). *The quality of qualitative research*. London, England: Sage Publications.

Seaman, A. T. (2010). "I hate to be caught in a lie": The ethics of therapeutic lying. Paper presented at the American Anthropological Association Annual Meeting, New Orleans, Louisiana.

Seaman, A. T., & Stone, A. M. (2012). Metasynthesis of deception in the context of Alzheimer's disease. Unpublished manuscript.

Smith, A. P., & Beattie, B. L. (2001). Disclosing a diagnosis of Alzheimer's disease: Patient and family experiences. *Canadian Journal of Neurological Science, 28*(Suppl. 1), S67–S71.

Stenbacka, C. (2001). Qualitative research requires quality concepts of its own. *Management Decision, 39*(7), 551–555.

Stern, P. (1980). Grounded theory methodology: Its uses and process. *Image: The Journal of Nursing Scholarship, 12*(1), 20–23.

Stern, P., & Harris, C. (1985). Women's health and the self-care paradox: A model to guide self-care readiness. *Health Care for Women International, 6*(1–3), 151–163.

Stern, P., Allen, L., & Moxley, P. (1982). The nurse as grounded theorist: History, process and uses. *The Review Journal of Philosophy and Social Science, 7*, 200–215.

Stone, A. M., & Jones, C. L. (2009). Sources of uncertainty: Experiences of Alzheimer's disease. *Issues in Mental Health Nursing, 30*(11), 677–686.

Strauss, A., & Corbin, J. (1990). *Basics of qualitative research: Grounded theory procedures and techniques*. Newbury Park, CA: Sage Publications.

Taylor, S. J., & Bogdan, R. (1998). *Introduction to qualitative research methods: A guidebook and resource* (3rd ed.). New York, NY: John Wiley.

Thorne, S. (1994). Secondary analysis in qualitative research: Issues and implications. In J. M. Morse (Ed.), *Critical issues in qualitative research methods* (pp. 263–279). London, UK: Sage Publications.

Thorne, S., Jensen, L., Kearney, M. H., Noblit, G., & Sandelowski, M. (2004). Qualitative metasynthesis: Reflections on methodological orientation and ideological agenda. *Qualitative Health Research, 14*, 1342–1365.

Tuckett, A. G. (2007). Stepping across the line: Information sharing, truth telling and the role of the personal carer in the Australian nursing home. *Qualitative Health Research, 17*(4), 489–500.*

Tuckett, A. G. (2012). The experience of lying in dementia care: A qualitative study. *Nursing Ethics, 19*(1), 7–20.*

Van Maanen, J. (1983). *Qualitative methodology*. Thousand Oaks, CA: Sage Publications.

Walsh, D., & Downe, S. (2005). Meta-synthesis method for qualitative research: A literature review. *Journal of Advanced Nursing, 50*(2), 204–211.

Zimmer, L. (2006). Qualitative meta-synthesis: A question of dialoguing with texts. *Methodological Issues in Nursing Research, 53*(3), 311–318.

Cultural, Population, and Critical Concerns

A MATTER OF INTERPRETATION

Rhetorical Criticism of Health Communication

Ashli Q. Stokes

An undergraduate student in the on-campus health center wonders why a brochure for the Gardasil cervical cancer vaccine, which protects against the sexually transmitted infection HPV, does not mention how the infection is contracted. A parent online tries to decide which medicine is right for treating her daughter's ADHD. Physicians around the United States observe that requests for a particular prescription allergy medication have increased significantly following a televised seasonal advertising campaign. A local health educator in a large Southeastern city wonders how to better reach its growing, young, Hispanic audience about the importance of monthly breast self-exams. MS sufferers celebrate the approval of a new oral drug to treat the disease following a woman's passionate testimony at a FDA hearing. Each of these scenarios highlights the importance of the study of rhetoric in health communication.

Though scholars define rhetoric in various ways, generally it refers to the study of persuasive discourses, be they spoken, written, mediated, or encountered face to face (Campbell & Burkholder, 1997). This chapter explains the uses of rhetorical criticism in the study of health communication, describing the nature of the method and providing instruction and examples in how to employ it. Rhetorical criticism of health communication might not be as well known as some of the other methods described in this volume, but a closer look illuminates how it can be invaluable in answering important questions about how best to communicate health information, the consequences of those messages, and how cultures come to understand and address particular health concerns.

Nature of Method

Description of Method

Health communication scholars employing rhetorical criticism may be concerned with the persuasive elements of texts (Segal, 2005), but how critics approach this analysis is incredibly varied. Critics are interested in how the use of persuasion shapes relationships, identity, and action (Burke, 1969; Lingard, 2007). Similarly, they rely on rhetorical analysis because it provides "judgment upon texts for their ability to persuade, narrative prowess, or ideological positioning" (Hess, 2011, p. 128). Analyses might show, then, how young women come to *identify* with the anorexic identity on Tumblr, analyzing how they relate to, or are inspired by, the rhetoric of "thinspo." They might explore how a campaign *persuades* men to go to the doctor more frequently. Critics might investigate the *ideological positioning* at work in how we come to think, as a culture, that vaccinating our children might lead to autism, for example, or how fitness ads targeted toward young women may contribute paradoxically to developing poor body image. In summary, then, rhetorical critics explore advocacy, and they do so by evaluating the quality of persuasion and argumentation and suggesting how it might be improved (Elwood, 1995; Hess, 2011).

Interpretation is a key word in the rhetorical criticism enterprise (Brock, Scott, & Chesebro, 1990). Therefore, if a text represents a speaker's choices, "the critic's job is to identify these rhetorical choices and then consider possible interpretative implications (not message effects per se) in light of relevant information about the audience and or/social context of the rhetorical act" (Kline, 2007, p. 87). This interpretation goes beyond what an individual reader or critic might take away, however, as the method is designed to suggest how a variety of audience members might make meaning from a text (Kline, 2007). Whether persuasion is addressed to an individual or particular group, and whether that discourse emanates from an organization (such as a hospital) or from an individual (such as a nurse or physician), rhetorical criticism is a method "that analyses discourse, and illuminates the process by which such discourse influenced the targeted publics" (Elwood, 1995, p. 8). Some of the purposes of using rhetorical criticism in health communication should be coming into focus, but there are others that deserve mention. Criticism might help shape or improve public taste, helping to educate audience members and/or helping them to be better judges or consumers of health communication (Jasinski, 2001). Criticism might also help fight oppression and injustice, helping less advantaged communities to organize for better health services, for example, or teaching college students to resist harmful health behaviors.

Jasinski (2001), drawing on Hart (1990) and others, offers a comprehensive description of the how rhetorical critics go about the various ways of employing the method. There are five crucial characteristics: definition, classification, analysis, interpretation, and evaluation. First, criticism *defines*, meaning that it must identify objects as rhetorical. Commonly, an object is seen as rhetorical if it responds to situational exigencies or constraints, possesses persuasive intent, or ties to induce identification (Jasinski, 2001). A rhetorical critic would argue, then, that a rally to protest proposed changes restricting abortion should be defined as a rhetorical event, one that seeks to persuade others to alter policy leading to behaviors.

Criticism also *classifies*, whereby a rhetorical act is placed into a particular category, and *analyzes*, where critics seek to learn how particular rhetorical strategies function (Jasinski, 2001). Examples of classification involve critics putting a rhetorical act into a type of genre, such as apologia, where a rhetor makes a speech of defense or epideictic, which praises or celebrates. Health scholars are frequently interested in rhetorical activity that is classified as deliberative, meaning they seek to understand how particular health policies or decisions come about. Criticism also analyzes, where critics describe how a rhetorical act or text is constructed and how it functions. Describing this crucial category in detail would require a separate essay, but, in general, analysis can draw on the once dominant neo-Aristotelian perspective, looking for the five traditional canons of rhetoric (invention, arrangement, style, memory, and delivery) and the three modes of proof (ethos, logos, and pathos). Today, critics might focus on understanding how texts and public action can function as types of social or political power. Health scholars engaged in this sort of analysis might look, for example, at how city policies regarding public transportation subtly discriminate against the disabled and how specific types of protest strategies and tactics seek changes in accessibility laws (Quinlan & Bates, 2012).

Criticism also *interprets* and *evaluates*, which are more disputed characteristics in the discipline (Jasinski, 2001). When engaged in interpretation, critics try to reflect on particular stylistic textual phenomena in order to show how or what a rhetor was doing in a particular rhetorical text. Also thought of as translating or decoding the rhetorical object, critics must be careful of noting the polysemous nature of a text, where one critic's interpretation might differ from another's, as well as one audience member's from another's. Whereas the Truth anti-smoking campaign is widely praised for reducing teen smoking by appealing to rebellion (Rosenberg, 2012), for instance, there are always those in the target audience who may find the campaign messages patronizing and ineffective. Critics of this step-wise process described here (looking first for style, argument, and structure, then interpreting) also argue that analysis and interpretation are unavoidably interwoven (see Fish, 1980, for more on this critique). Finally, during the evaluation process critics bring their own assumptions, beliefs, and political positions to a text in ways that should be acknowledged in a piece of criticism (Jasinski, 2001).

As there is disciplinary disagreement about various steps in the criticism process, there are also debates about the standards available for evaluation, with some looking for the effects of a rhetorical act and others more concerned with response, indicative of the challenge of determining rhetorical effectiveness (Jasinski, 2001). Noting that it is difficult to "prove" the outcome of a rhetorical act on an audience, critics should be most concerned with the quality of rhetorical effort. Critics can also look at the persuasiveness of a speech or employ a critical touchstone. There are ongoing concerns that rhetoricians be careful of claiming specific effects of rhetorical efforts, leading this characteristic to become somewhat downplayed in contemporary criticism. Today, scholars might focus more on interpretation and analysis in their pieces, with others looking at how messages perpetuate particular ideologies (Jasinski, 2001). Emmons (2010), for example, after providing analysis and interpretation of the "discourse of depression," such as metaphors like the "black dog of depression" and "the blues," contends that this language perpetuates contemporary attitudes toward mental health and illness. She argues that women, in particular, may come to self-medicate and describe themselves through gendered illness identities. Thus, like Emmons, many critics choose to examine gradual shifts in language patterns, preferences, or particular ideologies concerning health. Ultimately, however, when working on evaluation, critics still struggle with judging a text's ethical, aesthetic, logical, or effects standards.

Theoretical Assumptions

From the previous description of the method, it should be clear that rhetoricians do not "separate" themselves from their research in ways that social scientists might. There are four theoretical assumptions in rhetorical criticism that often create a closer relationship between critic and what is being critiqued. First, and most broadly, rhetoricians assume that reality is constructed through language and culture is perpetuated through discourse. As a result, they are interested not only in the measurable outcome of a particular campaign, but how that campaign might shift a culture's views about a particular health issue. Scholars using the rhetorical method to analyze recent anti-bullying campaigns like It Gets Better would be interested in the outcomes of the campaign (number of bullying instances decreasing against lesbian, gay, and transgender adolescents), but they would also look at how the campaign begins to shift our culture's understanding of lesbian, gay, and transgender people as a whole. Does the campaign help society to become more inclusive of gay lifestyles while reducing bullying instances?

Next, many rhetorical critics now also assume that they are unable to take a neutral, disinterested stance toward a critical object, with contemporary scholars arguing that this position is both impossible and unethical (see Jasinski, 2001, for an overview of this important debate). In general, debate over the role of a critic is central in rhetorical studies, but, today, they are less likely to believe that there is an object for study upon which particular theories can be simply brought to bear. Today's rhetorical critics recognize that they bring their own particular ideologies and biases into the study of a particular rhetorical phenomenon. In their book *Body Talk: Rhetoric, Technology, Reproduction*, for instance, the authors note that they use rhetorical analysis to reveal the gendered nature of societal and medical views about reproduction, arguing that their analysis is more inclusive of women's voices than once dominant neo-Aristotelian approaches (Brown, 2001; Lay, Gurak, Gravon, & Myntti, 2000).

Third, in the same way that many scholars recognize that they bring a set of ideological assumptions to a text, they also note that a text does not just have one meaning (see Jasinski, 2001). Rhetoric is polysemous, as discussed briefly above, meaning that any rhetorical act can be read in numerous ways, and, thus, the critic's perspective is selective (Brock et al., 1990). Critics do not determine a text's right or wrong meaning, but, rather, consider which meaning is privileged (Hall, 1997). Although critics may point out themes or types of representation not apparent to laypeople (Dow, 1996) and challenge "the obvious thinking about what a given text means" (Kline, 2003, p. 567), they recognize that audiences may take away different meanings from a particular health message.

Finally, rhetorical critics assume that there is an object they can critique, but what can constitute that object is increasingly debated (see Jasinski, 2001). Some scholars assume that rhetorical criticism analyzes an object of persuasive discourse, but others argue that critics assemble texts or artifacts out of a sea of discursive fragments (see Black, 1978, and McGee, 1990, for more on this important debate). In this tradition, a critic interested in the discourse of military veteran post-traumatic stress disorder might analyze transcripts from policy meetings, literature distributed to Veterans Affairs patients, and brochures given to family members. Still others study the rhetoric of health-related social movements (e.g., sustainable eating); controversy (vaccination); and particular genres (public awareness campaigns). Regardless of how this debate is engaged, rhetorical critics must study some type of persuasive object; in doing so, they must also decide how to engage its persuasive elements, a complex process described in the next section.

Applications and Exemplars

Broadly speaking, rhetorical criticism is ideal for understanding the implications of particular symbolic choices, the structure and sequence of arguments or narratives, and the way particular images resonate within cultures (see Brock et al., 1990; Kline, 2007; Lupton, 1992). Health communication scholars use the method for understanding how health messages induce cooperation or compliance as well as promote identification with a set of health beliefs or perspectives (Kline, 2007). To further demarcate the types of uses of rhetorical criticism in health communication, and recognizing there are exceptions, analyses tend to commonly take three forms. The majority of scholars use the method to: (a) critique campaigns, media representation of health or illness, or other mediated health communication form; (b) critique the patient–provider relationship and suggest ways to improve it; or (c) look more broadly at the formation of health policy, perspectives, and worldviews.

Representing the first broad category of health-related rhetorical analysis, Thornton (2010) analyzes the 2006 Depression is Real campaign. Critics increasingly engage there types of public awareness campaigns. Designed to counter misperceptions of depression among racial minorities—specifically, African and Latino Americans who may be reluctant to accept a depression diagnosis and pharmaceutical treatments—Thornton (2010) reveals how the Depression is Real campaign works to expand the boundaries of depression diagnosis in some problematic ways. The campaign, although sponsored by a number of patient advocacy groups, two social justice organizations, and financed by different pharmaceutical industries, ultimately articulates racial and cultural differences "as 'risks' in the context of illness that must be eradicated through individual initiatives via the agency of medical science" (Thornton, 2010, p. 311). That is, Thornton (2010) shows how racial identity is pathologized as a "barrier to empowerment and freedom" requiring consumption of pharmaceuticals as an attractive, and perhaps obligatory, choice as pathways to these ideals (p. 330).

Another example of the first broad type of criticism, like Thornton, Kline (2007) is interested in the implications of rhetorical choices, but she employs the method to help design health educational materials for specific audiences. She looks at the implications of rhetorical choices in breast cancer education materials for African American audiences, looking at whether the information is culturally sensitive. She examines the implicit values conveyed in the discursive choices of the materials, both visual and textual, and argues that, although some adaptations have been made in some pamphlets that acknowledge African American cultural values, many messages could be further revised to provide a more comprehensive, balanced, and accurate discussion of the breast cancer issue in this community. Perlmutter Bowen and Michal-Johnson (1990) take a similar approach in using the rhetorical perspective to help design HIV education for Black urban adolescents. They explore the rhetorical strategies used to persuade the adolescent audience, as well as the lines of argument more likely to be resonant with this target audience.

Representing the second most frequently used rhetorical method, Segal (2007) examines how the way that migraine patients build cases for their illnesses results in particular physician recommendation and treatment. She argues that we should view the patient–physician interview as an exchange of arguments to help physicians come away from viewing migraine sufferers, or sufferers of other types of "contestable" diseases, as particular "types" of patients. Doing so, she argues, moves attention away from what patients *are* to what they *say*, providing physicians another way to evaluate and adjudicate patient complaints (Segal, 2007). As she points out, physicians are "gatekeepers for the kingdom of the sick," and patients may only receive treatment when a physician has been persuaded that someone is indeed ill (p. 231). In cases of "contestable" diseases, such as migraine, fibromyalgia, and chronic fatigue syndrome, it falls to patients to persuade physicians that they have a "real disease" (Segal, 2007). She argues that the exchanges between patients and physicians are necessarily rhetorical, as each seeks (sometimes unconsciously) to persuade the other of something. Applying the rhetorical strategies of *kairos* and *pisteis*, she looks at how accounts of illness are both contingent and made of several types of persuasive appeals. In forwarding this view of the patient–physician relationship, she does not seek to compete with biomedical accounts of illness, but suggests that rhetorical ones offer the ability to study illness as argumentation.

The third tradition uses the method to examine the rhetoric of health and medicine and what it means for particular health policies (e.g., Condit, 1994, 1999; Hyde, 2001; Lay et al., 2000). For instance, Segal (2005) explores health and medicine issues such as norms and values in public health and the public debate on health policy through rhetorical principles. She examines the role of persuasion in hypochondria, the rhetoric of death and dying and the importance of end-of-life talks, and the use of metaphor in health policy, such as "medicine is a business," and "the person is genes." Segal (2005) shows how health policy debates can be constrained through such metaphors, and calls for new ones to be used. Other scholars working within this third area might specialize, such as Lay et al. (2000), who focus on feminist rhetorical criticism in matters of health and science, pointing out how women may be constrained by particular conceptions. In this tradition, for example, Britt (2001) shows how insurance companies construct medical definitions of "infertility" in ways that complicate the problem rather than ease it for women.

Condit's (1990) work provides another example of scholarship concerned with how health policy, perspectives, and worldviews form through the use of rhetoric. She studies how we arrived at current abortion laws and practices by tracing the public discourse surrounding the topic over several decades. Similarly, she explores how language patterns about genetics influences healthcare policy, looking at how genetics research affects women's reproductive options (Condit, 2000). Hyde (2001) examines the definitions, arguments, and narratives that shape the debate and practice of euthanasia and physician-assisted suicide. These scholars illustrate the complex relationship between the way we conceive, discuss, and implement policies surrounding health issues.

If it is possible to divide the use of rhetorical criticism in the three main types detailed in this section, it is not as easy to delineate the steps critics follow in employing the method, as practices vary widely. Nevertheless, this chapter now addresses the procedures used when employing the method of rhetorical criticism for analyzing health issues.

Employing the Method

Procedures

As there are many different approaches to rhetorical criticism, I "deconstruct" several examples in this section to illuminate its various procedures, strengths, and challenges. These examples show varying ways to engage in criticism, but they also illustrate that scholars are systematic, following a particular process or employing a particular critical touchstone. Still, the process of criticism has evolved over the years. Into the middle of the 20th century, neo-Aristotelian criticism was dominant (briefly described previously), and, today, there are more than 60 critical methods listed for rhetorical criticism, including archetype, Burkeian, fantasy theme, game theory, and Marxist critique. Some critics use what is called a "generative approach," whereby they generate units of analysis for criticism, rather than selecting them from formal developed methods of criticism (Kline, 2007). Critics choosing this approach do not use highly operationalized variables, with predetermined criteria, like those who do content analysis (Kline, 2007). Kline (2007) compares this process to that of an open-ended interview, where she uses an inductive approach to first read the text to isolate units of analysis. Often, once common forms of arguments, claims, and so on, are located, critics use a particular theoretical perspective to help glean insight into the implications of their use.

In general, scholars today resist too rigid a critical method, wanting to apply various approaches or techniques to best illuminate a text (Jasinski, 2001). Further, today's criticism is often more conceptual in nature, with critics moving away from illustrating particular motifs found in a set of rhetorical artifacts to showing how texts express power or ideology, for example (Jasinski, 2001). These more conceptual studies do not follow a series of set procedures, making them harder for budding critics to replicate or duplicate. As a result, it is helpful to think of rhetorical criticism as a process, or a set of steps, which I describe here.

One important part of conducting rhetorical criticism of a health issue is to locate a relevant, controversial, or otherwise interesting object for analysis. Over the years, for example, the author of the present chapter has been interested in the persuasive appeals and consumer health literacy implications of direct-to-consumer advertising (DTCA), or "any promotional effort by a pharmaceutical company to present prescription drug information to the general public and the lay media" (Huh, DeLorme, & Reid 2005, p. 569).[1] Approved since 1997, these prescription drug ads often appear on television or in magazines, with consumers encountering DTCA more than any other type of health communication (Kuehn, 2010).

Scholars and practitioners debate whether DTCA simply boosts prescription drug sales or strengthens health literacy, which can be thought of as the ability and knowledge to use health and medical information to promote and maintain physical health (Bell, Taylor, & Kravitz, 2010; Epps et al., 2007). Consumers' increasing reliance on the Internet for health information has refreshed the debate over DTCA, as consumers now consult the web more than their physicians about medical concerns (Weppner, Hollon, Chew, & Larson, 2009). Thus, to investigate how online DTCA (ODTCA) may play a significant role in how Americans think about their health, consume medical information and consider treatment, and understand health care (Heffernan, 2011), I decided to examine an ODTCA campaign addressing infertility, drawing on this example to contend that this type of web-based presentation of health information deserves greater scrutiny by regulatory agencies due to the strength of its persuasive appeals. In other words, I found the DTCA debate refreshed by companies' use of the Internet, building from this initial interest to then finding a relevant campaign to analyze. Those interested in the method should follow a similar process, becoming interested in a health question and then finding an object for analysis that provides a way to explore the concern. Sometimes, critics work the other way, however, finding themselves struck by a particular campaign and, through its analysis, connecting that campaign to a larger health concern or issue.

Whichever way an object is selected for analysis, critics look at how various types of persuasive strategies and/or symbolic communication make meaning about diseases, conditions, or other health issues (Foss, 1996; Heath, 2009). In my example, I wanted to see how online uses of DTCA made particular meanings about infertility. I chose to examine the Increase Your Chances (IYC) campaign, created by Merck's EMD Serono Division in 2010. The campaign provides a health information awareness site for infertility, which interested users can choose after typing "infertility" into a search engine. The site also offers a series of shareable videos about infertility; links to a site called Fertilitylifelines.com, a Merck-sponsored healthcare information site; and a one-click link to its Gonal-F infertility treatment information.

Whether investigating the IYC campaign or other artifact, in general, critics must explore the content of the communicative artifact itself, its context or occasion, the persons addressed, and the purpose of the message or artifact (Lingard, 2007). Especially critical is understanding the "exigence"or urgency rhetors face, a very important part in evaluating rhetorical efforts. As disciplinary pioneer Bitzer (1968) pointed out, each of these rhetorical situations presents an audience and a set of constraints that a speaker faces (including audience, occasion, speaker, speech). The rhetorical situation can be thought of as a "configuration of physical circumstances and earlier rhetorical attempts to shape perceptions" (Elwood, 1995, p. 12); how rhetors (corporate, organizational, institutional, individual, or otherwise) respond to the rhetorical situation forms the field of interest for critics.

As part of the critical process, critics must contextualize their campaigns, artifacts, or texts as a type of rhetorical form, ideally showing how the artifact is an example of a particular type of discourse. For example, Thornton (2010), in her analysis of the Depression is Real campaign, needed to present the campaign as an exemplar of what she calls "psychiatric governmentality," which erases racial identity in the pursuit of disease awareness. As such, she traces the history of disease awareness campaigns, showing how they instruct the public about diseases, help individuals to screen themselves and their loved ones, and, ideally, promote social acceptance as an alternative to stigma. To make the case for her argument about the negative implications of the Depression is Real campaign, she also must describe the origination and execution of the campaign, describe the groups involved in its production, and pay particular attention to the role of pharmaceutical industries in its construction. Since she is also describing the campaign as a type of governmentality rhetoric that controls people not by direct imposition but by aligning diverse agents through shared vocabularies (Thornton, 2010), she must trace the development of this type of psychiatric rhetoric as one that does not abandon appeals to race but constructs them in paradoxical fashion.

Critics then analyze how particular rhetorical strategies function in a key text or texts. In Thornton's (2010) example, she isolates the strategies of stigma and risk in the Depression is Real campaign, looking for ways that the campaign locates "stigma" within the African American community that are risks "best ameliorated through medical treatments" (p. 322). She then looks at how these strategies work in various campaign media, presenting typical examples of their wording, visuals, and how these strategies work to position race as "risk factor" that must be managed (Thornton, 2010, p. 326).

I followed a similar process to explore how persuasive strategies functioned in the IYC campaign. To explain how IYC and other ODTCA campaigns make meaning about particular health conditions, I first looked for its identifying features, noting there were three key strategies addressing consumer identity. I loosely relied on dramatistic criticism (thus doing a type of genre criticism mentioned earlier) to guide my analysis and help strengthen its claims about the strategy of identification. In the IYC campaign, reassurance, encouragement, and subtle promotion emerged as identification strategies that create common ground in order to shape consumer knowledge about diseases and health conditions, cultivate a positive image for particular products among consumers, and influence consumer purchasing decisions (Berkowitz, 2003; Condit, 1994; Foss, 1996; Stokes, 2005).

One part of my argument about ODTCA is that it cannot completely serve a health literacy purpose, often favoring promotion and sales over consumer education. So, in my analysis, for example, I first looked at how the Increaseyourchances.org website reassures infertility sufferers that they are not alone in dealing with complex emotions surrounding the condition, and provides a particular type of education for consumers that emphasizes drug sales. The story-based videos on Increaseyourchances.org take a different approach than is typical in addressing infertility. Instead of offering users dry statistics about the condition, or sharing patient stories about the often heartbreaking condition, Increaseyourchances.org addresses the subject through warmth, dark humor, and sarcasm. Featuring the tagline "Birds and bees can't always make babies," its five videos introduce site visitors to Neil and Karen, an "average" couple suffering from infertility. Site visitors can watch Neil and Karen deal with the problem through the series of videos each addressing a different facet of infertility, such as social pressure to conceive and feelings of helplessness. What makes the site distinctive is its emotional, but darkly comedic and absurdist approach: the videos have the couple discussing challenging infertility issues with Neal dressed as a bumblebee and Karen as a bluebird. They feature sarcastic dialogue such as the following:

> NEIL (*to his wife*): Oh, and Jane's pregnant again.
>
> KAREN (*after a stunned pause*): Whatevs.
>
> NEIL: What?
>
> KAREN: It's just? It seems like? It just seems like Jane can run into a pole and get pregnant. Y'know? And she has the nerve to ask me when we're going to start.
>
> NEIL: We have been trying for a while.
>
> KAREN: I hate her uterus.

Another video shows Karen miserably helping to record baby gifts at a friend's baby shower (in a voice-over, Karen complains, "Who has a shower for their fourth child, anyway?"). Another has Neil remarking, "They're pregnancy tests, they're not scratch-off tickets," after finding Karen's secret stashes of negative pregnancy tests that she insists must be wrong.

In my example, then, I argue that couples suffering from infertility can relate to Neil and Karen's experiences, the absurdist approach allowing them, perhaps oddly enough, to identify with the protagonists. That they are dressed in costumes allows anyone to identify with their experience, regardless if they don't look the same or talk exactly the same as the consumer might. Instead, their ridiculous appearance may provide catharsis, crystallizing the types of emotion couples may experience, with infertility presented as a common, but difficult, part of life. As Karen explains, "We take care of ourselves. We exercise (*flash to a shot of the two playing tennis in their costumes*), but we can't get pregnant." Between the relatable stories and educational content that, for example, informs consumers about the frequency of the infertility condition (1 in 8 women) and corrects myths (it is always easy to get pregnant), viewers may find the site affirming.

After illustrating how strategies work in the given artifact, critics must then present the implications of the use of these strategies in the health campaign or in other types of health media. In my example, I showed how, in addition to providing affirmation, the IYC site also begins to construct a tension, as infertility treatments, and particularly IVF, become the primary answers to the infertility problem. After consumers watch the identification-inducing videos with Neil and Karen, the site offers consumers messages that attempt to reassure them about infertility. One notes, for example, that, "Seeing a fertility specialist does not mean you've given up on Mother Nature. Up to 85–90% of fertility issues are treatable, and less than 5% lead to IVF (in-vitro fertilization)." Note how this statement references natural approaches to reassure consumers that their efforts may pay off, but then, by stressing how many issues are *treatable*, the inference is that something medical must be done for such couples to become pregnant. Ultimately, the site's messages reinforce an understanding of fertility that promotes expensive medical intervention, and work to heighten the sense of anxiety and urgency couples facing the condition have. Particularly since the messages stress the importance of time, couples may feel acutely the need to seek this particular medical intervention. The rest of my analysis showed how these strategies rely on identification to construct infertility as a condition that must be addressed quickly, and with a particular product and procedure, in order to increase chances of successful conception and reproduction (Stokes, 2005).

Similarly, Thornton (2010) must assess the implications of the rhetorical strategies used in the Depression is Real campaign. Instead of focusing on commercial implications, as I did, Thornton considers the potential racial consequences of the campaign's strategies. She argues that, despite a commitment to racial diversity, the campaign defines racial difference as pathology and illness, presents mental health as "color-aversive," and suggests that mental health is key to African American empowerment. However, she points out that this empowerment requires pharmaceutical consumption, a choice that carries both medical and moral implications. As Thornton (2010) does, critics must attempt to move beyond a particular campaign, suggesting how particular discourses function more broadly in our culture. The Depression is Real campaign, along with other disease awareness campaigns, then, help usher in more subtle forms of racism because they work collectively to privatize and individualize racial and economic problems. Thornton (2010) argues that we need sustained critiques of such contemporary psychiatric discourse in order to provide social critique and democratic engagement. Again, though, the point of criticism is to suggest how discourse—here, in the form of a campaign—may shift cultural patterns over time, not to claim that there is a clear, measurable effect of them. In this way, rhetorical critics address the ideals of reliability and validity in different ways than do social scientists.

Reliability and Validity

As Thornton's (2010) and my analyses show, the standard scientific concepts of reliability and validity are problematic for the rhetorician for two reasons. First, subjectivity is necessarily involved in rhetorical analysis, which challenges the strongly held value of objective assessment in social science research (Lingard, 2007). Rhetorical critics are not as concerned with reliability and validity in the same way a social scientist would be, but, nevertheless, they do follow steps so that their studies can be understood and/or followed by other interested scholars. In order to help assure that the results of the inquiry will be valid, rhetorical critics do have a process, such that someone following a recipe for chocolate cake will get a similar result, whether or not the individuals live in different parts of the country (Jasinski, 2001). More importantly, "measuring" the effects of a particular rhetorical effort is not the point of criticism, but, rather, the method seeks to offer a meaningful interpretation of a rhetorical act. Again, critics loosely follow certain steps to boost an analysis' strengths of claims and/or interpretation. Further, without attention to following certain steps or procedures traditional in the discipline, they may find themselves unable to convince others to read, interpret, or otherwise understand an object of study in the same way they do. In other words, argument is everything in rhetorical analysis, and critics must take care to ensure that they build a strong one to convince others to see the importance of, or agree with, their claims and analyses.

Strengths and Limitations of Method

Strengths

From our detailed look at the myriad examples of criticism in this chapter, one key benefit of conducing rhetorical criticism of health communication is that critics show how and why a particular persuasive effort functions and why it matters in terms of public health. Studies that seek to learn how language "facilitates and delimits human agency" (Brown, 2001, p. 2) in terms of health concerns function as a type of intervention; that is, when we understand how language works, we see how it can include or exclude certain groups or viewpoints in forming health policy and procedures. The scholars in *Body Talk* (Lay et al., 2000) show how this process works in controlling women's reproductive practices, encouraging women to re-appropriate control over these issues through language. Thornton's (2010) analysis highlights the danger in individualizing health campaigns, and how "blaming the victim" is a problematic part of contemporary psychiatric discourse. Similarly, my analysis of the IYC campaign (Stokes, 2005) illustrates that promotion and education may be conflated in ODTCA campaigns in general, which adds to the overall scholarly concerns about the role of DTCA in American pharmaceutical marketing. Users may be empowered and encouraged to take action about infertility, but, between the featured videos and other vignettes, pursuing prescription treatment becomes the primary reaction couples should have when faced with the infertility problem. In this way, the rhetorical strategies offered favor particular prescription treatments, and encourage a commercial worldview for approaching health, which echoes the assessment of traditional DTCA (Stokes, 2005). Further, since currently pharmaceutical companies have a good deal of leeway in marketing their products in the online environment, analysis of the IYC campaign suggests that closer regulatory attention to ODTCA is incredibly important. Consumers are not going online to research cars or buy household supplies; rather, they use the information they find to make important health decisions.

In addition to revealing how public health policy and worldviews form, rhetorical analysis has other strengths in studying health communication. It can help "translate" scientific information to lay publics and audiences, such as risk communication scholars using rhetoric to examine how various publics respond to different messages (see Schwartzman, Ross, & Berube, 2011). For example, Amberg and Hall (2010) argue that journalists' rhetorical practices offer conflicting information about the dangers of contamination in eating farmed salmon, suggesting that even the use of highly precise numerical data is presented to readers in likely confusing ways. It can show how risk categories form, and how these categories frame the way research is conducted, money is allocated, and policies are created. For instance, since the AIDS risk was categorized early on as largely affecting homosexuals, Haitians, and hemophiliacs, as a result, women, infants, and other "unclassified" groups did not receive as much attention in the medical literature, research, and treatment (Preda, 2005). Another strength of rhetorical analysis is that it can showcase how health policy and prevention efforts are targeted incorrectly because they are shaped by particular social values, as McKenna (2011) does in her study of methamphetamine abuse. On the whole, the strength of the rhetorical enterprise is in showing how language used in health communication includes and excludes, highlights and downplays, praises and criticizes—often with significant implications in making health decisions.

Limitations

For all its usefulness, rarely can rhetorical critics claim that their analyses alone reveal or guarantee how a particular persuasive phenomenon functions; instead, they must argue that, taken as a whole, in concert with other strategies, or on the basis of certain things that seemingly shift in culture, their explanation is valid. For example, although I examined an example of ODTCA that includes each of the main types of the genre found on the Internet today by analyzing the IYC campaign, my findings are limited because these may not represent the full range of ODTCA. My example also represents another common limitation of rhetorical criticism of health issues; like mine, many applications of rhetorical criticism focus on analyzing Western medicine and health systems. Further, rhetorical studies are sometimes critiqued for being too abstract, theoretical, culturally biased, or esoteric, and, as such, scholars should take care that their work addresses, or is grounded in, practical health problems and concerns (Messner, 2006).

Challenges

It is important that critics do more than think about how particular rhetorical strategies are at work in an object of analysis; they must also explain why the use of particular rhetorical strategies matter, or what their consequences might be. They need to suggest why we should take note, as health scholars and practitioners, of how a persuasive strategy is operating in our culture. For example, my analysis of the IYC campaign raises a red flag about how well ODTCA campaigns can serve a health literacy function in general. The campaign may use reassurance, empowerment, and education strategies, but the use of the subtle promotion strategy, where content functions as narrative-based, relatable entertainment rather than direct, sales-driven pitches, provides a particular, corporately influenced way of shaping consumers' perceptions.

Similarly, it is helpful when critics use their rhetorical skills to offer grounded practical suggestions in improving health communication efforts. Landau (2011), for instance, does more than just critique the rhetorical strategies at work in Merck's 2006 Tell Someone, direct-to-consumer advertising campaign to educate about the human papillomavirus (HPV). She first observes that the campaign problematically presents middle- to upper-middle-class adult women as the only people who contract HPV, amplifies the equation that HPV equals cancer, and functions with other campaigns to present women's bodies as inherently diseased. Then, however, she offers an improved video for a public health campaign about HPV. This effort to translate interpretive skills into informed healthcare practice and policy formation is also seen in a number of recent developments and foci within the field.

Recent Developments

There are three broad categories that represent recent trends and developments in employing the rhetorical method in health communication. Some scholars in medical communication and education, of late, are teaching rhetoric to complement medical training, using its tenets to help teach novice medical students, to explain the nature of socialization on clinical teams, and to explore communication patterns and patient safety (see Lingard, 2007, for a detailed description of this use of rhetoric).

Another developing use of the method is in exploring the "everydayness" of rhetorical discourses, with scholars combining the method with ethnography. The critic still seeks to explain advocacy or argumentation, but here she might travel with or otherwise experience an organization's ideals and events. Hess (2011) calls this approach "embodied advocacy," where researchers are interested in, and participate in, deliberation as it occurs (see Blair, 2011; Brummett, 2008; Dickinson, 2002; Dickinson, Ott, & Aoki, 2006, for examples of criticism of local discourses). Hess (2011) uses this approach to make drug safety advocacy in the Rave scene more effective, for example, structuring messages as a result of his experience in the community.

Rhetorical analysis is also being used to enhance knowledge about bioterrorism and pandemic communication, genetic testing and research, and reproductive choices and challenges. Keränen (2011) examines the rhetorics of science and medicine that support the development, proliferation, and potential use of biological weapons agents, cautioning against the buildup of biodefense. Angeli (2012) uses rhetorical analysis to understand the metaphors surrounding H1N1 and swine flu. Lynch (2011) uses rhetorical analysis to examine genetic testing and research. Gronnvoll and Landau (2010) follow a similar metaphoric approach to examine the consequences of three common genetic metaphors, (1) genes as a disease or problem, (2) genes as fire or bomb, and (3) genes as gambling, to suggest implications for public health. Finally, genetic models of health are playing roles in scholars' work on issues of women's reproductive choice and decision making. Silva (2011) argues that a cultural focus on the individual can make abortion seem like the only moral, and responsible, choice for families facing the possibility of a disabled child. Weingarten (2012) also examines the role of choice surrounding abortion and reproductive technologies, arguing that relying on the discourse of "choice" may limit women's ability to make choices about abortion freely because of social and political pressures, economic inequalities, and insufficient knowledge.

The variety of recent developments and trends in rhetorical criticism of health suggests the field is headed in some exciting directions. Far from being merely a theoretical pursuit or abstraction, the use of criticism in health communication yields important insights in the study of health communication. Rhetorical criticism may be a matter of interpretation, but its skilled application helps drive message development, policy formation, and patient/consumer decision making in invaluable ways.

Note

1. The extended example used in this section was first published in *The Routledge Companion to Advertising and Promotional Culture*. The author has received publisher permission to use the excerpts included here.

References

Amberg, S., & Hall, T. (2010). Precision and rhetoric in media reporting about contamination in farmed salmon. *Science Communication, 32*(4), 489–513.

Angeli, E. L. (2012). Metaphors in the rhetoric of pandemic flu: Electronic media coverage of H1N1 and swine flu. *Journal of Technical Writing and Communication, 42*(3), 203–222.

Bell, R. A., Taylor, L. D., & Kravitz, R. L. (2010). Do antidepressant advertisements educate consumers and promote communication between patients with depression and their physicians? *Patient Education and Counseling, 81*(2), 245–250.

Berkowitz, S. J. (2003). Originality, conversation and reviewing rhetorical criticism. *Communication Studies, 54*(3), 359–363.

Bitzer, L. F. (1968). The rhetorical situation. *Philosophy and Rhetoric, 1*(1), 1–14.

Black, E (1978). *Rhetorical criticism: A study in method.* Madison, WI: University of Wisconsin Press.

Blair, C. (2011). Reflections on criticism and bodies: parables from public places. *Western Journal of Communication, 65*(3), 271–294.

Britt, E. C. (2001). *Conceiving normalcy: Rhetoric, law, and the double binds of infertility.* Tuscaloosa, AL: University of Alabama Press.

Brock, B. L., Scott, R. L., & Chesebro, J. W. (1990). *Methods of rhetorical criticism: a twentieth century perspective* (3rd ed.). Detroit, MI: Wayne State University Press.

Brown, D. (2001). Review of "Body talk: Rhetoric, technology, reproduction." *Kairos, 6.2* (Fall). Available from http://english.ttu.edu/kairos/6.2/binder.html?reviews/brown/index.html

Brummett, B. (2008). *A rhetoric of style.* Carbondale, IL: Southern Illinois University Press.

Burke, K. (1950). *A rhetoric of motives.* Berkeley, CA: University of California Press.

Burke, K. (1969). *A grammar of motives.* Berkeley, CA; University of California Press.

Campbell, K. K., & Burkholder, T. R. (1997). *Critiques of contemporary rhetoric* (2nd ed.). Berkeley, CA: Wadsworth Publishing Company.

Condit, C. M. (1990). *Decoding abortion rhetoric: Communication social change.* Urbana, IL: University of Illinois Press.

Condit, C. M. (1994). Hegemony in a mass mediated society: Concordance about 'reproductive technologies'. *Critical Studies in Mass Communication, 11*(3), 205–230.

Condit, C. M. (1999). *The meaning of the gene: Public debates about human heredity.* Madison, WI: University of Wisconsin Press.

Condit, C. M. (2000). Women's reproductive choices and the genetic model of medicine. In M. M Lay, L. J. Gurak, C. Gravon, & C. Myntti (Eds.), *Body talk: Rhetoric, technology, reproduction.* Madison, WI: University of Wisconsin Press.

Dickinson, G. (2002). Joe's rhetoric finding authenticity at Starbucks. *Rhetoric Society Quarterly, 32*(Pt. 4), 5–28.

Dickinson, G., Ott, B., & Aoki, E (2006). Spaces of remembering and forgetting: The reverent eye/I at the Plains Indian Museum. *Communication and Critical/Cultural Studies, 3*(1), 27–47.

Dow, B. (1996). *Prime-time feminism: Television, media, culture, and the women's movement.* Philadelphia, PA: University of Pennsylvania Press.

Elwood, W. (1995). *Public relations inquiry as rhetorical criticism: Case studies of corporate discourse and social influence.* Westport, CT: Praeger.

Emmons, K. (2010). *Black dogs and blue words*. Rutgers, NJ: Rutgers University of Press.

Epps, C. S., Armstrong, M. I., Davis, C. S., Massey O. T., McNeish, R., & Smith, R. B. (2007). *Development and testing of an instrument to measure mental health literacy*. Tampa, FL: Louis de la Parte Florida Mental Health Institute, University of South Florida.

Fish, S. (1980). *Is there a text in this class? The authority of interpretive communities*. Cambridge, MA: Harvard University Press.

Foss, S. (1996). *Rhetorical criticism: Exploration and practice* (2nd ed.). Prospect Heights, IL: Waveland Press.

Gronnvoll, M., & Landau, J. (2010). From viruses to Russian roulette to dance: A rhetorical critique and creation of genetic metaphors. *Rhetoric Society Quarterly*, *40*(1), 46–70.

Hall, S. (1997). *Representation: Cultural representations and signifying practices*. Thousand Oaks, CA: Sage Publications.

Hart, R. (1990). *Modern rhetorical criticism*. Glenview, IL: Scott Foresman, and Company.

Heath, R. L. (2009). The rhetorical tradition: Wrangle in the marketplace. In R. L. Heath, E. L. Toth, & D. Waymer (Eds.), *Rhetorical and critical approaches to public relations II* (pp. 17–47). New York, NY: Sage Publications.

Heffernan, V. (2011). A prescription for fear. *New York Times*, February 4, 2011. Retrieved November 9, 2011, from http://www.nytimes.com/2011/02/06/magazine/06FOB-Medium-t.html

Hess, A. (2011). Critical-rhetorical ethnography: Rethinking the place and process of rhetoric. *Communication Studies*, *62*(2), 127–152.

Huh, J., DeLorme, D. E., & Reid, L. N. (2005). Factors affecting trust in on-line prescription drug information and impact of trust on behavior following exposure to DTC advertising. *Journal of Health Communication*, *10*(8), 711–731.

Hyde, M. (2001). *The call of conscience: Heidegger and Levinas, rhetoric and the euthanasia debate*. Columbia, SC: University of South Carolina Press.

Jasinski, J. (2001). *Sourcebook on rhetoric: Key concepts in contemporary rhetorical studies*. Thousand Oaks, CA: Sage Publications.

Keränen, L. (2011). Concocting the viral apocalypse: Catastrophic risk and the production of bio (in)security. *Western Journal of Communication*, *75*(5), 451–472.

Kline, K. N. (2003). Popular media and health: Images, effects, and institutions. In T. L. Thompson, A. M. Dorsey, K. I. Miller, & R. Parrott (Eds.), *Handbook of health communication* (pp. 557–582). Mahwah, NJ: Lawrence Erlbaum Associates.

Kline, K. N. (2007). Cultural sensitivity and health promotion: assessing breast cancer education pamphlets designed for African American women. *Health Communication*, *21*(1), 85–96.

Kuehn, B. M. (2010). FDA weighs limits for online ads. *JAMA (The Journal of the American Medical Association)*, *303*(4), 311–313.

Landau, J. (2011). Women will get cancer: Visual and verbal presence (and absence) in a campaign about HPV. *Argumentation and Advocacy*, *48*(1), 39–54.

Lay, M., Gurak, L. Gravon, C. & Myntti, C. (2000). *Body talk: Rhetoric, technology, reproduction*. Madison, WI: University of Wisconsin Press.

Lingard, L. (2007). The rhetorical "turn" in medical education: What have we learned and where are we going? *Advances in Health, Science Education Theory and Practice*, *12*(2), 121–133.

Lupton, D. (1992). Discourse analysis: A new methodology for understanding the ideologies of health and illness. *Australian Journal of Public Health, 16*(2), 55–67.

Lynch, J. (2011). Information at the intersection of the public and technical spheres: A reply to Majdik. *Rhetoric & Public Affairs, 14*(2), 369–378.

McGee, M. C. (1990). Text, context, and the fragmentation of contemporary culture. *Western Journal of Speech Communication, 54*(3), 274–289.

McKenna, S. A. (2011). Maintaining class, producing gender: Enhancement discourses about amphetamine in entertainment media. *International Journal of Drug Policy, 22*(6), 455–462.

Messner, D. H. (2006). Rhetoric as practice: Framing AIDS knowledge. *Metascience, 15*(2), 353–357.

Perlmutter Bowen, S., & Michal-Johnson, P. (1990). A rhetorical perspective for HIV education with black urban adolescents. *Communication Research, 17*(6), 848–866.

Preda, A. (2005). *AIDS, rhetoric, and medical knowledge.* New York, NY: Cambridge University Press.

Quinlan, M. M., & Bates, B. R. (2012). "Walking in the city": Performance of strategies and tactics in the 1985 bus accessibility protests. *Disability Studies Quarterly*, 32(1). Available from: http://dsq-sds.org/article/view/1636/3059

Rosenberg, T. (2012). For teenage smokers, removing the allure of the pack. *New York Times*, August 1, 2012. Available from: http://opinionator.blogs.nytimes.com/2012/08/01/for-teenage-smokers-removing-the-allure-of-the-pack/

Schwartzman, R., Ross, D. G., & Berube, D. M. (2011). Rhetoric and risk. *Poroi*, 7(1), 1–9.

Segal, J. (2005). *Health and the rhetoric of medicine.* Carbondale, IL: Southern Illinois University Press.

Segal, J. (2007). Illness as argumentation: A prolegomenon to the rhetorical study of contestable complaints. *Health, 11*(2), 227–244.

Silva, V. T. (2011). Lost choices and eugenic dreams: Wrongful birth lawsuits in popular press narratives. *Communication and Critical/Cultural Studies, 8*(1), 22–40.

Stokes, A. Q. (2005). Healthology, health literacy, and the pharmaceutically empowered consumer. *Studies in Communication Sciences, 5*(2), 129–146.

Thornton, D. J. (2010). Race, risk, and pathology in psychiatric culture: Disease awareness campaigns as governmental rhetoric. *Critical Studies in Media Communication, 27*(4), 311–335.

Weingarten, K. (2012). Impossible decisions: Abortion, reproductive technologies, and the rhetoric of choice. *Women's Studies, 41*(3), 263–281.

Weppner, W. G., Hollon, M., Chew, L. D., & Larson, E. B. (2009). Direct-to-consumer offers for free and discounted medications on the Internet: A content analysis of "e-samples." *Archives of Internal Medicine, 169*(21), 2024–2039.

METHODOLOGICAL CHALLENGES FOR HEALTH RESEARCH WITH STIGMATIZED POPULATIONS

Kathryn Greene and Kate Magsamen-Conrad

Health researchers continue to study an ever-widening range of stigmatized populations, providing valuable information for health prevention, treatment, and utilization. This chapter focuses on how best to adapt methodologies for research with stigmatized groups. We begin with one distinction: stigma that emerges as a research theme during a study and stigma as a component of the sampling plan. This chapter focuses on the latter. In certain studies, some but not all participants report stigmatizing experiences, yet, in some of these studies, population segmentation is not a driving impetus for the study. This type of stigma research is markedly different from cases where a specific group is sampled in order to investigate a phenomena related to a uniting stigmatizing factor. This chapter examines the challenges researchers encounter when they choose to focus on stigmatized populations, as well as recommendations for addressing those problems. It begins by defining *population* more broadly, and then narrows to define stigmatized populations. The chapter continues with conceptualizations of stigma and stigmatized populations, before turning to four recommended methodological practices and final comments.

Stigmatized Populations

One issue that affects research broadly, and health communication research more specifically, is sampling the particular population of interest. Although some fields are dominated by college student samples and associated limited generalizability, researchers increasingly conduct studies using sites such as schools, organizations, hospitals, clinics, medical offices, and service organizations. A research population is a collection of individuals who have some consistent characteristic or trait defined as "the theoretically specified aggregation of the elements in a study"

(Babbie, 2004, p. 190). Kindig and Stoddart (2003) more specifically define population health as "the health outcomes of a group of individuals, including the distribution of such outcomes within the group" (p. 380). Some health issues are relevant to specific populations, groups, or segments of the population, for example, overrepresentation of a group with a particular disease or differential access to prevention or treatment for a specific group. The National Institutes of Health (NIH) created the Division of Special Populations to strengthen their "commitment to ensuring the health and well-being of children, adults, families, and communities by addressing and eliminating health disparities through the participation of diverse populations in biomedical and behavioral research within the United States and abroad" (NIH, 2012). Further, the NIH highlights population segments within particular research areas (e.g., vulnerable populations within alcohol health or cancer control). Some of these groups are stigmatized, and the following sections define stigma and stigmatized populations.

Some segments of the population are considered stigmatized because of an identifying characteristic, studied under the label "stigma." This characteristic may manifest as a mark or a deviation from a prototype (see Jones et al., 1984). Goffman (1963) is credited with early conceptualizations of the notion of stigma by focusing on how the reaction of others spoils normal identity, and he defined stigma as an "attribute that is deeply discrediting" (p. 3). Goffman (1990) identified three primary sources of stigma. The first source includes visible deformities of some kind (e.g., scarring, physical manifestations of anorexia, leprosy, obesity). The next stigma source includes personal or social aberrations (e.g., mental illness, drug abuse, alcoholism, criminal behavior). The final source of stigma, "tribal stigma," represents traits that deviate from what is considered normative for a particular group (i.e., ethnic group, nationality, religious group; see Rush, 1998, for social stigma).

Goffman's work, although well cited and useful as a research framework, is not well formulated for use in health contexts. More specifically for health, Leary and Schreindorfer (1998) described how individuals are stigmatized to the extent that their identifying traits or characteristics lead to avoidance or rejection from others, and their view is rooted in interaction and perception of others. They suggest four stigma characteristics that can be better utilized to consider methodological challenges for health research: individuals pose a threat to others' health and safety; deviate from group standards; fail to contribute; and create negative emotional reactions in others.

In their conceptualization, developed for the context of HIV/AIDS stigma, Leary and Schreindorfer (1998) highlight the effects of multiple sources of stigma (i.e., more than one stigmatizing trait/characteristic), stigma attribution, and social contagion. They identify the concept of "master status" that arises when multiple factors coalesce to intensify stigma and therefore increase the negative effects of stigma. Considerable research also addresses the effect of attribution on stigma; that is, the degree to which the stigmatized individual is perceived to be "responsible" for the acquisition of their condition (e.g., DeJong, 1980; Levine & McBurney, 1977). Researchers may also study partners or family of people with a stigmatized condition or those who work with stigmatized populations (see AIDS volunteers; Frey, Query, Flint, & Adelman, 1998) and should be aware that stigma may "rub off" onto these groups (see "courtesy stigma" in Leary & Schreindorfer, 1998; Alzheimer's patients' caregivers in Blum, 1991).

Stigma often creates a sense of "us versus them" that may be used to bolster identity, studied within the model of social comparison (Taylor & Lobel, 1989) or downward comparison theory (Wills, 1981). To cope with uncertainty-related stigma, people may compare themselves with others. For example, Derlega, Greene, Henson, and Winstead (2008) had people with HIV read vignettes manipulated to test social upward affiliation and cognitive downward evaluation processes for other HIV patients' physical and psychological status. The researchers reported that participants negatively evaluated the patients doing poorly physically (downward comparison) and would avoid patients doing poorly psychologically; however, they also found that the participants wanted to affiliate with patients doing well physically. Another study of these comparison phenomena interviewed people who trade sex for drugs, referred to as "skeezers" in street language (Elwood & Greene, 2003). African American crack smokers (N = 200) were interviewed, including the "johns" who traded crack for sex and the women. The first finding was that the men believed that women who trade sex for crack are at the bottom of the social hierarchy (and cannot transmit disease to higher social members). Another finding was that men who used condoms—and many did not—did so to increase social distance. This study illustrated how one group denigrated another group engaged in markedly similar behavior (trading crack and sex), yet this comparison was one-sided: the women described the interaction in economic terms but reported little power in condom negotiation. Overall, these comparison theories demonstrate how people cope with stigma in part by seeing themselves as superior even to similar others. Along with theories of social comparison, Leary and Schreindorfer's conceptualization of characteristics of stigma and other stigma-related phenomena allow researchers to better plan and execute projects with stigmatized populations. The next section reviews research within populations that have been stigmatized historically.

Examples of Stigmatized Populations

Stigma research transcends disciplines, methodologies, and national borders. Scholars from medical and social sciences (including psychology, anthropology, sociology, social work, public health, and communication) investigate stigma. Some of this research clearly fits into one of the three primary sources of stigma derived from Goffman's work or Leary and Schreindorfer's more specific health stigma conceptualization. For example, researchers have studied stigma related to visibility or creating negative reactions of others, such as with obesity (e.g., Lawrence, 2010; Teixeira & Budd, 2010), including in Germany (Sikorski et al., 2011), and physical disability (e.g., Barg, Armstrong, Hetz, & Latimer, 2010; Kwong, Chung, Cheal, Chou, & Chen, 2012), including in Canada (Bahm & Forchuk, 2009). Homosexuality may be considered within the framework of deviating from group standards or social aberration. Perceptions of homosexuality may be confounded by disease-related stigma (e.g., HIV, see Crandall, 1991; e.g., Cain, 1991; see also stigma of children with lesbian mothers, Gershon, Tschann, & Jemerin, 1999; suicide and transgender stigma, Clements-Nolle, Marx, & Katz, 2008), including research with men who have sex with men (MSM) in China (Neilands, Steward, & Choi, 2008) and Taiwan (Wang, Bih, & Brennan, 2009). Other examples of social aberration or deviating from group standards may include the stigma associated with alcoholism (Keyes et al., 2010), illicit drug use (Palamar, 2012), criminal behavior (Schnittker & John, 2007), or a combination of these (Room, 2005). The distinctions between sources of stigma may be less applicable as a frame because the sources of stigma frequently overlap, and elements of a "master status" (Leary & Schreindorfer, 1998) affect manifestations of stigma. Therefore, rather than review stigmatized populations from the perspective of stigma source, the following sections review examples of research with stigmatizing conditions.

Mental Illness-Related Stigma

Mental illness is highly stigmatized and encompasses a wide range of conditions such as schizophrenia, depression, post-traumatic stress disorder (PTSD), and dementia. Researchers study mental illness stigma (see Herman, 1993; Shaw, 1991), including with Arab participants (Dalky, 2012a), and in Europe (Evans-Lacko, Brohan, Mojtabai, & Thornicroft, 2012) and India (Tirupati, Rangaswamy, & Raman, 2004). Schomerus et al.'s (2011) review of research on mental illness attitudes found increased public knowledge/literacy about mental illness and increased acceptance of mental illness treatment. However, they found no evidence of reduction of stigmatization of people with mental illness (see also Dalky, 2012b, for a review of mental illness stigma intervention trials).

In the past decade, increasing research in the United States has focused on the mental health of veterans returning from deployment. Depression, PTSD, and substance abuse are common in military populations, especially among soldiers returning from combat (American Psychiatric Association, 2012); these effects also have an impact on military families, including spouses. Much of this research on veterans focuses on PTSD. The U.S. Army Office and Surgeon General define a PTSD case as "an individual having at least two outpatient visits or one or more hospitalizations at which PTSD was diagnosed" (Fischer, 2010, p. 2). A combined diagnosis figure (across deployed and non-deployed soldiers) is

88,719 diagnosed cases in all branches of military service between 2000 and 2010, with the highest concentration among the Army (Fischer, 2010). This figure must be considered an underestimate, given the pressure in military organizations to avoid mental health labeling. Mental illness stigma is "especially pronounced in the military, where the pervasive culture is one of mental and physical toughness, 'pushing through the pain'" (Office of the Vice Chief of Staff (Army), 2012, p. 69).

Military populations may be particularly affected by stigma within the context of help-seeking behaviors (e.g., Hoge et al., 2004; see also Hooyer, 2012). The heightened stigma acts as a barrier to pursuing or maintaining care or therapy and thus would inhibit research. Nearly two-thirds (60%) of military members believe that seeking help for mental health concerns would negatively affect their careers (American Psychiatric Association, 2012). The military supports anti-stigma campaigns specifically designed for military populations (e.g., Real Warriors, http://www.realwarriors.net), yet mental illness stigma remains in the military, and, more broadly, in the United States and other countries. The following section explores a second stigmatized population well represented in the literature: physical illnesses.

Physical Illness-Related Stigma

Considerable research also investigates stigma related to specific health or medical conditions. Much of this research examines stigma related to sexually transmitted infections (STIs) such as HIV/AIDS (e.g., Florom-Smith & De Santis, 2012; Sowell & Phillips, 2010), including several meta-analyses (see Logie & Gadalla, 2009, for a meta-analysis of HIV and health and demographic correlates of stigma; Smith, Rossetto, & Peterson, 2008, for a meta-analysis of HIV stigma, social support, and disclosure). Other topics include hepatitis C (for a review, see Paterson, Backmund, Hirsch, & Yim, 2007) and behaviors associated with STIs, such as with male sex workers in Bangladesh (Khan, Bhuiya, & Uddin, 2004), or sex workers and injection drug use in Scotland (Bloor, Leyland, Barnard, & McKeganey, 1991). However, research in this area also examines other issues related to health and stigma, such as infertility in the United States (Steuber & Solomon, 2011), the Middle East (Ahmadi, Montaser-Kouhsari, Nowroozi, & Bazargan-Hejazi, 2011), and Ghana (Donkor & Sandall, 2007; Miall, 1986); chronic pain (Goldberg, 2010); and epilepsy (Schneider & Conrad, 1980), including epilepsy in Zambia (Atadzhanov, Haworth, Chomba, Mbewe, & Lano Birbeck, 2010).

Stigma related to a physical condition is a central concern in health management. Golden, Conroy, O'Dwyer, Golden, and Hardouin (2006) conducted clinical interviews at a hospital with 87 patients awaiting treatment for hepatitis C and discovered a strong fear of illness discovery as well as social isolation and rejection. They also found that perceptions of stigmatization were higher among persons who had contracted hepatitis C through injection drug use and contaminated blood transfusion (for hemophiliacs) than for those who did not know how they contracted the disease. These findings are consistent with Leary and Schreindorfer's (1998) notions of attribution and blame and the source of the disease.

Attribution issues, such as blame for method of disease contraction, are common among stigmatized illnesses, especially STIs such as HIV and hepatitis C. In some instances, the health of the patient is compromised because of beliefs about their degree of "fault" in acquiring their illness. For example, some health practitioners stigmatize persons with hepatitis C, in part because of the associations with drug use (see Corrigan, 2004). This behavior is consistent with reports of medical personnel who refuse to treat HIV+ patients. One emerging area of stigma research is with lung cancer and cancer stigma. Some people who disclose that they have lung cancer report being asked, "Were you a smoker?", similar to questions in response to sharing an HIV+ diagnosis, such as "How did you get it?". These questions also focus attention on how a condition was contracted (see Leary & Schreindorfer, 1998). For some receivers, perceived patient responsibility is key in responding to disclosure of a health diagnosis (see Greene, Derlega, Yep, & Petronio, 2003). People who engage in behavior that could lead to risk are more stigmatized than those termed "innocent victims," who are viewed as having no role in their diagnosis/infection (see Leary & Schreindorfer, 1998).

Patients devote tremendous energy to avoiding these types of stigma, and report stigma is one of their greatest concerns. Many patients choose not to share with others to avoid stigma (e.g., hemophiliacs, adoptees, or parents with children having lice). People also avoid telling others about stigmatized medical procedures (e.g., abortions or cosmetic surgery). Even physicians who perform abortions and clinic staff often do not widely publicize this practice.

Race/Ethnicity and Group Stigma

Researchers have extensively investigated the stigma surrounding race/ethnicity (e.g., African Americans, Latinos, Native Americans), much of which is relevant for health research, such as health disparities. Race/ethnicity disparities are rampant in American healthcare. As an example, even controlling for factors such as health status, insurance, income, and disease severity (Smedley, Stith, & Nelson, 2003), elderly Latinos have higher rates of diabetes and disability than elderly Whites (Wallace & Villa, 2003), and elderly African Americans report more chronic health conditions than elderly Whites (Centers for Medicare & Medicaid Services, 2000). These disparities may also have implications for treatment-related attitudes and help-seeking behaviors (see Brown et al., 2010). For example, Matthews, Sellergren, Manfredi, and William (2002) reported that African American cancer patients' embarrassment with cancer stigma was as high as was cancer-related fear.

A variant of group stigmatization research focuses on population segments that are stigmatized for reasons such as extreme poverty, homelessness, or living in remote areas. Research explores Appalachian stigmatization (e.g., Jones, 1997; Latimer, 2006; Zaheer et al., 2011), for example, as it relates to human papillomavirus (HPV) vaccination appraisals (Smith & Parrott, 2012). Other research focuses on the stigma of poverty itself (e.g., Mickelson & Williams, 2008; Reutter et al., 2009; see Waxman, 1983, for a review). For example, Collins (2005) conducted interviews with women from low-income families who expressed a common theme of feeling that others "looked down on them." This stigmatization is even more pronounced for those who utilize public assistance (e.g., Kerbo, 1976; Stuber & Kronebusch, 2004) or the homeless (e.g., Roschelle & Kaufman, 2004; Snow & Anderson 1993). Researchers have also investigated the intersection of poverty stigma and AIDS/HIV stigma as a barrier to care or treatment adherence (see Coetzee, Kagee, & Vermeulen, 2011), poverty stigma and mental health stigma in Uganda (see Ssebunnya, Kigozi, Lund, Kizza, & Okello, 2009), and poverty and HIV stigma in Tanzania (Amuri, Mitchell, Cockcroft, & Andersson, 2011) and in Zimbabwe (Campbell et al., 2012).

Multiply Stigmatized

Some research examines individuals at the intersection of several different sources of stigma that may compound difficulties with research due to the intensity of the stigma (see Leary & Schreindorfer, 1998). For example, Hartwell (2004) compared the issues of mentally ill persons in the criminal justice system that had or were struggling with substance abuse ("dually diagnosed") to mentally ill persons involved with the criminal justice system. Hartwell reported that individuals battling both mental illness and drug abuse stigma were more likely to be homeless, violate the terms of their probation, and recidivate.

Researchers should attend to the presence of multiple forms of stigma that can confound and compound both participants' experiences and research participation. Leary and Schreindorfer (1998) described this as "master status," and others have referred to "double disclosure," when one person shares a diagnosis and also (by choice or not) shares another stigmatized trait. For example, in order to share their HIV status, some people with HIV must also disclose homosexuality, injection drug use, or infidelity. In these cases, sharing the information becomes a kind of dialectical "double-edged sword," where participants may be seeking to access support yet the sharing exposes them to potential negative outcomes.

Lessons for Research with Stigmatized Health Populations

This chapter focuses on methodological considerations and adjustments researchers should make when studying stigmatized populations. Based on the existing research on stigma and our team's research, four recommendations are proposed to consider when working with stigmatized populations. These include consideration of language use, threat to reputation, legal status, and illegal behaviors. The recommendations include review of best practices and features to avoid, supplemented by examples from published research or our research projects. We begin with the first recommendation, caution surrounding language use.

Language Use

Researchers working with stigmatized populations should have heightened awareness of how language is used in all stages of research projects, from recruitment through data collection, analyses, and presenting results. Because of the very nature of their status, stigmatized populations may have very strong reactions to use of specific labels. More obvious examples include the terms "faggot" or "dyke" or derogatory racial, ethnic, or religious references (e.g., "nigger," "WOP," and "kyke"). Researchers should note, however, that the very nature of in-group dynamics and identification may lead participants to embrace these terms and utilize them during interviews and focus groups, in a process similar to Leary and Schreindorfer's (1998) description of "stigma avowal." We caution, however, that, even if participants use a particular term and have reframed it, researchers should be wary of adopting parallel language and using these terms. Use of particular terms by members outside of a community or group—even if the researchers are generally viewed positively or as members of the same group—can backfire and damage relationships (and, potentially, the quality of data). Risks include participants withdrawing from research, avoiding participation generally, and/or responding in socially desirable or perhaps shallow and limited ways.

We have encountered people choosing to identify themselves in particular ways through labeling. First, health researchers increasingly study men who have sex with men (MSM), and some of these men vehemently reject the labels "gay," "homosexual," "bisexual," and "MSM." Some of these men—for example, heterosexually identified, married, African American men we interviewed in the southeastern United States—described their sexual behavior with men as "just playing around" or a "way to release stress." These "behaviorally bisexual" men did not acknowledge the sexual acts as relationships but would discuss their sexual behavior; these men emphasized being married and having children as why they were not part of "that group," rejecting the terms MSM, gay, or bisexual. Thus, some members of this group use certain markers to reject specific labels and avoid potential stigma.

Perceptions of group labels may be especially intense for stigmatized groups, leading to recommendations that researchers be sensitive to participant preferences. In our interviews with women who have sex with women (WSW), we encountered similar cases where people rejected the term "WSW" for lesbian, and others who rejected both "lesbian" and "WSW," despite being in a same-sex relationship for more than 10 years (some of these women strongly identified as "bisexual"). Related to these challenges is sensitivity to terms used to describe same-sex partners (i.e., "partner" versus "husband"/"wife"). Partners are crucial in many aspects of health research, not limited to sexual health but also more broadly for social support for a wide range of health conditions where behavior changes are recommended (e.g., cardiac or diabetes patients). The inconsistencies currently created by varying current national and state marriage and civil union laws add tension to an already loaded topic, and researchers may choose to ask participants "Are you in a relationship?" and "How do you refer to him/her?"

Another emerging example is related to transgendered participants (historically "LGB," now commonly referred to as "LGBT" or "LGBTQ"). When interviewing a participant in sexual transition and/or who presents androgynously or with physical or social markers of both genders, researchers may have difficulty determining which pronoun to use. One participant we interviewed described how hurtful it was that some healthcare staff referred to him as "her" repeatedly, even after specific requests. Although the participant perceived that many staff at this location were sensitive and adapting, some staff appeared resistant to using language other than "legally defined biological gender." This kind of illustration provides an opportunity for studying factors that affect transgender people's utilization of health services beyond perception of stigma. In similar cases, one previously successful approach is to ask the participant how s/he would like to be referred ("What name would you like to be called?" and/or "Do you like to be referred to as 'he' or 'she'?"). In our research, this issue has also arisen when interviewing drag queens. In one instance, it was important to refer to the participant by stage name and as "she" when presenting in that identity (i.e., in costume); on follow up, the participant self-identified as "he" and by his birth name rather than performance name.

Finally, our last example is where people misuse terminology related to diseases. We see this repeatedly in our HIV disclosure research. One African American woman described how language use caused her to withdraw and not share with others: "My husband died from AIDS in the early '80s. And so automatically, you know, they going to say I got it, if I tell them or not, you know, 'She got the AIDS.' It is always 'the AIDS,' it's never HIV." Participants may be hurt or frustrated with lack of education related to some diseases, but they also seek to avoid stigma. Researchers should recall that the original acronym for acquired immunodeficiency syndrome (AIDS) was "GRID" (gay-related immunodeficiency disorder), despite the presence of heterosexual patients even at the outset of the epidemic. Similarly sexually-transmitted disease (STD) became sexually-transmitted infection (STI), focusing on "infection" rather than using the more emotionally charged term "disease." Changes in terminology occurred in the sexual assault community, where many issues including stigmatization lead to underreporting of this crime (Egan & Wilson, 2012).

Individuals once commonly labeled "rape victims" are now referred to as "sexual assault survivors."

Language is a reflection of group values, and effective researchers will immerse themselves in the environment and observe/listen prior to engaging in any type of formal research that would include key informant contact, interviews, surveys, or even focus groups. This kind of reflection is important at early stages, including with recruitment and flyers: researchers are unlikely to recruit effectively if they are using the wrong labels (and, in some cases, if using any labels). Our team regularly uses key informants (members of the stigmatized group) to review recruitment material, scripts, surveys, and interview and focus group protocols. We increase the levels of research material review when participants are multiple stigmatized. Also, we caution that some "key informants" may be more active or open with their condition and may not best represent the population of interest.

Threat to Reputation

Because of the very nature of their status, stigmatized populations may be concerned about threats to their reputation or others finding out either about a health condition (e.g., STI) or some other stigmatized information. This concern may lead stigmatized participants to avoid research altogether or be especially sensitive about location, recording, or note taking. As one example, our team conducts interviews for people with HIV and sexual minorities in coffee shops, nightclubs, and religious institutions if requested by participants, even though most of this research occurs in private offices at AIDS Service Organizations (ASOs). Some participants report that, if they were seen in a specific building in a community such as the AIDS service organization or the public health department, "then everyone would know." For some of these participants, these avoidance strategies included traveling to different cities or counties to receive treatment and services. The choice of location can increase participant comfort but can also introduce challenges such as maintaining privacy (booths close together at a diner) or noise interfering with audio recording (e.g., at a nightclub or restaurant). Researchers should reflect on how the use of an ASO as location, or a gay bar or public health department, for example, results in oversampling people using these particular resources and underrepresents avoiders who may be the population of interest.

Another example that we have encountered related to threat to reputation is hidden information that may be revealed during the research, such as a participant with multiple sexual partners whose primary partner (e.g., wife or husband) is unaware of the other's sexual behavior. At times, both participants may be in a research program (i.e., being interviewed), and the staff must be extremely careful not to inadvertently share the partner's information. We separately interviewed a couple where one described their relationship as "I see us buying a house together this fall," yet his partner reported, "I'm not sure where this relationship is going or if we'll be together in six months." A more amusing example involved interviewing couples in which one had a heart condition about how they share information and reinforce the patient's behavioral changes (e.g., increase exercise and modify diet). In this instance, the wife proudly described how her husband (the cardiac bypass patient) was now walking for an hour every morning. The husband, however, separately described that each morning he puts on his sneakers, leaves the house, goes several blocks away to buy a newspaper and spends 45 minutes reading on what he described as "a lovely park bench." It may seem obvious that interviewing this couple separately was important, but we would recommend a combination of separate and couple interviews if the focus is on relational dynamics affecting health. For this couple, the joint interview portion of the study also provided valuable information where they clarified perspectives of the other's narrative.

A large pharmaceutical company in the northeastern United States banned smoking not just in their buildings but also within their physical property; smokers cannot smoke outside the buildings or in parking lots. The company also implemented widespread programs for decreasing employee smoking, in addition to encouraging other health benefits such as cholesterol screenings and weight-loss programs. Some employees have successfully quit, yet, for others, there is a great deal of pressure to hide any evidence of smoking or tobacco use. In this kind of case, interviewing tobacco users through this company (unless former tobacco users) is likely to create challenges if interviews occur on site.

Many phenomena are "hidden" to protect people's reputations from stigma, and this occurs for employment and in families where people seek to avoid loss of job or perhaps child custody. For example, some websites offer strategies for concealing anorexia (see Harshbarger, Ahlers-Schmidt, Mayans, Mayans, & Hawkins, 2009), and smoker stigma remains high (Graham, 2012). Extensive research exists on sharing for recovery in Alcoholics Anonymous, yet there remain millions of alcoholics in the United States alone, many of whom hide their drinking patterns (see Schomerus et al., 2011, for a review). A final example is widespread underreporting of sexual harassment (McDonald, Charlesworth, & Cerise, 2011; Vijayasiri, 2008) when people may fear job loss or injury to career path.

Researchers should be cautious with choosing locations and contacting participants, whether at work or even at home (especially if the partner is unaware). Recommendations include using audio-recording rather than videotaping, or taking notes rather than recording the conversations. Make conscious decisions and ensure participants know that they are being protected. Although sometimes an unpopular recommendation, researchers should work with Institutional Review Boards (IRBs), which may have useful and creative suggestions for protecting participants. Overall, researchers should consider the potential effects of the research on employment, spouses, and families.

Legal Status

If researchers are interested in specific populations (e.g., undocumented immigrants, people not paying child support, parolees), there are additional considerations. The very nature of their status may put some populations at risk of legal consequences which vary by country but could include deportation or arrest. The stigma attached to some of these groups includes portraying them as a drain on the public and not contributing to society (see Leary & Schreindorfer, 1998). For example, undocumented workers are abundant in the United States but they may be reticent to participate in research. These millions of undocumented workers may be relevant for studying a wide range of health issues such as utilization of healthcare services, vaccination, or prenatal nutrition.

For some research, any form of linkage with the research project could put the participant at risk. For example, a researcher may be interested in children's health coverage in families where one participant owes child support, yet identifying the "delinquent parent" could put the individual at risk of incarceration. In these cases, researchers should request waivers of written consent, which removes the requirement for documentation such as a recorded signature, yet retains the elements of consent. Where needed, researchers should also obtain federal Certificates of Confidentiality to ensure that the risk posed by participating in the research is minimized (e.g., no list of names/addresses is tied to the study, even for payment). Researchers should take maximum precautions to keep confidential any list or data that includes identifying information. It is possible that the risks to participants (and, potentially, to researchers) outweigh the potential gain from the research. In some countries, certain behaviors, such as being raped, committing infidelity, or being homosexual, remain punishable by death.

In some cases in the United States and other countries, researchers may consider notifying police of an ongoing research project. This is a difficult decision requiring evaluation of benefits with potential risks. As an example, researchers have interviewed mobile commercial street workers (i.e., prostitutes) about how they negotiate condom use. One potential risk to these researchers is that, if a raid or "sweep" occurs, the researchers and/or participants may be detained or arrested. Some researchers send pairs of staff and/or women to interview female prostitutes (or male prostitutes) because they are less likely to be perceived as "johns." In these cases, researchers should carry copies of research documentation (e.g., IRB approval) and the minimum cash or gift cards possible. Some researchers do choose to identify the research project to local police units. This decision, however, must be balanced against the potential to generate distrust with participants and potentially put participants at risk for identification (e.g., recordings could be seized). If a participant was arrested during or right after an interview, beyond the impact for the participants, a sense of distrust will spread quickly and endanger the project. Some of these concerns about legal status are also relevant for studying illegal behaviors.

Illegal Behaviors

Beyond legal status, researchers may be interested in specific populations engaged in illegal behavior. This is a related but separate question from the participant's legal status, and, in many cases, the two are completely unrelated. Additionally, some definitions of "illegal behavior" are fluid. For example, the behavior of anal intercourse has been selectively prosecuted in the southeastern United States for MSM but not for heterosexual couples. For other behaviors, and research, however, the distinctions are clearer. We earlier described examples of trading sex for crack (Elwood & Greene, 2003), and drug use is an example more generally. The specific case of marijuana in the United States (not just medical marijuana) is an emerging challenge, because as of January 2014 several state laws allowing marijuana sales contradict federal legislation.

Consider the research on needle exchange programs, a successful public health approach to reducing the spread of STIs including HIV (see MacNeil & Pauly, 2011; Strike, Myers, & Millson, 2004). Despite tremendous, documented program success in decreasing transmission of HIV, program funding remains politically contested. Participation in these exchange programs identifies the person as using injection drugs. In one case for our team, law enforcement officers followed a needle exchange worker over a period of several weeks. Police have arrested needle exchange workers in states where this public health practice is illegal. These challenges put participants at risk—and, potentially, the researcher(s) as well.

One understudied area that may receive increased attention is injection drug use, including performance-enhancing drugs or steroids (and potential for disease transmission, beyond other effects). This practice has increased among athletes at many levels and receives some very public scrutiny (e.g., the Major League Baseball controversy surrounding the record for home runs in a baseball season, or Lance Armstrong's doping scandal in cycling). Many of these athletes would reject labeling as "injection drug users," and access to these drugs is often illegal and vigorously hidden from reviewing committees such as the NCAA or Olympics.

Recommendations for research with illegal behaviors are similar to those for legal status mentioned above. Additionally, researchers should consider using "fake names," and, in instructions, ensure that participants do not share certain behaviors, such as robbing a store for drug money or plans to kill a drug supplier to take a stash. If any questionable statements are recorded, researchers should stop taping immediately, rewind the recorder, and record over the statement (and later notify the relevant reviewing body). Researchers could also consider asking participants to "share what others you know do," rather than reporting their own behavior. Any tapes should be transcribed quickly, de-identified, and destroyed. Researchers should also seek expert input on electronic file storage (encryption is one option, but password protection and limited copies also increase protection).

Final Comments

Health research with stigmatized populations presents a unique set of methodological challenges. Lest we forget, some of these populations have very negative perceptions of research and researchers generally. Tuskegee, for example, was active as a research project in the United States into the 1970s, yet many people consider it "ancient history." For some African Americans, however, the distrust remains. Other communities may have similar reticence and question the research or researcher goals. Thus, researchers must be especially vigilant in establishing rapport with communities who may have heightened reactions to potential stigma. This process of establishing relationships, however, can be painstakingly slow. Researchers should observe the group, behavior, or community to the extent possible before embarking on a research project. This requires time and careful planning. Some researchers choose to volunteer for a long period of time before seeking access to participants, and that is one approach. Other teams might hire staff that better blend with the population based on age, gender, race, sexual orientation, or language fluency.

Relationships with both staff and clients can be crucial to successfully complete research projects. Staff may serve as access points, and this can be complicated if there are competing goals. We conducted one study with an ASO in a large city, and one staff member was so motivated for participants to "get the incentive" that she consistently misrepresented inclusion criteria to our staff, even after repeated clarification. Although this action may have been beneficial for participants, it created chaos for the project.

Researchers should also consider what they are giving back to the particular community prior to study onset or recruiting. Besides payment for participation, what would be productive for the group? We provide training sessions for staff, such as with ASOs, yet these approaches only indirectly assist the target population (i.e., clients). To more directly affect communities, researchers working with economically distressed populations could provide a training session on job interviewing or writing a resume. Researchers should reflect on—and may be asked by human subject review committees—what level of incentive is coercive for an economically distressed group?

For some participants, the reason for participating in the study may not be known to others and identification of even participating in the study will concern some participants (e.g., writing the participant a check for payment or signing a list or consent form). Some studies require a "cover story," and we recommend planning a backup story before embarking on research with stigmatized populations. We interviewed a MSM at a local restaurant regarding condom use and risk behaviors, and, when leaving, ran into a friend of his who wanted to know what we were doing. The participant identified the researcher as "a researcher studying African Americans trying to quit smoking." The researcher was able to cover and go along with the story by asking the friend if he was a smoker and wanted to participate (thankfully not, in this case, or we would have had to report the incident, and likely tell the "friend" that "the study is full").

Focus group methods create unique challenges in research with stigmatized populations: people who hear things may not respect confidentiality. Most focus group protocols directly address this concern in instructions, but participants should be reminded that others might not respect their information (increasingly, this may be included as a warning on a consent form). Researchers should not assume that, because all participants are similar in status (e.g., not in a country legally or hiding their drinking), others will respect their privacy. This circumstance may lead researchers to allow participants to choose other names, similar to what may be done with interviews. In other cases, focus groups are simply not appropriate given the added risk, and individual interviews are more appropriate.

Less seasoned researchers or those accessing a new population should partner with experienced researchers; even a brief consulting meeting could dramatically improve a project. We encourage researchers to thoughtfully consider how their research can decrease—or at least not increase—participants' stigmatizing experiences. Research can be beneficial for participants, sometimes by asking about positive experiences and providing efficacy and skill training at study conclusion to ensure that the research does not contribute to perceptions of stigmatization. Research with stigmatized populations creates unique challenges and opportunities. Successfully navigating these challenges can provide rich data, and also has the potential to decrease some health disparities.

References

Ahmadi, H., Montaser-Kouhsari, L., Nowroozi, M. R., & Bazargan-Hejazi, S. (2011). Male infertility and depression: A neglected problem in the Middle East. *Journal of Sexual Medicine*, *8*(3), 824–830.

American Psychiatric Association. (2012). Military. Retrieved from http://www.healthyminds.org/More-Info-For/Military.aspx

Amuri, M., Mitchell, S., Cockcroft, A., & Andersson, N. (2011). Socio-economic status and HIV/AIDS stigma in Tanzania. *AIDS Care*, *23*(3), 378–382.

Atadzhanov, M., Haworth, A., Chomba, E. N., Mbewe, E. K., & Lano Birbeck, G. (2010). Epilepsy-associated stigma in Zambia: What factors predict greater felt stigma in a highly stigmatized population? *Epilepsy & Behavior*, *19*(3), 414–418.

Babbie, E. R. (2004). *The practice of social research* (10th ed.). Belmont, CA: Wadsworth/Thompson Learning.

Badgett, M. V. L. (1995). The wage effects of sexual orientation discrimination. *Industrial and Labor Relations Review*, *48*(4), 726–739.

Bahm, A., & Forchuk, C. (2009). Interlocking oppressions: The effect of a comorbid physical disability on perceived stigma and discrimination among mental health consumers in Canada. *Health & Social Care in the Community*, *17*(1), 63–70.

Barg, C. J., Armstrong, B. D., Hetz, S. P., & Latimer, A. E. (2010). Physical disability, stigma, and physical activity in children. *International Journal of Disability, Development & Education*, *57*(4), 371–382.

Blascovich, J., Mendes, W. B., Hunter, S. B., Lickel, B., & Kowai-Bell, N. (2001). Perceiver threat in social interactions with stigmatized others. *Journal of Personality and Social Psychology*, *80*(2), 253–267.

Bloor, M., Leyland, A., Barnard, M., & McKeganey, N. (1991). Estimating hidden populations: A new method of calculating the prevalence of drug-injecting and non-injecting female street prostitution. *British Journal of Addiction*, *86*(11), 1477–1483.

Blum, N. S. (1991). The management of stigma by Alzheimer family caregivers. *Journal of Contemporary Ethnography*, *20*(3), 263–284.

Brown, C., Conner, K. O., Copeland, V. C., Grote, N., Beach, S., Battista, D., & Reynolds, C. F. (2010). Depression stigma, race, and treatment seeking behavior and attitudes. *Journal of Community Psychology*, *38*(3), 350–368.

Cain, R. (1991). Stigma management and gay identity development. *Social Work*, *36*(1), 67–73.

Campbell, C., Skovdal, M., Mupambireyi, Z., Madanhire, C., Robertson, L. L., Nyamukapa, C. A., & Gregson, S. S. (2012). Can AIDS stigma be reduced to poverty stigma? Exploring Zimbabwean children's representations of poverty and AIDS. *Child: Care, Health and Development*, *38*(5), 732–742.

Centers for Medicare & Medicaid Services. (2003). *The characteristics and perceptions of the Medicare population: Data from the 2000 Medicare current beneficiary survey*. Baltimore, MD: U.S. Dept. of Health and Human Services, Centers for Medicare and Medicaid Services. Retrieved from http://www.cms.gov/Research-Statistics-Data-and-Systems/Research/MCBS/Data-Tables-Items/CMS1253271.html

Clements-Nolle, K., Marx, R., & Katz, M. (2008). Attempted suicide among transgender persons. *Journal of Homosexuality*, *51*(3), 53–69.

Coetzee, B., Kagee, A., & Vermeulen, N. (2011). Structural barriers to adherence to antiretroviral therapy in a resource-constrained setting: The perspectives of health care providers. *AIDS Care*, *23*(2), 146–151.

Collins, S. (2005). An understanding of poverty from those who are poor. *Action Research*, *3*(1), 9–11.

Corrigan, P. W. (2004). Target-specific stigma change: A strategy for impacting mental illness stigma. *Psychiatric Rehabilitation Journal*, *28*(2), 113–121.

Crandall, C. S. (1991). Multiple stigma and AIDS: Illness stigma and attitudes toward homosexuals and IV drug users in AIDS-related stigmatization. *Journal of Community & Applied Social Psychology*, *1*(2), 165–172.

Dalky, H. F. (2012a). Perception and coping with stigma of mental illness: Arab families' perspectives. *Issues in Mental Health Nursing*, *33*(7), 486–491.

Dalky, H. F. (2012b). Mental illness stigma reduction interventions: Review of intervention trials. *Western Journal of Nursing Research*, *34*(4), 520–547.

DeJong, W. (1980). The stigma of obesity: The consequences of naïve assumptions concerning the causes of physical deviance. *Journal of Health and Social Behavior*, *21*(1), 75–87.

Derlega, V. J., Greene, K., Henson, J. M., & Winstead, B. A. (2008). Social comparison activity in coping with HIV. *International Journal of STD & AIDS*, *19*(3), 164–167.

Donkor, E. S., & Sandall, J. (2007). The impact of perceived stigma and mediating social factors on infertility-related stress among women seeking infertility treatment in Southern Ghana. *Social Science & Medicine*, *65*(8), 1683–1694.

Egan, R., & Wilson, J. C. (2012). Rape victims' attitudes to rape myth acceptance. *Psychiatry, Psychology & Law, 19*, 345–357.

Elwood, W. N., & Greene, K. (2003). Desperately seeking skeezers: Downward comparison theory and the implications of HIV/STD prevention among African American crack users. *Journal of Ethnicity in Substance Abuse, 2*, 15–33.

Evans-Lacko, S., Brohan, E., Mojtabai, R., & Thornicroft, G. (2012). Association between public views of mental illness and self-stigma among individuals with mental illness in 14 European countries. *Psychological Medicine, 42*(8), 1741–1752.

Fischer, H. (2010). *U.S. military casualty statistics: Operation New Dawn, Operation Iraqi Freedom, and Operation Enduring Freedom*. Washington, D.C.: Congressional Research Service.

Florom-Smith, A. L., & De Santis, J. P. (2012). Exploring the concept of HIV-related stigma. *Nursing Forum, 47*(3), 153–165.

Frey, L. R., Query, J. L., Flint, L. J., & Adelman, M. B. (1998). Living together with AIDS: Social support processes in a residential facility. In V. J. Derlega, & A. P. Barbee (Eds.), *HIV and social interaction* (pp. 129–146). Thousand Oaks, CA: Sage Publications.

Gershon, T. D., Tschann, J. M., & Jemerin, J. M. (1999). Stigmatization, self-esteem, and coping among the adolescent children of lesbian mothers. *Journal of Adolescent Health, 24*(6), 437–445.

Goffman, E. (1963). *Stigma: Notes on the management of spoiled identity*. Englewood Cliffs, NJ: Prentice-Hall.

Goffman, E. (1990). *The presentation of self in everyday life* (rev. ed.). New York, NY: Penguin.

Goldberg, D. S. (2010). Job and the stigmatization of chronic pain. *Perspectives in Biology and Medicine, 53*(3), 425–438.

Golden, J., Conroy, R. M., O'Dwyer, A. M., Golden, D., & Hardouin, J.-B. (2006). Illness-related stigma, mood and adjustment to illness in persons with hepatitis C. *Social Science & Medicine, 63*, 3188–3198.

Graham, H. (2012). Smoking, stigma and social class. *Journal of Social Policy, 41*(1), 83–99.

Greene, K., Derlega, V. J., Yep, G. A., & Petronio, S. (2003). *Privacy and disclosure of HIV in interpersonal relationships: A sourcebook for researchers and practitioners*. Mahwah, NJ: Lawrence Erlbaum Associates.

Harshbarger, J. L., Ahlers-Schmidt, C. R., Mayans, L., Mayans, D., & Hawkins, J. H. (2009). Pro-anorexia websites: What a clinician should know. *International Journal of Eating Disorders, 42*(4), 367–370.

Hartwell, S. (2004). Triple stigma: Persons with mental illness and substance abuse problems in the criminal justice system. *Criminal Justice Policy Review, 15*(1), 84–99.

Herman, N. J. (1993). Return to sender: Reintegrative stigma-management strategies of ex-psychiatric patients. *Journal of Contemporary Ethnography, 22*(3), 295–330.

Hoge, C., Castro, C., Messer, S., McGurk, D., Cotting, D., & Koffman, R. (2004). Combat duty in Iraq and Afghanistan: Mental health problems and barriers to care. *The New England Journal of Medicine, 351*(1), 13–22.

Hooyer, K. (2012). Going AWOL: Alternative responses to PTSD stigma in the U.S. military. *Field Notes: A Journal of Collegiate Anthropology, 4*(1), 106–128.

Jones, P. S. (1997). Dialect as a deterrent to cultural stripping: Why Appalachian migrants continue to talk that talk. *Journal of Appalachian Studies, 3*(2), 253–261.

Jones, E. E., Farina, A., Hastorf, A. H., Markus, H., Miller, D. T., & Scott, R. A. (1984). *Social stigma: The psychology of marked relationships*. New York, NY: W. H. Freeman.

Kerbo, H. (1976). The stigma of welfare and the passive poor. *Sociology and Social Research, 60*(2), 173–187.

Keyes, K. M., Hatzenbuehler, M. L., McLaughlin, K. A., Link, B. B, Olfson, M. M., Grant, B. F., & Hasin, D. D. (2010). Stigma and treatment for alcohol disorders in the United States. *American Journal of Epidemiology, 172*(12), 1364–1372.

Khan, S. I., Bhuiya, A., & Uddin, A. S. (2004). Application of the capture-recapture method for estimating number of mobile male sex workers in a port city of Bangladesh. *Journal of Health, Population and Nutrition, 22*(1), 19–26.

Kindig, D., & Stoddart, G. (2003). What is population health? *American Journal of Public Health, 93*(3), 380–383.

Kwong, K., Chung, H., Cheal, K., Chou, J. C., & Chen, T. (2012). Disability beliefs and help-seeking behavior of depressed Chinese American patients in a primary care setting. *Journal of Social Work in Disability & Rehabilitation, 11*(2), 81–99.

Latimer, M. (2006). "We have never asked for help that was not desperately needed": Patterns of stigma management among former welfare recipients in West Virginia. *Journal of Appalachian Studies, 12*(2), 88–109.

Lawrence, S. (2010). The impact of stigma on the child with obesity: Implications for social work practice and research. *Child & Adolescent Social Work Journal, 27*(4), 309–321.

Leary, M. R., & Schreindorfer, L. S. (1998). The stigmatization of HIV and AIDS: Rubbing salt in the wound. In V. J. Derlega & A. P. Barbee (Eds.), *HIV and social interaction* (pp. 12–29). Thousand Oaks, CA: Sage Publications.

Levine, J. M., & McBurney, D. H. (1977). Causes and consequences of effluvia: Body odor awareness and controllability as determinants of interpersonal evaluation. *Personality and Social Psychology Bulletin, 3*, 442–445.

Logie, C. C., & Gadalla, T. M. (2009). Meta-analysis of health and demographic correlates of stigma towards people living with HIV. *AIDS Care, 21*(6), 742–753.

MacNeil, J., & Pauly, B. (2011). Needle exchange as a safe haven in an unsafe world. *Drug & Alcohol Review, 30*(1), 26–32.

Matthews, A. K., Sellergren, S. A., Manfredi, C., & Williams, M. (2002). Factors influencing medical information seeking among African American cancer patients. *Journal of Health Communication,* 7(3), 205–219.

McDonald, P., Charlesworth, S., & Cerise, S. (2011). Below the "tip of the iceberg": Extra-legal responses to workplace sexual harassment. *Women's Studies International Forum, 34*(4), 278–289.

Miall, C. E. (1986). The stigma of involuntary childlessness. *Social Problems, 33*(4), 268–282.

Mickelson, K. D., & Williams, S. L. (2008). Perceived stigma of poverty and depression: Examination of interpersonal and intrapersonal mediators. *Journal of Social and Clinical Psychology, 27*(9), 903–930.

National Institutes of Health. (2012). *Division of special populations.* Bethesda, MD: National Institutes of Health. Retrieved from http://www.nichd.nih.gov/about/org/dsp/

Neilands, T. B., Steward, W. T., & Choi, K. (2008). Assessment of stigma towards homosexuality in China: A study of men who have sex with men. *Archives of Sexual Behavior, 37*(5), 838–844.

Office of the Vice Chief of Staff (Army). (2012). *Army 2020: Generating Health & Discipline in the Force Ahead of the Strategic Reset.* Washington, D.C.: Headquarters, Department of the Army.

Palamar, J. J. (2012). A pilot study examining perceived rejection and secrecy in relation to illicit drug use and associated stigma. *Drug & Alcohol Review, 31(4)*, 573–579.

Paterson, B. L., Backmund, M., Hirsch, G., & Yim, C. (2007). The depiction of stigmatization in research about hepatitis C. *International Journal of Drug Policy, 18*, 364–373.

Reutter, L. I., Stewart, M. J., Veenstra, G., Love, R., Raphael, D., & Makwarimba, E. (2009). "Who do they think we are, anyway?": Perceptions of and responses to poverty stigma. *Qualitative Health Research, 19*(3), 297–311.

Room, R. (2005). Stigma, social inequality and alcohol and drug use. *Drug & Alcohol Review, 24*(2), 143–155.

Roschelle, A. R., & Kaufman, P. (2004). Fitting in and fighting back: Stigma management strategies among homeless kids. *Symbolic Interaction, 27*, 23–46.

Rush, L. L. (1998). Affective reactions to multiple social stigmas. *The Journal of Social Psychology, 138*, 421–430.

Schneider, J. W., & Conrad, P. (1980). In the closet with illness: Epilepsy, stigma potential and information control. *Social Problems, 28*, 32–44.

Schnittker, J., & John, A. (2007). Enduring stigma: The long-term effects of incarceration on health. *Journal of Health & Social Behavior, 48*(2), 115–130.

Schomerus, G., Lucht, M., Holzinger, A., Matschinger, H., Carta, M. G., & Angermeyer, M. C. (2011). The stigma of alcohol dependence compared with other mental disorders: A review of population studies. *Alcohol and Alcoholism, 46*(2), 105–112.

Shaw, L. L. (1991). Stigma and the moral careers of ex-mental patients living in board and care. *Journal of Contemporary Ethnography, 20*, 285–305.

Sikorski, C., Luppa, M., Kaiser, M., Glaesmer, H., Schomerus, G., König, H.-H., & Riedel-Heller, S. G. (2011). The stigma of obesity in the general public and its implications for public health—a systematic review. *BMC Public Health, 11*(1), 661–668.

Smedley, B. D., Stith, A. Y., & Nelson, A. R. (Eds.). (2003). *Unequal treatment: Confronting racial and ethnic disparities in health care*. Washington, D.C.: National Academies Press.

Smith, R. A., & Parrott, R. L. (2012). Mental representations of HPV in Appalachia: Gender, semantic network analysis, and knowledge gaps. *Journal of Health Psychology, 17*, 917–928.

Smith, R., Rossetto, K., & Peterson, B. L. (2008). A meta-analysis of disclosure of one's HIV-positive status, stigma and social support. *AIDS Care, 20*(10), 1266–1275.

Snow, D. A., & Anderson, L. (1987). Identity work among the homeless: The verbal construction and avowal of personal identities. *American Journal of Sociology, 92*, 1336–1371.

Sowell, R. L., & Phillips, K. D. (2010). Understanding and responding to HIV/AIDS stigma and disclosure: An international challenge for mental health nurses. *Issues in Mental Health Nursing, 31*, 394–402.

Ssebunnya, J., Kigozi, F., Lund, C., Kizza, D., & Okello, E. (2009). Stakeholder perceptions of mental health stigma and poverty in Uganda. *BMC International Health and Human Rights, 9*, 5–14.

Steuber, K. R., & Solomon, D. H. (2011). Factors that predict married partners' disclosures about infertility to social network members. *Journal of Applied Communication Research, 39*, 250–270.

Strike, C. J., Myers, T., & Millson, M. (2004). Finding a place for needle exchange programs. *Critical Public Health, 14*(3), 261–275.

Stuber, J., & Kronebusch, K. (2004), Stigma and other determinants of participation in TANF and Medicaid. *Journal of Policy Analysis and Management, 23*, 509–530.

Taylor, S. E., & Lobel, M. (1989). Social comparison activity under threat: Downward evaluation and upward contacts. *Psychological Review, 96*, 569–575.

Teixeira, M. E., & Budd, G. M. (2010). Obesity stigma: A newly recognized barrier to comprehensive and effective type 2 diabetes management. *Journal of the American Academy of Nurse Practitioners, 22*(10), 527–533.

Tirupati, N. S., Rangaswamy, T., & Raman, P. (2004). Duration of untreated psychosis and treatment outcome in schizophrenia patients untreated for many years. *Australian and New Zealand Journal of Psychiatry, 38*, 339–343.

Vijayasiri, G. (2008). Reporting sexual harassment: The importance of organizational culture and trust. *Gender Issues, 25*(1), 43–61.

Wallace, S., & Villa, V. (2003). Equitable health systems: Cultural and structural issues for Latino elders. *American Journal of Law and Medicine, 29*, 247–267.

Wang, F. Y., Bih, H., & Brennan, D. J. (2009). Have they really come out: Gay men and their parents in Taiwan. *Culture, Health & Sexuality, 11*(3), 285–296.

Waxman, C. I. (1983). *The stigma of poverty: A critique of poverty theories and policies.* New York, NY: Pergamon Press.

Wills, T. A. (1981). Downward comparison principles in social psychology. *Psychological Bulletin, 90*, 245–271.

Zaheer, J., Links, P. S., Law, S., Shera, W., Hodges, B., Tsang, A. K. T., . . . Liu, P. (2011). Developing a matrix model of rural suicide prevention. *International Journal of Mental Health, 40*, 28–49.

METHODOLOGICAL APPROACHES WHEN INVESTIGATING HEALTH DISPARITIES

Lisa Sparks and Michelle Miller-Day

The shifting landscape of populations in the United States challenges investigators to adapt existing research efforts to reflect the needs of an increasingly diverse society (Nápoles-Springer & Stewart, 2006) and to reduce health disparities (Smedley, Stith, & Nelson, 2003). The term "health disparity" connotes difference, inequality, and unfairness in the quality and access to healthcare among different population groups (LeCook, McGuire, & Zaslavsky, 2012). This involves not just differences in direct health care, but the operation of healthcare systems, the legal and regulatory climate, discrimination, and other factors (Institute of Medicine, 2003; LeCook et al., 2012). While much of the literature on health disparities focuses on race, ethnicity, and socioeconomic status, there are a variety of other cultural groups that are subject to inequities in healthcare such as age, sexual orientation, disability, and geography (Bushy, 2008). As the demographic trends in the United States change, meeting the needs of diverse cultural groups when conducting research becomes more challenging, and adaptations to traditional design and methodological approaches are warranted. This chapter argues for culturally grounding research efforts as a way to reflect cultural diversity and enhance representativeness of samples; describes relevant definitions and characteristics important to consider in conducting health disparities research; and provides methodological suggestions for culturally grounding research efforts to reduce disparities.

Culturally Grounded Research

Culture shapes worldviews, norms, rules, attitudes, values, and beliefs, and, thereby, influences the perceptual processes by which messages are sent and received (Baldwin, Faulkner, & Hecht, 2006). As a result, research efforts (e.g., recruitment and retention strategies and materials) that adjust to and accommodate a person's culture are likely to be received more positively than efforts that do not. With federal guidelines mandating the inclusion of diverse cultural groups in research (e.g., National Institutes of Health, 2001), scientists must learn to adapt traditional approaches to conducting research with diverse populations in culturally competent ways. Acknowledging diversity and approaching research in a culturally competent fashion foregrounds the role of culture (e.g., socioeconomic status, ethnicity, age, gender, sexuality, geographic area) in research development and implementation.

Hecht and colleagues (Hecht & Krieger, 2006; Hecht & Miller-Day, 2009) argue concepts such as "cultural sensitivity" and "cultural appropriateness" may present a limited notion of culture, placing it outside the research (e.g., something to bring in through being sensitive or appropriate to the "other"), but the concept of "cultural grounding" recognizes that culture is a complex, multilayered phenomenon and that these layers of complexity should be integrated into designing and implementing health research from "the ground up." Culturally grounding research acknowledges that research participants who are part of cultural group memberships have personal concepts of self that cut across layers of identity (Ndiaye, Krieger, Warren, Hecht, & Okuyemi, 2008). So, a culturally grounded approach to conducting health research involves the complex process of representing and expressing relevant culture(s) in creative and meaningful ways to the design, implementation, interpretation, and dissemination of research products to meet the needs of individuals or groups for health promotion, prevention, or care.

Definitions of Interest When Conducting Health Disparities Research

Health Disparities

According to the *Unequal Treatment* report (Institute of Medicine, 2003), disparities are differences in healthcare services received by two groups that are not due to differences in the underlying healthcare needs or preferences of members of the groups. So, to better be able to identify disparities in populations, researchers must first develop a more complete understanding of the values, preferences, and needs of different populations, including underserved groups.

At Risk

The term "at risk" is used by researchers interested in potential health problems affecting our most vulnerable populations. At-risk populations are vulnerable to serious health disparities, with many immigrants experiencing significantly worse health outcomes, such as higher rates of morbidity and mortality, than other segments of society. At-risk groups disproportionately suffer from heart attacks, cancer, diabetes, strokes, HIV/AIDS, and many other serious diseases.

Ethnicity

The term "ethnicity" includes labels such as "Hispanic," "African American," "Asian," "Caucasian," and/or "Native American," as defined by the Bureau of the Census, with national origin or ancestry viewed as establishing group membership (Marín & Marín, 1991). While it may be appropriate to compare and contrast responses or behaviors of African American, Hispanics, Caucasians, or Asians, researchers should not assume that these labels are necessarily mutually exclusive. It is possible for an individual to be ethnically non-Hispanic White/Caucasian, but be culturally Hispanic from growing up in the Mexican border town of Brownsville, Texas. An individual could be ethnically Hispanic, but racially Black or White at the same time (Marín & Marín, 1991). Moreover, researchers must be cautious about cross-group comparisons without first considering within-group diversity (Swanson et al., 2003).

Cultural Competence

The term "cultural competence" in the health context refers to awareness of unique and defining characteristics of the populations for which health professionals provide care and from which they wish to enroll research participants (O'Brien, Kosoko-Lasaki, Cook, Kissell, Peak, & Williams, 2006). Cultural competence in research is the explicit use of culturally based knowledge in sensitive ways to address the needs of cultural group members, researchers, and other stakeholders. To collect and analyze meaningful data, researchers need an understanding of the importance of social and cultural influence on patients' health beliefs and behaviors (Betancourt, Green, Carrillo, & Ananeh-Firempong, 2003). Cultural competency in research moves beyond sensitivity or awareness to action (Shiu-Thornton, 2003).

Collectivism

Collectivism describes members of a cultural group who emphasize the needs, objectives, and points of view of an in-group emphasizing interdependence, field sensitivity, conformity, mutual influence and empathy, sacrifice and trust of in-group members (e.g. Hispanic cultures), while more individualistically oriented members of a cultural group determine their social behavior primarily in terms of objectives, attitudes, and values that reflect more individualistic, competitive, and achievement-oriented cultures (e.g., American or German cultures; Hofstede, 1980; Marín & Triandis, 1985). Further, research indicates that collectivistic cultures prefer interpersonal relationships in in-groups that are nurturing, loving, show intimacy, and respect, whereas individualistic cultures prefer super-ordinated, hierarchical, and confrontational interactions (Triandis, Marín, Hui, Lisansky, & Ottati, 1984). Understanding these preferences and patterns toward interpersonal relationships and preferences for personal contact can be of great importance in designing effective research projects with members of more collectivistic-oriented cultures as well as tapping into distinct cultural and health beliefs that may impact the effectiveness of the health-care intervention. One caveat to also keep in mind is that these same characteristics and preferences toward a nurturing encounter situation may lead respondents to provide researchers with socially desirable or biased responses (e.g. Hofstede, 1980). For instance, "simpatica" is a cultural script likely derived from collectivistic value orientation as it emphasizes the need for interactions promoting empathy, conformity, and pleasant social relationships that avoid conflict and negativity. Simpatica may play a role in low refusal rates and participant drop out in returning for follow-up interviews from members of more collectivistic cultures. In addition, small talk before and after an interview is generally preferred by members of collectivistic-oriented cultures as it can facilitate respondent satisfaction and cooperation and build an empathic relationship between the researcher and respondent (Marín & Marín, 1991).

Familialism

"Familialism," or "*familismo*" in Hispanic cultures, is a cultural value involving strong identification with and attachment to families, with feelings of reciprocity, loyalty, and solidarity holding high importance for family members (Marín & Marín, 1991). The notion of familialism typically is not generation dependent, and includes orientations about perceived obligations to provide financial and emotional support within the family; reliance on relatives for support and help when needed; and the perceptions of relatives as behavioral and attitudinal referents throughout the life span (Marín & Marín, 1991). Researchers working with Hispanic populations will find that gaining a strong understanding and respect for the important role of familialism in these families will be very helpful. For example, behavior change smoking cessation research has shown that identifying particular consequences of behavior change on the family is often a crucial component in motivating behavior change (Marín, Marín, Pérez-Stable, Sabogal, & Otero-Sabogal, 1990). Such family-related reasons for behavior change, as well as appeals to family values and/or small incentives, can motivate these respondents to participate in research projects.

Power Distance

"Power distance" is defined as a measure of interpersonal influence or power existing between two individuals, and is another important cultural value that differentiates cultural groups (Hofstede, 1980). An assumption of power distance is that societies have powerful individuals resulting from acquired or inherited characteristics, such as education or financial means, or traits, such as intelligence. Such individuals strive to retain their power in relationship to those less powerful, and societies lean toward supporting such power differences, which has huge implications in terms of barriers and access to health information and health care, and, arguably, increases health disparities. Individuals from low power-distance cultures accept power relations that are more democratic and consultative, whereas individuals from high power-distance cultures tend to accept more autocratic, paternalistic, and hierarchical relations. Hofstede's (1980) power distance index (ranging from 1 to 120) demonstrates higher scores for Latin and Asian countries, African areas, and the Arab world, whereas Anglo and German countries indicate lower power distance scores. For instance, Austria = 11, Denmark = 18, Israel = 13, the United States = 40, the United Kingdom = 35, and Sweden = 31 on the cultural scale of Hofstede's analysis, yet southern and eastern European countries tend to have higher scores; for example, Romania = 90 and Spain = 57. Thus, if you are working with individuals with lower power distance, one can expect less respect, deference, and consideration of titles (e.g. MD or PhD), preference for more informal interaction or small talk with little etiquette or protocol, and preference for more involvement and joint decision-making. If you are working with individuals with higher power distance cultures, be sure to give clear, direct directions, explicit deadlines taking an authoritarian research approach, show respect and deference to those in positions higher than you, and expect higher levels of bureaucracy in the organization. Health communication scholars interested in effective implementation of health disparities research projects must design research procedures that respect and recognize the differential social power levels of participants and integrate face-saving conversations and messages when dealing with disclosure of personal information.

Personal Space

Personal and physical space interaction preferences differ for people of different cultures. For decades, anthropologists have been studying similarities and differences among people from "contact cultures," who prefer physical closeness, shorter interpersonal distances, and personal contact (e.g. Hispanic cultures), and those from non-contact oriented cultures, who prefer a bit more distance (Hall, 1969). Implications for health disparities researchers' ability to navigate personal space, in terms of establishing affinity and connections with participants, are important to consider.

Time Orientation

In the early 1960s, Kluckhohn and Strodtbeck observed that cultures have different time orientation, with certain cultures more future-oriented and others more present-oriented (1961). Future-oriented cultures, such as the United States, emphasize efficiency, planning, and punctuality, with an overall ability to delay gratification, whereas present-oriented cultures are less able to be on time, tend to be less efficient, and have a more flexible attitude toward time. For example, Hispanics' emphasis on relationship quality is a cultural trait that can impact time orientation. Thus, researchers who are highly efficient and time conscious should be aware when participants have cultural traits leaning toward present orientation.

Gender Roles

Although gender roles are shifting dramatically in most societies, these stereotypic perceptions between male and female roles can still differ in more traditional cultures (Marín & Marín, 1991). For instance, a male Hispanic may be suspicious of an interviewer of either gender who wishes to speak with his wife or daughter and may not allow her to participate in the study. This machismo attitude could have important implications for health-care communication studies dealing with sexually transmitted diseases or other sensitive health topics. Such gender roles can also impact participant selection and sampling issues. Involving the entire family in sensitive health-care studies may help to reduce health disparities in terms of selection and sampling of segmented populations of interest.

Finally, it is important to understand that, within cultural groups, there are also individual differences to consider among subgroups based on background characteristics such as national origin, religion and faith preferences, migration and generational history, and language use and preferences, as well as unique cultural values and norms (Marín & Marín, 1991). The information included here can serve as a set of definitional tools to more effectively understand and conduct health disparities research.

Conducting Culturally Grounded Health Communication Research: Suggestions for Design and Methodology

To engage and more meaningfully incorporate diverse populations of interest in health research, we need to make sure that the experiences of the cultural group members are valued in the development and implementation of research. Trust is an essential ingredient for collecting valid data, yet an ongoing issue is lack of trust for research and researchers, due to a variety of reasons, such as limited understanding of the need for research, negative experiences with previous research groups, or perceptions of the research agency possessing power over research participants (Cardona & Joshi, 2007). Hence, methods for accessing diverse groups must include steps aimed at enhancing trust among study participants, researchers, and key stakeholders. Culturally grounding research efforts by employing a participatory action research approach is one way in which cultural group members can collaborate with researchers and other stakeholders in designing and implementing health research. This approach heightens the potential for the next generation of health communication researchers to execute health disparities research that is important, practical, and will resonate with different populations. Suggestions are illustrated in Figure 16.1.

Suggestions for Design

When designing culturally grounded research, the design must reflect more than just surface structure elements of culture (Colby et al., 2013). There are two primary dimensions of culture (Resnicow, Baranowski, Ahluwalia, & Braithwaite, 1999) that should be addressed when enhancing cultural sensitivity in research efforts: surface structure and deep structure. Surface structure refers to observable, superficial characteristics of a cultural group (e.g., people, places, language, settings) while deep structure refers to the underlying elements of culture, such as values and meanings. An example of deep structure is illustrated in a case study reanalyzed by Trickett (2011), where women in a Peruvian village refused to boil water because of a cultural belief that cooked water (regardless of its temperature when consumed) was linked with illness. Cooked water held cultural significance for these women. This is an example of a deep structure. Incorporating deep structure into research is more complex and requires an understanding of cultural, social, historical, environmental, and psychological forces that influence target health behavior (Colby et al., 2013). Yet, both surface and deep structure information can be included into the research process by integrating this cultural information into research materials (e.g., recruitment materials, consent documents, instruments) and procedures (e.g., recruitment procedures, researcher training, data collection and analysis procedures, and research dissemination).

A strategy for enhancing understanding of both surface and deep structure dimensions of culture is to authentically engage the targeted research community in the design of research efforts. The first step in this process is to establish partnerships and *solicit community members and community groups to assist in study design*. In the design stage, researchers must first become familiar with the target group's needs, socio-demographic, cultural, power differentials, and health-related characteristics as well as preferred communication and health information channels. Such community information is crucial in terms of contacting potential participants, but also in obtaining community support for the project and data collection. Targeting and talking with community opinion leaders is a great place to start in terms of breaking into the community and beginning to think about an appropriate research design strategy that will work with the target audience. Constituting a formal *research advisory board* is an excellent way to

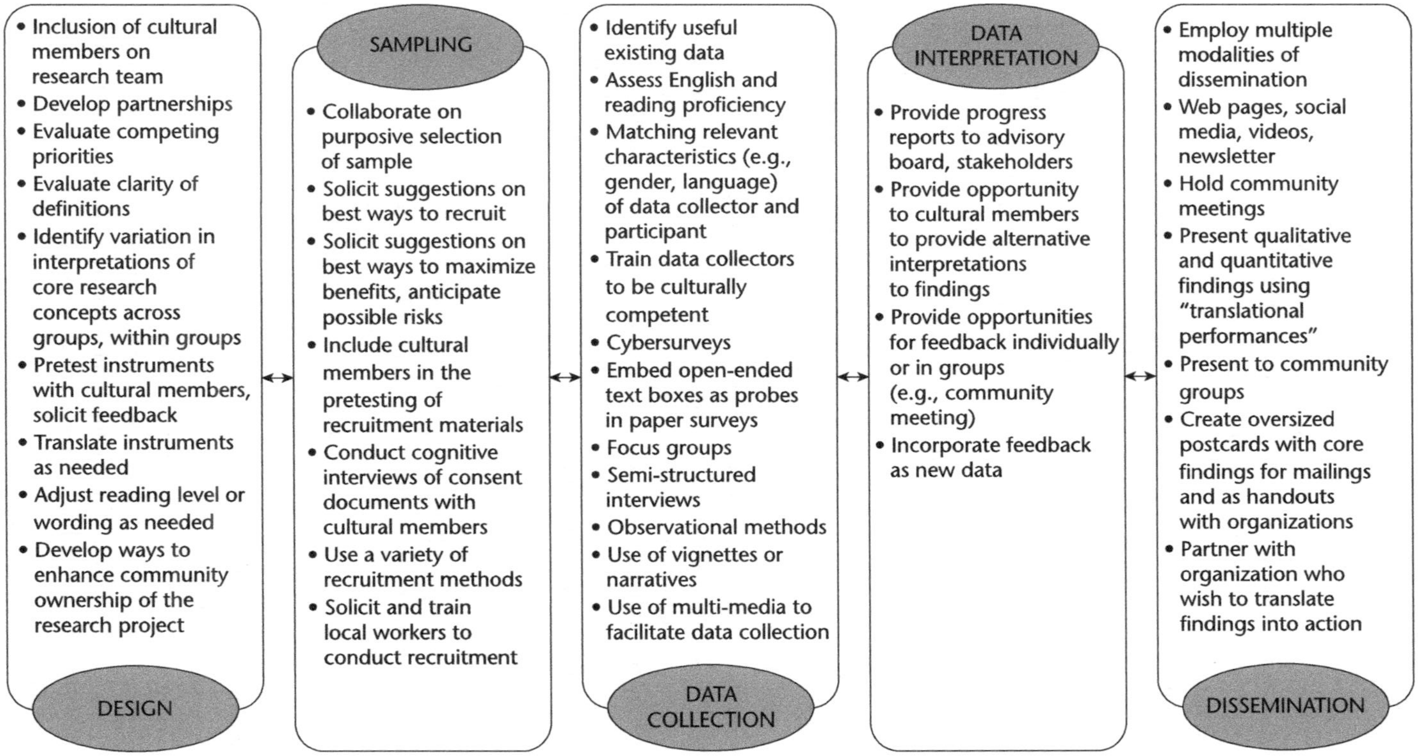

DESIGN

- Inclusion of cultural members on research team
- Develop partnerships
- Evaluate competing priorities
- Evaluate clarity of definitions
- Identify variation in interpretations of core research concepts across groups, within groups
- Pretest instruments with cultural members, solicit feedback
- Translate instruments as needed
- Adjust reading level or wording as needed
- Develop ways to enhance community ownership of the research project

↔

SAMPLING

- Collaborate on purposive selection of sample
- Solicit suggestions on best ways to recruit
- Solicit suggestions on best ways to maximize benefits, anticipate possible risks
- Include cultural members in the pretesting of recruitment materials
- Conduct cognitive interviews of consent documents with cultural members
- Use a variety of recruitment methods
- Solicit and train local workers to conduct recruitment

↔

DATA COLLECTION

- Identify useful existing data
- Assess English and reading proficiency
- Matching relevant characteristics (e.g., gender, language) of data collector and participant
- Train data collectors to be culturally competent
- Cybersurveys
- Embed open-ended text boxes as probes in paper surveys
- Focus groups
- Semi-structured interviews
- Observational methods
- Use of vignettes or narratives
- Use of multi-media to facilitate data collection

↔

DATA INTERPRETATION

- Provide progress reports to advisory board, stakeholders
- Provide opportunity to cultural members to provide alternative interpretations to findings
- Provide opportunities for feedback individually or in groups (e.g., community meeting)
- Incorporate feedback as new data

↔

DISSEMINATION

- Employ multiple modalities of dissemination
- Web pages, social media, videos, newsletter
- Hold community meetings
- Present qualitative and quantitative findings using "translational performances"
- Present to community groups
- Create oversized postcards with core findings for mailings and as handouts with organizations
- Partner with organization who wish to translate findings into action

FIGURE 16.1 Suggestions for Culturally Grounding Research Design and Implementation

include members of a target population in research design to enhance the cultural representativeness of research efforts. Depending on the complexity of the target population, one or more groups may be necessary, each reflecting a homogenous layer of culture (e.g., a youth advisory team, a Latino advisory team). Additionally, broader community involvement may be solicited through town hall meetings, individual or group interviews, and/or observations.

At the design stage, it is necessary to identify the needs and concerns of the community prior to deciding on the study research questions. Conducting a *needs assessment* within the target population serves to situate the research activity in the real-life needs of the participants, making the research responsive to those needs, ensuring greater investment of the community to accomplish the research goals. In doing so, it is important for researchers to ascertain if there is dissonance between the research agenda and the local social and service delivery priorities. Will the research interfere with ongoing activities in the community? Will it be perceived as threatening to planned or existing activities? Do the community members understand why the proposed research is important?

Once it is determined that the planned research is understood by cultural group members, perceived to be responsive to the needs of the community, and not in conflict with existing or other planned activities, members can assist the research team in *developing and refining clear research objectives*, research questions or hypotheses, and conceptual definitions. Following from a clear research purpose are research objectives and questions or hypotheses. Cultural group members can assist in the development or provide reactions to and refinement of existing objectives and research questions, adding insight into important wording and key concepts, variables, or even methods that may have been overlooked. Are the operational definitions in line with the conceptual definitions group members hold? Do different cultural groups interpret concepts similarly or differently? Do the proposed measures meet the basic psychometric criteria for this group?

Consultation with indigenous groups serves to assist with research design, but also *the protection of human participants*. In some American Indian research, sacred knowledge, objects, and sites have been violated in the name of research (An-Na'im, 1992). Inclusion of indigenous members in the design of research can help protect participants and make the research more attractive to potential participants. Cultural group members can serve to generate convincing language to use in recruitment efforts and consent documents, and assist researchers in identifying how the research might cause undue burden on the target population in terms of approach, effort required, travel required, interruption of the daily routine, and/or length of procedures. Feedback at this stage can evaluate if measures need to be translated, assist in necessary translations, and determine if materials need to be adjusted for reading level. Moreover, design phase feedback can identify ways the research team might enhance community ownership of the research project.

Suggestions for Sampling

Population-based methods often generate extremely small samples of some cultural groups (e.g., sexuality, age) who are geographically dispersed, precluding their use in examining possible differences (Braveman, 2006). Sampling inclusion of cultural groups may need to be accomplished through stratified sampling or maximum variation sampling techniques, and inclusion of feedback from advisory board members can assist in this process. Cultural group members can suggest where to recruit participants, who might be the gatekeepers to useful samples, and the best way to maximize benefits and anticipate possible risks with the population. Additionally, opinion leaders in the community can open doors to places frequented by the target population, such as shopping and dining areas, church, social, or community activities and organizations.

Group members can also provide valuable feedback in terms of whether recruitment procedures are culturally appropriate or might not be effective. For example, within a particular community, word of mouth and personal contact may be perceived by possible participants as much more persuasive and credible. The use of varied recruitment procedures is also recommended.

Cultural group members in advisory positions can assist in pretesting recruitment materials, forms, protocols, and materials. Cognitive interviews are recommended to assess the sensitivity and readability of consent documents. For the conduct of the cognitive interview, volunteer subjects are recruited and are interviewed about the cognitive processes that respondents use when reading materials, such as what the respondent believes the sentence/document is asking or what comes to mind when certain risks are described. Finally, cultural group members can assist with soliciting local workers to do recruitment during the normal course of their personal or professional activities.

Suggestions for Data Collection

Existing Data

The quality of any research is determined, in part, by the information obtained and analyzed. Before considering suggestions for data collection, we suggest that researchers consider *existing data sources* in order to access information from and about a variety of cultural group members. One rich source of information that researchers are not always aware of is the electronic health record (EHR), sometimes referred to as the electronic medical record. The EHR is an enabling technology that allows physician practices and hospitals to manage the health information of individual patients. Electronic, rather than paper and pencil, records are supposed to help improve the quality of medical care in the United States (Blumenthal & Tavenner, 2010). To this end, the federal government is providing financial incentives for their adoption (see the Health Information Technology for

Economic and Clinical Health Act 2009). This includes incentives to purchase, install, and use the software. This has enhanced the amount and quality of health data potentially available to health research, such as ethnicity, age, disability, chronic care status, vital signs, active medications and allergies, up-to-date problem lists of current and active diagnoses, clinical decisions, laboratory results, and reporting of data on the quality of care (Blumenthal & Tavenner, 2010). The information generated by EHRs can be extremely valuable to study and address disparities; however, a lag in EHR adoption by medical institutions might further exacerbate disparities in the quality of health care (Jha et al., 2006). Large-scale national surveys are also resources that are often overlooked and can be highly useful in mining existing data for useful information about specific populations. For further discussion on large-scale studies, see examples from the Health Information National Trends Survey (HINTS), National Health Interview Survey (NHIS), National Health and Nutrition Examination Survey (NHANES), or Hispanic Health and National Nutrition Examination Survey (H-HANES).

Qualitative Approaches

One method for tapping into the shared experiences of a cultural group is to conduct a reactance format *focus group*, which provides instruction in basic concepts and scenarios to which lay people can react, as well as a superior method for ascertaining public preferences and the unique needs of an at-risk group (see also Ndiaye et al., 2008). Focus groups also allow participants to respond to issues with their own preferences, concerns, and language, as opposed to survey research, which typically requires participants to select from a closed, and often limited, set of options that might reflect the researcher's world views rather than those of the participants. Focus group methodology allows for exploration and understanding of motivations for behaviors and behavioral processes, moderators can encourage participants to articulate their own choices, but also the reasons behind those choices. Yet, Greene and Magsamen-Conrad (this volume) state that focus group methods can create unique research challenges as some individuals are likely to respect confidentiality more than others, even when focus group protocols directly address this concern in instructions. When a sufficient number of focus groups are chosen carefully to represent target audiences, however, focus groups can provide a solid understanding of cross-cutting patterns within cultural groups regarding general health beliefs, attitudes, intentions, and perceptions.

Semi-structured, face-to-face interview with cultural group members are also a valuable tool for gathering in-depth and nuanced information about culturally held health beliefs, preferences, and perceptions. Semi-structured interviews can tap into participants' perceptions of who they define themselves to be (social identity) and how they orient to others, as well as individual knowledge, attitudes, and beliefs toward the often-sensitive health-care topic. Most importantly, individual interviews provide the researcher with the opportunity to follow up on comments and probe for more detailed explanation, prompting discussion of topics of interest and also new, emergent, ideas. Novel information generated in individual and group interviews can expand the scope of any investigation into new and exciting directions. When conducting individual or group interviews, it is wise to involve cultural group members in the development of the interview schedule, including possible prompts and probes, as well as the interview protocol itself, regarding social and cultural expectations to develop rapport and disclosure.

Another tool used to enhance the reach of research efforts and validity of results is the use of *vignettes*, or narratives crafted to facilitate participant identification with a story through realism (Hecht & Miller-Day, 2009; Lapatin et al., 2012). Vignettes can be shaped to reflect a variety of cultural elements such as race, ethnicity, gender, age. In Colby et al. (2013), narrative data were crafted into written and video vignettes that reflected both the surface and deep structure of the targeted rural youth culture in their study. Vignette drafting is an iterative process, where narratives are generated, select narratives are crafted into a coherent story or example, pilot tested, and group feedback is obtained on images and wording, calibrating the vignettes based on feedback (Lapatin et al., 2012). Research using this approach reports that narrative vignettes serve to overcome resistance to health messages, facilitate information processing, provide surrogate social connections, and address emotional (not just cognitive) issues (Kreuter et al., 2007; Miller-Day & Hecht, 2013).

Observational research is often time intensive and expensive to conduct; however, there has been increased interest in conducting cyber-ethnographies—observation in chatrooms, discussion boards, and on blogs—to document both surface and deep structural elements to culture. Researchers attempting to "write culture" (ethnography) have traditionally conducted fieldwork by living in distant cultures, conducting interviews, and observing participants. As people conduct more and more activities online and leave digital tracks (e.g., pictures, blogs, public posts, tweets), researchers have begun to study human behavior in cyberspace. By documenting and analyzing online data, researchers can identify cultural concepts relevant to a specific research topic, but also gain insight into the best ways to solicit research participation and query group members.

Quantitative Approaches

Certain quantitative methods, such as structured telephone interviews and surveys, may not be appropriate to reach certain populations because of limited English proficiency or reading literacy. Involving community member advisory members in the process of pilot testing any instrument is crucial for the effectiveness of this research. Instruments may need to be translated and all translations must be reviewed before implementation to identify mistakes and disfluencies. Moreover, when conducting closed-ended or forced-choice surveys, several researchers have suggested the inclusion of open-ended text boxes to probe for additional comments and thoughts on a response.

Cyber surveys (Mathy, Schillace, Coleman, & Berquist, 2002) are becoming increasingly popular to reach diverse and targeted populations. Using technology to conduct survey research can involve sending surveys via electronic mail, posting a link to the survey on websites, or even on online discussion boards. There are even services such as Datafield that provide phone applications for survey responses. These technological advances allow researchers to widen their reach and access diverse populations that might be difficult to access using other means, but they also allow the research to specifically target under-represented populations at the locations where they might naturally coalesce.

General Procedural Concerns

In addition to incorporating the voices of cultural members on advisory boards to assist in the development of data-collection materials and using methods that are sensitive to capturing cultural differences, research procedures may need to be adapted. Alegria (2009) stated that researcher training of new investigators is a particularly important issue when conducting research with diverse populations. Researchers should learn "atypical" research strategies, such as community-based participatory research, and strategies for integrating community members into research teams (Minkler & Wallerstein, 2008). Additional researcher training is needed to enhance cultural competence, reduce what might be perceived as patronizing behaviors, increase sensitivity to issues such as matching staff with participant ethnicity or language, increase skill in modifying or translating traditional study methods, instruments, and interventions, and provide resources for the exploration of new innovative research methods and data-collection methods that might fit the needs of diverse multicultural populations.

Suggestions for Data Interpretation and Feedback

The history of research in many at-risk populations (e.g., African Americans) is fraught with abuses and deceit. See, for example, the description of the Tuskegee syphilis study (Centers for Disease Control and Prevention, 2011). Once data are collected and analyzed, traditional research practice involves publication in peer-reviewed journals, chapters, or books, and the community members hear nothing more about the research. In the traditional model of research, feedback on research progress and findings is virtually non-existent and most certainly insufficient for community members to use to address real-life problems or concerns. Withholding information—especially health-related information—from the very groups who might use it may intensify disparities. The following suggestions may assist researchers, as they move forward and embrace community-based involvement of target populations, to maintain community partnerships and gain additional insights into study findings.

The first suggestion is to provide progress reports to stakeholders and/or advisory boards across the life of the project. Progress reports can be in the form of academic reports, newsletters, or oral presentations during meetings or town hall gatherings. Reports should be devoid of "academic speak" and summarize key accomplishments, challenges, and any preliminary findings. Final reports should also be devoid of academic language, and it is often useful to hire or seek a volunteer community member to edit these reports for a more general audience.

As findings emerge, provide opportunities for cultural group members to supply alternative interpretations to findings. For statistical results, group members might add insight into significant findings or question the generalizability of the results using researcher interpretations. For qualitative research, soliciting additional interpretations can illuminate things previously unseen, uncover novel findings, and reveal information about negative cases.

Provide opportunities for cultural group members to provide feedback individually or in groups (e.g., community meeting) about the ongoing research efforts and findings. These opportunities provide a way for cultural group members to join the academic conversation in a way that is meaningful to them. Feedback and interpretations collected during this process can then be treated as new data; that is, new information, new insights into the phenomenon, and new directions for future research.

Suggestions for Dissemination

Petronio (2002) argued that 21st-century scholars must reconceptualize the research enterprise to effectively accomplish translation of scientific research. She argued that contemporary scholars must reconsider current definitions of evidence and develop ways to bring information more effectively to those who desire, are in need of, and can make use of this scientific knowledge. Despite this call for translational research, there seems to be a "health research information disparity" in the United States. Using the definition of disparity we posed at the beginning of this chapter, we argue that there is difference, inequality, and unfairness in the quality and access to health research information among different population groups in the United States. Specifically, up-to-date health research information is typically only available to highly educated, mostly Caucasian, literate individuals who have access to scholarly publications.

Many have noted that translational research that is accessible to many is a very real need, especially for marginalized or at-risk populations (Kreps, Neuhauser, Sparks, & Villagran, 2008; Kreps & Sparks, 2008; Miller-Day, 2008a, 2008b). Indeed, the National Institutes of Health have charged researchers with the tasks of speeding up the use of research findings within applied settings, and facilitating partnerships between research, practice, and policy constituencies in ways to enhance the relevance of scientific research (Miller-Day, 2008a).

Traditional research views written reports as the preeminent medium for information dissemination, and practitioners, policy makers, and community members remain relatively unaware of these written reports or of their importance. In an effort to enhance the relevance of social and health sciences, and honor myriad audiences who might be interested in research findings, we pose the following suggestions for disseminating research information. These suggestions are not intended to replace traditional written reports, but to supplement them and expand the visibility of health information research to different audiences by creating diverse products for distinct audiences through the use of multiple delivery systems.

The first suggestion for researchers is to consider the different audiences for the research during the design phase of the study. Including cultural group members in this discussion may generate some audiences that the researchers would not have thought of otherwise. In addition to an academic audience, other audiences might be practitioners, policy makers, community developers, and individual community members. Different aspects of the study might be relevant or useful to different groups. Research products can be developed specifically for each audience.

As humans are increasingly connected by technology, they are becoming more visual and cinematic (Denzin, 2003). Therefore, we suggest that researchers make an effort to develop multiple products employing a variety of communication modalities. Designing oversized postcards and visually attractive handouts for community groups, creating web pages, social media pages (e.g., Facebook), Twitter accounts for the project securing "followers" for the research and creating an ongoing flow of information about process and findings, and YouTube videos reflecting major findings are just some of the ways multimedia formats can be used to engage groups other than researchers in the research process.

Miller-Day (2008a, 2008b) argued for "translational performances," combining theatrical practices with social science discovery in an evocative public presentation that has the potential to be educational and emancipatory; a performative social science approach that acknowledges scholarly articles. This method of research dissemination is live performance based and is intended to decode and render accessible the research process and findings. While qualitative findings based on in-depth individual interviews, observations, and focus group interviews lend themselves more naturally to this type of dissemination practice, quantitative findings can also be represented, using projection screens, programs, and other written texts along with the presentation. Inviting community members, research stakeholders, policy makers, and opinion leaders to these performances can promote agency–community relations and serve to contribute to a rapid diffusion of the information.

Public presentations of the research to community groups beyond the academic audience are another excellent way to engage community members in the research process. Volunteering to speak in town hall meetings, to specific community groups, or educating and training community advocates to speak on your behalf to groups is time consuming but highly rewarding. These presentations sometimes require the researcher to partner with community organization and consult with them on ways to translate findings into action.

In the end, this chapter pointed out the necessity of adapting traditional research design and methodological approaches to accommodate an increasingly diverse national and international population. Whether diversity is defined in terms of ethnic, racial, economic, gender, age, geographic, or other characteristics, a culturally grounded approach to conducting social scientific research offers cultural group members a "seat at the table" to participate in research design, implementation, and dissemination. By culturally grounding our research efforts, we can reduce disparities in our research efforts and move toward more representative findings that, in turn, may assist in reducing health disparities for these cultural group members.

References

Alegria, M. (2009). Training for research in mental health and HIV/AIDS among racial and ethnic minority populations: Meeting the needs of new investigators. *American Journal of Public Health, 99*(1), S26–S30.

An-Na'im, A. A. (Ed.). (1992). *Human rights in cross-cultural perspectives: A quest for consensus.* Philadelphia, PA: University of Pennsylvania Press.

Baldwin, J. R., Faulkner, S. L., & Hecht, M. L. (2006). A moving target: The illusive definition of culture. In J. R. Baldwin, S. L. Faulkner, M. L. Hecht, & S. L. Lindsley (Eds.), *Redefining culture: Perspectives across the disciplines* (pp. 3–26). Mahwah, NJ: Lawrence Erlbaum Associates.

Betancourt, R. J., Green, A. R., Carrillo, J. E., & Ananeh-Firempong II, O. (2003). Defining cultural competence: A practical framework for addressing racial/ethnic disparities in health and health care. *Public Health Reports, 118*(4), 293–302.

Blumenthal, D., & Tavenner, M. (2010). The "Meaningful Use" regulation for electronic health records. *New England Journal of Medicine, 363*(6), 501–504.

Braveman, P. (2006). Health disparities and health equity: Concepts and measurement. *Annual Review of Public Health, 27*, 167–194.

Bushy, A. (2008). Conducting culturally competent rural nursing research. *Annual Review of Nursing Research, 26*, 221–236.

Cardona, M., & Joshi. R. (2007). The challenge of balancing methodological research rigour and practical needs in low–income settings: What we are doing and what we need to do better. *Critical Public Health, 17*(1), 81–89.

Centers for Disease Control and Prevention. (2011). *The U.S. Public Health Service syphilis study at Tuskegee.* Washington, D.C.: U.S. Department of Health and Human Services. Available from: http://www.cdc.gov/tuskegee/timeline.htm/

Colby, M., Hecht, M., Miller-Day, M., Krieger, J., Syvertsen, A., Graham, J., & Pettigrew, J. (2013). Adapting school-based substance use prevention curriculum through cultural grounding: An exemplar of adaptation processes for rural schools. *American Journal of Community Psychology, 51*(1–2), 190–205.

Denzin, N. (2003). *Performance ethnography.* Thousand Oaks, CA: Sage Publications.

Hall, E.T. (1969). *The hidden dimension.* Garden City, NY: Doubleday.

Hecht, M. L., & Krieger, J. L. (2006). The principle of cultural grounding in school-based substance abuse prevention. *Journal of Language and Social Psychology, 25*(3), 301–319.

Hecht, M. L., & Miller-Day, M. (2009). The drug resistance strategies project: Using narrative theory to enhance adolescents' communication competence. In L. R. Frey & K. N. Cissna (Eds.), *Routledge handbook of applied communication* (pp. 535–557). New York, NY: Routledge.

Hofstede, G. (1980). *Culture's consequences.* Beverly Hills, CA: Sage Publications.

Institute of Medicine. (2001). *Crossing the quality chasm: A new health system for the 21st century.* Washington, D.C.: National Academy Press.

Institute of Medicine. (2003). *Unequal treatment: Confronting racial and ethnic disparities in healthcare.* Washington, D.C.: National Academy Press.

Jha, A. K., Ferris, T. G., Donelan, K., DesRoches, C., Shields, A., Rosenbaum, S., & Blumenthal, D. (2006). How common are electronic health records in the United States? A summary of the evidence. *Health Affairs, 25*(6), 496–507.

Kluckhohn, F. R., & Strodtbeck, F. L. (1961). *Variations in value orientations.* New York, NY: Row, Peterson.

Kreps, G. L., & Sparks, L. (2008). Meeting the health literacy needs of immigrant populations. *Patient Education and Counseling, 71*(3), 328–332.

Kreps, G. L., Neuhauser, L., Sparks, L., & Villagran, M. (Eds.) (2008). The power of community-based health communication interventions to promote cancer prevention and control for at-risk populations. *Patient Education and Counseling, 71*(3), 315–318.

Kreuter, M.W., Green, M. C., Cappella, J. N., Slater, M. D., Wise, M. E., Storey, D., Clark, E. M. et al. (2007). Narrative communication in cancer prevention and control: A framework to guide research and application. *Annals of Behavioral Medicine, 33*(3), 221–235.

Lapatin, S., Goncalves, M., Nillni, A., Chavez, L., Quinn, R. L., Green, A. et al. (2012). Lessons from the use of vignettes in the study of mental health service disparities. *Health Services Research, 47*(3)(Pt. 2), 1345–1362.

LeCook, B., McGuire, T. G., & Zaslavsky, A. M. (2012). Measuring racial/ethnic disparities in health care: Methods and practical issues. *Health Services Research, 47*(3)(Pt. 2), 1232–1254.

Marín, G., & Triandis, H. C. (1985). Allocentrism as an important characteristic of the behavior of Latin Americans and Hispanics. In R. Díaz-Guerrero (Ed.), *Cross-cultural and national studies in social psychology* (pp. 85–104). Amsterdam, Netherlands: Elsevier Science Publishing Company.

Marín, G., & Marín, B. V. (1991). *Research with Hispanic populations.* Newbury Park, CA: Sage Publications.

Marín, G., Marín, B.V., Pérez-Stable, E. J., Sabogal, F., & Otero-Sabogal, R. (1990). Changes in information as a function of culturally appropriate smoking cessation community intervention for Hispanics. *American Journal of Community Psychology, 18*(6), 847–864.

Mathy, R. M., Schillace, M., Coleman, S. M., & Berquist, B. E. 2002. Methodological rigor with Internet samples: New ways to reach underrepresented populations. *Cyberpsychology and Behavior, 5*(3), 253–266.

Miller-Day, M. (2008a) Translational performances: Toward relevant, engaging, and empowering social science. *Forum: Qualitative Social Research*, *9*(2), Art. 54.

Miller-Day, M. (2008b). Performance matters. *Qualitative Inquiry*, *14*(8), 1458–1470.

Miller-Day, M., & Hecht, M. L. (2013). Narrative means to preventative ends: A narrative engagement framework for designing prevention interventions. *Health Communication*, *28*(7), 657–670.

Minkler, M., & Wallerstein, M. (2008). *Community-based participatory research for health*. San Francisco, CA: Jossey-Bass.

Nápoles-Springer, A. M., Santoyo-Olsson, O'Brien, H. (2006). Using cognitive interviews to develop surveys in diverse populations. *Medical Care*, *44*(Suppl. 3), S21–S30.

National Institutes of Health. (2001). *NIH policy and guidelines on the inclusion of women and minorities as subjects in clinical research*. Bethesda, MD: National Institutes of Health, Office of Extramural Research. Available from: http://grants.nih.gov/grants/funding/women_min/guidelines_amended_10_2001.htm/

Ndiaye, K., Krieger, J. L., Warren, J. R., Hecht, M., & Okuyemi, K. (2008). Health disparities and discrimination: Three perspectives. *Journal of Health Disparities Research and Practice*, *2*(3), 51–71.

O'Brien, R. L., Kosoko-Lasaki, O., Cook, C. T., Kissell, J., Peak, F., & Williams, E. H. (2006). Self-assessment of cultural attitudes and competence of clinical investigators to enhance recruitment and participation of minority populations in research. *Journal of National Medical Association*, *98*(5), 674–682.

Petronio, S. (2002). The new world and scholarship translation practices: Necessary changes in defining evidence. *Western Journal of Communication*, *66*(4), 507–512.

Resnicow, K., Baranowski, T., Ahluwalia, J. S., & Braithwaite, R. L. (1999). Cultural sensitivity in public health: Defined and demystified. *Ethnicity and Disease*, *9*(1), 10–21.

Shiu-Thornton, S. (2003). Addressing cultural competency in research: Integrating a community-based participatory research approach. *Alcoholism: Clinical and Experimental Research*, *27*(8), 1361–1364.

Smedley, B. D., Stith, A. Y., & Nelson, A. R. (Eds.). (2003). *Unequal treatment: Confronting racial and ethnic disparities in healthcare*. Washington, D.C.: National Academy Press.

Swanson, D.P., Spencer, M.B., Harpalani, V., Dupree, D., Noll, E., Ginzburg, S., & Seaton, G. (2003). Psychosocial development in racially and ethnically diverse youth: Conceptual and methodological challenges in the 21st century. *Development and Psychopathology*, *15*(3), 711–743.

Triandis, H. C., Marín, G., Hui, C. H., Lisansky, J., & Ottati, V. (1984). Role perceptions of Hispanic young adults. *Journal of Cross-Cultural Psychology*, *15*(3), 297–320.

Trickett, E. J. (2011). From "Water boiling in a Peruvian town" to "Letting them die": Culture, community intervention, and the metabolic balance between patience and zeal. *American Journal of Community Psychology*, *47*(1), 58–68.

Method Reflections

REFLECTIONS ON HEALTH COMMUNICATION RESEARCH METHODS

Joan A. Jurich, Austin S. Babrow, Lindsey M. Rose, and Spencer D. Patterson

> In a famous parable, the Buddha imagines a group of blind men who are invited to identify an elephant. One takes the tail and says it's a rope; another clasps a leg and says it's a pillar; another feels the side and says it's a wall; another holds the trunk and says it's a tube.
>
> *(Batchelor, 1997)*

"Reality," "Knowledge" of Reality, and Research Methods

Like the blind men in the Buddhist parable, when we choose a research method, we shape what we come to know about health communication (see Thompson, Cusella, & Southwell, this volume). Look to the left, and what is to our right vanishes. Look ahead, and what is behind is out of view. Writing as a rhetorical critic, Kenneth Burke (1984/1935) expressed this point quite elegantly when he said, "a way of seeing is also a way of not seeing" (p. 49). A bit more technically, frames make frame-congruent perception and sensemaking easy at the same time that they obscure other perceptions and meanings. For instance, a metaphor clarifies whatever is consistent with it and ignores whatever is not (Lakoff & Johnson, 1980). Another example is the parable of the elephant; even as it helps us to see the limits of perception, the parable emphasizes variation in the surfaces of a unitary reality, obscuring the idea of multiple realities.

The idea of a single reality is often attributed to "material realists," those who believe that all of reality will ultimately be reducible and describable in terms of material elements and forces. This view is contrasted with the idea that there are multiple realities, such as the worlds of matter (physics and chemistry), living things (biology), and meaning (the semiotic world; see Anderson, 1996). Another interesting way to understand the distinction between unitary and multiple realities is given by Berger and Luckmann (1967); the commonsense "here and now" of everyday life is taken by most people, most of the time, as the paramount reality, although it suggests within it a variety of distinguishable alternatives (e.g., dreaming, fantasy, theater or fiction, play, transcendent religious experience, hypothetical or theoretical thought). In this chapter, we write from the standpoint that "reality" is everything that omniscience can grasp. In other words, whatever reality is, it exceeds finite human grasp. We will never know more than those parts of the elephant within our reach.

When we put together these ideas—that reality exceeds human intelligence, and that the frames by which we attempt to understand reality shape what we understand—we arrive at a useful way of understanding and reflecting on the many methods of health communication research that comprise this book. Each method is a way to approach and gain knowledge about health communication. Each privileges its own way of seeing, making aspects of health communication that are consistent with the frame easiest to see and think about, just as the method obscures aspects that fall outside of the methodological frame. A researcher taking up a method in response to the impulse to study health communication is comparable to an artist attempting to render her conception of a landscape. The rendering will differ depending on whether the artist uses pencil, charcoal, pastels, watercolors or oil-based paints, or black and white or color film. And lest we think that one or another of these media allows for more or less accurate representation of reality, we should keep in mind a story about Pablo Picasso. The great Cubist painter was speaking with a critic who expressed a preference for photographic realism. Subsequently, when the critic shared a picture of his girlfriend, Picasso quipped, "My, is she really that small?" (quoted in Gunderman, 2008, p. 57). In other words, every rendering is its own way of seeing, one of a potentially infinite number of possible renderings. Extending the previous example, the landscape will have still different meanings to a poet, composer, botanist, geologist, environmentalist, logger, architect, and so on. Similarly, every understanding of health communication is necessarily shaped into the features or meanings evoked by the method we use to study it. And different methods will offer different understandings.

The ideas we have been pursuing can be brought to further important points by linking them with the general semanticist Alfred Korzybski's (1994/1933) famous dictum, "the map is not the territory." We have, until now, emphasized that ways of seeing, just like the representations that result, are never "complete." Innumerable maps, and innumerable map-making approaches, are possible. We must add here the social constructionist insight that there is nothing inherent in any aspect of reality that *requires* it to be understood—mapped—in any particular way (Gergen, 2000). For example, there is nothing about a landscape that requires the artist to use watercolors or charcoal. And add to this the pragmatist insight that the knowledge we seek about health communication is not some timeless Truth; rather, we seek knowledge that serves our purposes. Knowledge about health communication is functional, useful, and practical for purposes at hand.

Health communication is among the most elemental of human experiences, so it is not surprising—and, indeed, it is fortunate—that the field has come to value a wide variety of methods serving a rich array of research and practical/applied interests.

Methods differ not only in terms of aims and procedures for conducting research, but also in terms of what the methods imply about the nature of communication ("ontological" assumptions) and what it means to attain knowledge about communication ("epistemological" assumptions). Although there are a wide range of distinctly different assumptions in these areas (see Anderson, 1996; Klein & Jurich, 1993), they are often reduced to contrasts between qualitative and quantitative methods, or between empirical (i.e., based on observation) and non-empirical methods of research. This chapter will avoid these usages because they obscure more than they clarify. Instead, we will boil down the complexities to the distinction between post-positivist and interpretive methods. However, to understand and appreciate this distinction well, it is useful to understand its genesis.

A Very Brief History of Human Inquiry

From the moment human beings emerged as entities capable of thinking beyond the instant of experience, beyond our immediate response to sensory stimuli, we have been faced with the question of what to believe. In our late modern world, it is nearly impossible to imagine the profundity of this question. Today, particularly as people in the Western world, we rarely face serious or sustained questions about where to find safe food and drink now or in the coming days and months, where and how to cleanse ourselves or dispose of our bodily waste, how to shelter and clothe ourselves, how to organize ourselves with others, including who presents a threat to our existence, how to control pregnancy and achieve safe childbirth, or what to think and do about smoking, an infected toe, or a mysterious lump on the breast or testicle. This is not to say that we always know precisely what to think and how to act; rather, it is to recognize that humans have collectively achieved so much comprehension of the workings of the world and so much control in so many domains of experience that we take for granted the enormous stores of knowledge at our command. We also take for granted the vague understanding we have about how to attain knowledge. However, particularly *when there is a great deal at stake*, when we think more carefully about what we know and how to attain knowledge, we are soon confronted with this most basic challenge of human being: what to believe (see Babrow, 1992, 2007). We find ourselves faced with the same quandary that has vexed humanity since thought emerged.

One simple but instructive way to characterize potential sources of knowledge is to distinguish among knowledge that comes from direct experience, information from others, and knowledge derived from inference[1] (Fishbein &

Ajzen, 1975). Each of these sources of knowledge has strengths and limits. For instance, direct sensory experience confers knowledge of reality by making it palpable and hence more credible than second-hand reports from others who could be less competent observers than you might be or could be untrustworthy for many other reasons. Of course, another person could be a better observer than you are (e.g., he could be less invested than you are in seeing the world in a particular way), and, more generally, the senses are notoriously fallible (e.g., magic depends on the limits of sight). Inference, reason, or logic might free us from the limitations of direct sensory experience or information from others, but inference or reasoning has its own weaknesses. For instance, reasoning cannot overcome the limitations of faulty premises ("garbage in–garbage out"), can be led astray by bias (indeed, self-interest often determines what we take to be reasonable), and frequently yields contradictory or paradoxical results. So, over the millennia, humans have struggled with the question of how to study and understand the world, at times refining, and at times privileging one or another of the three sources of knowledge.

For much of human history, traditional knowledge, or what we have called knowledge based on information from others (ancestral teachings, God, the Church, the king), was dominant. In the West, the Renaissance (roughly, the 14th to 17th centuries CE) and Enlightenment (approximately, the 17th to 18th centuries CE) ignited confidence in the human intellect, thus de-emphasizing traditional (at the time, largely church) doctrine. Observation (direct experience) and reason, working together, were seen as the most effective engines of knowledge creation. To this day, rigorous reasoning combined with careful observation is taken by most researchers to be absolutely required of research method. The specific methods discussed in this book reflect developments or refinements of our understanding of these pathways to knowledge. To understand some of the variations in these methods, it is useful to briefly track the evolution and divergence of post-positivist and interpretive inquiry.

Post-Positivism

The Genesis of Post-Positivism

Following the (re)discovery of the glorious capacities of humankind during the Renaissance, the Enlightenment gave rise to the modern conception of science. But what is science? Many consider the defining feature of science to be its commitment to observation or "empiricism" (sensory experience), but, as noted above, rigorous reasoning is also an absolute requirement. Beyond these very general commitments, understandings of science and the scientific method have been evolving over time. The dominant conception and practice of scientific inquiry today is called "post-positivism." Knowing how this perspective evolved is useful not only for understanding it but also for grasping alternatives.

Briefly, post-positivism emerged in the latter half of the last century, when a variety of assumptions underlying traditional conceptions of science (especially a philosophy of science known as "logical positivism"; see O'Keefe, 1975) began to be relaxed. As just one example, in the strict formulation, logical positivist philosophers insisted that science requires observation to be "theory free," or completely free of any biases. Particularly in the second half of the 20th century, it became clear to most philosophers of science that this assumption was unsupportable.

We have come to realize that it is impossible to observe the world without our observations being colored by the observer's point of view, including theoretical language. As we said earlier in this chapter, the very act of observing requires a point of view, an interpretive lens that allows us to see some aspect of reality even as it obscures other aspects. Our senses are surely our most basic lenses, and every one of our senses reflects our unique point of view. For example, natural sensory acuity varies from person to person; color blindness and tone deafness are moderately striking examples. Unique experiences introduce still other variations in individuals' sensory equipment. For example, people's capacity to sense the qualities of fine wine, Japanese 7-tone music, and Cubist sculpture and painting change substantially with personal experience. Our unique experiences also cause variations in sensory habituation; continued stimulation of a sense will eventually lead to desensitization, which is why you don't notice the distinctive smell of your own home but do notice the peculiar odor when you enter another person's house or apartment (Ackerman, 1991).

Layered almost seamlessly atop the senses, language itself provides the lenses by which we pick out aspects of experience for conscious attention and thought. As a thought experiment, it is instructive to imagine what your consciousness would consist of if you had no words for any aspects of the reality that engulfs you (also see Taylor, 2009). Of course, our linguistic tools vary considerably, not only between but within language communities. For example, when confronted with a table covered with items, what one person sees as the specific components of a computer, another, less knowledgeable person sees as an undifferentiated pile of "computer parts," and a still less knowledgeable person sees as a "bunch of junk." Language and the conceptual systems it makes possible are tools we use to observe the world; what we see depends on the conceptual system invoked. For example, recall the painter, poet, botanist, geologist, and logger looking at the very same landscape discussed above. Or consider the differences in how you would analyze health problems such as obesity and anorexia nervosa depending on whether you are a communication, economics, psychology, or nutrition major.[2] Obviously, then, when we turn to investigate some aspect of reality, we are guided from the moment of our conception of the project to see what our concepts incline us to see. In other words, there is no possibility of language- or theory-free observation.

As researchers in the latter half of the 20th century began to relax the logical positivist assumption that science *requires* theory-free observation and other highly restrictive and unsupportable views, alternative ways of understanding science began to emerge. Notably, one loosely unified alternative labeled "post-positivism" now roughly characterizes the underlying philosophy of science associated with many of the methods described in this book: especially the chapters on surveys, content analysis, conversation analysis, direct observation and coding of patient–physician interaction, network analysis, experimentation, and meta-analysis. Post-positivism is also the dominant mode of thought underlying the approaches taken in the chapters on stigmatized populations and health disparities.

Post-Positivist Commitments

Following Guba (1990; also see Phillips, 1990), post-positivist methods are unified by several commitments or assumptions. In one, which Guba termed "critical realism" (to contrast it with material realism, as described above), post-positivists assume that the reality of communication phenomena exists "but can never be fully apprehended" or completely understood because of our inability to perceive this reality through our limited senses and inability to fully control our biases (p. 23). Some critical realist researchers believe laws of nature determine the structure of health communication phenomena independent of any human knowledge or intention. For example, content analytic and experimental researchers have examined what they take to be the inborn psychological disposition to either like or dislike highly stimulating message features, such as loud, fast-paced driving music, fast camera shot changes, and unusual camera angles (Morgan, Palmgreen, Stephenson, Hoyle, & Lorch, 2003). Other critical realist post-positivists, including some experimentalists, content analysts, and survey researchers, believe that the forces shaping communication are not so much laws of nature that are independent of human knowledge and intention as they are so deeply embedded in human knowledge as to be relatively difficult to access and therefore quite stable. Conversation analysts are particularly likely to hold to this view.

Guba (1990) identified a second post-positivist assumption in what he termed "modified objectivism." In this view, objective understanding of reality, free from any bias or theory, is understood to be impossible, but "objectivity remains a regulatory ideal" (p. 23). To enforce the ideal, the community of scholars/experts essentially polices research reports submitted to conferences and journals for any signs of bias.

Third, whereas the narrowest view of science held experimentation to be the only legitimate form of empirical (observational) method, a third characteristic of post-positivism relaxes this requirement by accepting and attempting to synthesize data from a variety of research methods (see the Thompson et al. chapter discussion of "triangulation"). Guba (1990) explains the reasoning behind this as follows:

> If human sensory experience and intellective mechanisms cannot be relied upon, it is essential that the "findings" of an inquiry be based on as many sources—of data, investigators, theories, and methods—as possible. Further, if objectivity can never be entirely attained, relying on many different sources makes it less likely that distorted interpretations will be made.
>
> *(p. 21)*

In sum, many contemporary research methods are unified by sharing the post-positivist assumptions and commitments noted here. As the associated chapters in this text make clear, the specific methods have been developed to answer particular questions, but often these questions can themselves be answered using more than one method, or the methods can be used as complementary approaches to formulating answers. For example, experiments are considered the gold standard for testing small clusters of causal relations,[3] whereas surveys can probe causal structures involving larger numbers of variables (although the causal tests are more ambiguous than experiments; again, see note 3). As another example, direct observation and coding of patient–physician interaction, content analysis, and conversation analysis represent alternative and potentially complementary ways of analyzing health care and other health- and illness-related interaction. In all of these post-positivist projects, researchers proceed under the critical realist assumption that health communication phenomena reflect either laws of nature or dynamics so deeply ingrained in human habits of thought and action as to be highly reliable. Although we may never completely understand these dynamics, post-positivists assume that knowledge can come ever closer to an accurate understanding of communication processes. Moreover, post-positivists believe that strenuous efforts to reduce observational and inferential biases, or holding objectivity as a regulative ideal that is upheld by the community of researchers, will improve our research and bring us closest to accurate knowledge. So, too, will reconciling and synthesizing the findings from multiple studies using varied methods. Finally, as the amount and accuracy of our knowledge increase, experts will gain ever greater ability to predict and control the outcomes of health communication of all sorts. This increasing knowledge will improve our ability to promote health and reduce human suffering.

Interpretive Methods

Post-positivism is often contrasted with interpretive, hermeneutic, or constructionist approaches to research methods. Although significant nuances differentiate specific perspectives, we will use the phrase "interpretive methods" to refer to approaches that share more or less fully in several common assumptions about the research enterprise. These assumptions or rough approximations underlie the methods discussed in this book's chapters on in-depth interviews, case study, ethnography, narrative analysis, meta-synthesis, and rhetorical criticism[4] (Thompson, Cusella, and Southwell's introductory chapter to this volume attempts to bridge the post-positivist/interpretive method divide).

Earlier in this chapter, we said that post-positivism arose in part as a response to the recognition that we never observe the world directly—the idea that all observation is filtered through sensory and conceptual–linguistic filters. Post-positivists insist that, by striving for the ideal of objectivity, they can largely overcome these perceptual and conceptual limits and study communication processes and principles that exist independent of these filters (e.g., independent because these phenomena are governed by our biology or very strong habits of thought and action). Interpretive researchers reject this perspective. They make the interpretive process and its products the heart of research. For instance, Anderson (1996) argues that when we give up the idea that we engage with the world through "brute sense data—that one-to-one relationship between 'out there' and 'in the head—we are forced into the semiotic domain" (p. 50). In other words, most interpretive methods are based on the idea that humans live in a world made meaningful by acts of interpretation, acts in which we understand the world in and through words and other signs (e.g., figures, pictures). Researchers thus use interpretive methods (there are no other methods, after all) to study the processes of interpretation and their products.

As suggested in the preceding paragraph, interpretive methods generally reject the critical realism of post-positivism. Instead, they assume that reality is comprised of multiple realms, such as the purely material, biological, and semiotic, and focus on the latter. They also assume that the semiotic realm is plural. In other words, "realities" arise in the great variety of communicative constructions that emerge at different times and in different places and cultures (Guba, 1990). The general terms "health" and "illness," and specific aspects of well-being and forms of sickness, are made meaningful by the communicative acts and other practices in which they are lived.

The preceding should not to be taken to mean that physical states and processes, such as pain, pregnancy, and childbirth, are not real for interpretivists. It is, rather, to recognize that all such states are experienced subjectively. Realities such as pain in childbirth are shaped perhaps by inborn pain tolerance and idiosyncratic experience as well as sociocultural layers of meaning. For example, think of the history of paternalistic efforts to protect women from physical strain and pain in countless domains, and think too of the maternal quip that humans would soon be extinct if men rather than women had to bear the pain of childbirth. Whether or not there are any sex-linked differences in pain tolerance, there can be no doubt that gender expectations—and countless other sociocultural meanings—shape the ways we bear the trials of pain. The same might be said for heart disease, cancer, dementia, and every other widely accepted diagnosis. What these conditions mean, how they are experienced, how we actually talk—or believe we ought to talk—about them varies with individuals and cultures, time and place. If the reader can see this is true of well-defined health and illness processes and conditions, it should be even easier to see in relation to contested illnesses, such as chronic fatigue syndrome, fibromyalgia, Gulf War syndrome, and sicknesses attributed to environmental causes; debates about over-prescription (e.g., of drugs ostensibly meant to treat ADD and ADHD); and medicalization of mood, diet, substance abuse, sexuality, conception, pregnancy, and childbirth. These and countless other examples suggest that there is no single reality awaiting discovery by health communication researchers. Rather, there are multiple realms, interrelated in complex ways, and any one understanding of any aspect of this complexity is an ongoing accomplishment of people struggling to figure out what to believe and what to want in the context of their lives (i.e., their historical time, social location, and culture; see Babrow, 2007).

Given that interpretive methods assume humans construct and live in multiple realities, it should not be surprising to learn that these methods reject the modified objectivism of post-positivism. In other words, objectivity is not held to be an unreachable but still ideal achievement. Interpretive researchers embrace subjectivity, both their own and that of the people they study. As Guba (1990) expressed it, interpretations of the researcher and those of the people she or he studies are fused in the process of conducting an in-depth interview, case study, ethnography, or narrative analysis; "facts," says Guba, are a product of these interactions.

And here complications arise. Perhaps the most important is the question of how the researcher should integrate her or his interpretations with those of the study participants. If the researcher aims to represent the world only as participants see it, the researcher is essentially treating himself as a flawless mirror or frictionless conduit through which participant meanings are made available to readers of the research report, and the project slides into a post-positivist work; respondents' meanings are real and knowable to the extent the researcher's subjectivity is kept from contaminating representations of respondent meanings. By contrast, it should be easy to see the problems in allowing the researcher's point of view to dominate constructions of participants' interpretations. Therefore, as Guba says, knowledge of whatever reality is under study must somehow be constructed out of the researcher and participants' interpretations (for specific suggestions on how to manage this synthesis, see the chapters on in-depth interviews, case study, ethnography, narrative analysis, meta-synthesis, and rhetorical criticism).

In short, interpretive methodologists believe there is no single reality; rather, there are constantly emerging realities that are created in the very processes of communication. We construct reality by naming, forming analogies and other forms of metaphor, narrating, dialoging, debating, promising (and more formal contracts), threatening, describing, questioning, praising, and blaming; these and countless other acts and activities are performed no other way than by communicating. Out of these acts and interactions, the human world arises. (If the idea that reality is communicatively constructed is still difficult to understand or accept, try the following thought experiment in two parts: (a) imagine how you would perform any of the preceding acts without verbal—aural, written, or sign—language; (b) try to imagine a human world without the aforementioned acts. Or, recall the earlier thought experiment of trying to imagine what consciousness would consist of if you had no words for any aspects of the reality that engulfs you.) In any given time and place, reality "appears" to us only through our ways of seeing, through our conceptual or theoretical orientations, and never immediately and directly.

If reality is multiple, if it is a matter of interpretation, does this mean that all interpretations are equally worthy of belief? This question is frequently asked by people who fear that interpretivism is merely relativism[5] under a new label. The concern is ill-founded. As suggested earlier in this chapter, all interpretive researchers, no less than their post-positivist counterparts, believe that careful reasoning is essential to research. Moreover, many interpretive researchers are empiricists in believing that observation—of texts, discourse, naturally occurring interaction—is essential to knowledge; without these observations, the researcher's only source of knowledge would be her or his own thoughts and reflections (see Anderson, 1996, for a discussion of hermeneutic empiricism).

Although many interpretive methodologists are empiricists in the sense noted above, they disagree with their post-positivist counterparts' idealization of objectivity. Not only is objectivity impossible, argue interpretive researchers, but sometimes the very point of research is to understand the world from another's very particular point of view: so the healthy can understand the reality of sickness, so the diet and exercise and healthcare utilization choices of well-educated and affluent people are not taken for the choices of the less educated and poor, so the health challenges of heterosexuality are not taken to be everyone's or the only challenges of sexuality, so men might understand what it is like to live in a woman's body, and so on. But, again, interpretive research methods require not only great sensitivity, perspective-taking, empathy, and the like, but also very careful argument to justify interpretations. This is why interpretive researchers generally include not only explanations of the methods used to gather texts, but also frequent and, at times, lengthy quotations so that readers can judge the quality of the researcher's interpretations and related inferences.

Whereas post-positivists police research reports for inescapable influences of the observer's point of view, with objectivity held as the ideal toward which researchers aim, interpretive investigators evaluate their colleagues' constructions in terms of the sensitivity and sensibility of their synthesis of researcher and research participants' (natural actors') interpretations of reality. Moreover, interpretive researchers discuss the relationships between the understandings emerging in a study and past research, just as post-positivists judge the consistency of any new research report with past findings. Post-positivists assess this consistency in order to overcome the limits of any one study (its partiality, its inescapable point of view) to achieve an ever more accurate grasp of a reality that will nonetheless always exceed our complete understanding.[6] By contrast, interpretive methodologists consider the relationships of meanings emerging in a current investigation to those presented in past research not to assess validity or better capture a singular reality but as part of an ongoing dialogue about what we have reason to believe. In this way, papers reporting interpretive research contribute to what Guba (1990) referred to as "hermeneutic dialectic," or the ongoing, careful questioning and answering that constitutes the interpretive literature in an area of research (also see Bochner's 1985 notion of "juridical validation").

The contrast between post-positivist discussion about the validity of research findings and the hermeneuticist dialectic about the credibility of interpretive research reveals a vital difference in approaches to the question of what to believe. It is, however, not the only vital way to understand the difference between the methods. This is because it emphasizes a relatively conservative way of thinking about the issue of what to believe. In other words, when we ask "What is true?" or "What do I have good reason to believe?", the questions incline us to think about *the world as it is.* There is, of course, nothing wrong with this. Indeed, as we said earlier, these questions have bedeviled the species since we became creatures capable of a mental life outside of the moment of sensory experience. There is, however, another way to think about the issue of what to believe. That is the question, "What might the world be?" Or, "What is possible?" Like the more conservative understanding, this more liberating way of thinking brings to light contrasts between post-positivist and interpretive methods. Here, too, we see differences in motives for research, bases for choosing one or another method, and criteria for evaluating the quality of a study. But, as with the more conservative issue of validity of truth claims versus credibility of interpretations, the distinctions are both important and subtle. We will use this final contrast as a way to wrap up and conclude the chapter.

A Care-ful Conclusion

As we have said, post-positivist research aims to achieve ever more accurate understanding of a reality that exists largely, if not totally, independent of human intention. This does not mean, however, that post-positivists are necessarily focused on the world as it exists rather than the world as it might be. Indeed, as we said earlier, much of the reason for post-positivists' interest in understanding reality is so that they might predict and control it, and thereby reduce suffering and contribute to human flourishing. Still, critics of post-positivism might be tempted to say that its emphasis on understanding reality *as it is* can blind researchers to reality *as it might be*. This criticism is appealing to interpretive researchers because they insist that reality is largely what we make it to be through our sense-making and action guided by this understanding. This line of criticism suggests that we should beware of the delusion that reality is singular, that the world is and must be understood in only one way.

Thoughts such as these lead to a very important debate. Every health communication researcher necessarily takes a position in this debate, although often this is not a conscious decision, and one may later change her mind. Thoughtful students of research methods are aware of the debate, think about where they stand within it, and understand and appreciate why others take an alternative stance.[7]

The debate proceeds something like this. Based on their commitment to the idea that reality is plural, interpretive researchers tend to see post-positivist methods as imposing an inherently narrow, limiting view (reality is, after all, singular from this view). By contrast, interpretive methods are thought to be both broadening and potentially liberating. They are broadening in the sense of illuminating more than one way of conceiving and living reality; they are liberating in the sense that those who previously saw only one reality come to see new possibilities. Post-positivists counter by asking whether alternative "constructions" bear any relation to enduring, stable reality, and whether alternative possibilities have any real prospects of being achievable and sustainable. Although participants or researchers can conceive of reality in some counter-normative or novel way, how do we know that anyone else can or that this new way of understanding reality is sustainable or beneficial? To answer any of these questions, insists the post-positivist, we need to know what is true, what is our best warranted belief about what is true—both in current actuality and in possibility. We come to the most forcefully warranted answers to these questions by striving for objectivity, overcoming the limits of perception, and chasing out as many obvious biases as possible.

Interpretive researchers respond to the foregoing by arguing that, no matter what safeguards we put in place, our understandings will always be partial, dependent on what we choose to look at, how we choose to look, and indeed on who is doing the looking. The interpretive researcher will insist, there are several decisive reasons to believe that both reality *as it is* and reality *as it might be* are not reducible to facts existing in the world independent of human point of view, intention, and intervention (i.e., that facts are "out there" waiting to be discovered). One reason is the constructive power of communication, which we have been discussing in much of the chapter. A second reason is the apparent limitlessness of human imagination. A third reason to insist that reality does not exist independent of human construction is the very history of human discovery: in the realm of matter, we have developed nanotechnology, which involves engineering at the level of atoms and molecules, so it extends human imagination and ingenuity into a previously inaccessible realm, and we built the Large Hadron Collider, thought to be capable of recreating conditions that have not existed since the Big Bang. In the biological realm, the human imagination has penetrated and now manipulates the genome, bringing with it the promise/threat of re-engineering life. In the semiotic realm, we have seen the vast reaches and incomprehensible variety of human meanings that comprise all of human history to this point and anticipate going forward till we no longer exist. When we put all of these accomplishments of human imagination–knowledge together, we can better understand how human activity is now so powerful that it has brought about climate destabilization, with its global-scale impacts on matter, life, and meaning. In sum, for these many reasons, interpretive researchers insist that both reality *as it is* and reality *as it might be* are not reducible to facts existing in the world independent of human point of view, intention, and intervention (i.e., again, that facts are "out there" waiting to be discovered). Humans are continually reinventing not only what exists but what is possible. Research can be liberatory and empowering, to reduce suffering and promote the good, such as human health in all its many meanings (just as research can lead to devastating destruction, as some of our examples suggest).

Post-positivists counter that the amazing accomplishments of human discovery and invention have been made possible not merely by imagination and desire, but also by learning the truths of reality that are not determined by human desire and imagination—that is, laws of nature and the most deeply embedded habits of thought and action, those that simply do not change at our will. As we have penetrated these truths, we have used this understanding to predict and control experience in new ways. Our most powerful discoveries are made possible, they will insist, by methods of research that strive for objectivity by minimizing the influence of human preconceptions, theoretical and other commitments, and particularly our desires, on what we take to be true. Interpretivists respond by pointing to one more reason to believe that human imagination and desire simply must be part of all research efforts; every area of discovery and invention inhibits attention to alternative areas awaiting discovery and invention. In other words, interpretivists return to the Burkean (1984/1935) chestnut: "a way of seeing is also a way of not seeing" (p. 49). Post-positivists counter by arguing that their approach is well capable of noticing and addressing neglected areas of research, as illustrated by the chapter on health disparities in this book—and so the debate continues.

The question of what we ought to believe about the world—*as it is* and *as it could be*—is vital to all human beings. Researchers are simply people who are not content with beliefs rooted in tradition or beliefs based on the typical level of care that goes into everyday observation and inference. This is, for many people, the very reason we do research: to learn with greater confidence what we can and ought to believe. However, as the debates sketched above should make clear, there are important and difficult choices to be made. The best path forward is not obvious to all who would conduct research. For some, of course, there can be no single best path forward. If there was a best path that all agreed on, there would be no need for a book surveying a quite wide variety of methods, such as this one. We would need only a book focused on the one, undoubtedly best approach. Of course, we would then be a lot less vexed by the question of what to believe. We would know.

Because we so often do not know what to believe about the world, we are faced with a choice that might be formulated in one final way: We either satisfy ourselves with the truths given to us by tradition or everyday experience and common sense, or we take up the reflection and debates sketched in this chapter, and, in so doing, hope to come to better, more useful, more edifying understandings. Such is the purpose of all health communication research, and so various research methods are crafted in the ways they are.

Notes

1. Some might add intuition or (a sudden) flash of insight as a fourth source of knowledge, but we will not include it here. The main reason for this exclusion is that intuition and the sudden illumination of a flash of insight are notoriously fickle, well beyond intentional control, and thus unsuited to development as a dependable method of inquiry and knowledge attainment. Still, we are not completely comfortable with this omission, because, for the very same reason, we might be tempted to exclude inference. Like the flash of insight, inference also arises, at times, not necessarily under our willful control.
2. A related challenge to perception rooted in one's conceptual system is commonly called the "law of the hammer": If the only tool in your toolbox is a hammer, the whole world will look like a nail. The significance of this phenomenon is developed quite well in rhetorical scholar Kenneth Burke's (1984/1935) writing on "trained incapacity" and "occupational psychosis."
3. By "small clusters of causal relations," we mean causal systems involving two, three, four, or, rarely, five causally related variables. Of all known empirical methods, experiments provide the most compelling data bearing on three criteria thought to be necessary for inferring that a causal relationship exists between any two variables: establishing whether there is an empirical covariation (or systematic correlation) between the two variables, establishing the temporal order of covariation (i.e., that the "causal" variable changes prior to the "effect" variable), and ruling out the widest variety of alternative explanations for the empirical covariation (threats to validity; see the chapter on experiments).
4. Although here and above we have categorized particular methods as typical of one or the other orientation, there can be exceptions. Post-positivists, at times, use methods here considered primarily interpretive, and it is possible that interpretivists might use the methods we categorized as typically used by post-positivists. When this occurs, the same methods and results of their use will be understood differently, depending on the researcher's orientation.
5. Relativism is widely rejected, although the reasons are often overly simple (see Swoyer, 2010).
6. Inconsistencies between present and past work are irreducibly ambiguous: one can never know if one finding is accurate and the other inaccurate, or if there is an as-yet-unnoticed variable responsible for the inconsistency. Consistency is preferred because it suggests validation. Inconsistencies, however, can open doors to new ways of thinking

(Kuhn, 1970).

7. Researchers often say that they use whatever method is necessary to fit a given question. It is tempting to take a parallel stance relative to the post-positivist versus interpretivism debate, with researchers choosing the approach that best reflects the type of knowledge sought. It is just as tempting to say that such flexibility leads to incoherence; it undermines the meaningfulness of both positions by ignoring the incompatibility of the assumptions underlying the positions as articulated above. We offer no resolution, believing the choice must be the reader's. However, it would not be surprising if the reader has not decided these issues by the time she or he finishes undergraduate or graduate studies, or for a researcher to change outlook at some point.

References

Ackerman, D. (1991). *A natural history of the senses*. New York, NY: Vintage Books.

Anderson, J. A. (1996). *Communication theory: Epistemological foundations*. New York, NY: Guilford Press.

Babrow, A. S. (1992). Communication and problematic integration: Understanding diverging probability and value, ambiguity, ambivalence, and impossibility. *Communication Theory, 2*(2), 95–130.

Babrow, A. S. (2007). Problematic integration theory. In B. B. Whaley & W. Samter (Eds.), *Explaining communication: Contemporary theories and exemplars* (pp. 181–200). Mahwah, NJ: Lawrence Erlbaum Associates.

Batchelor, S. (1997). *Buddhism without beliefs: A contemporary guide to awakening*. New York, NY: Riverhead Books.

Berger, P. L., & Luckmann, T. (1967). *The social construction of reality: A treatise in the sociology of knowledge*. New York, NY: Anchor Books.

Bochner, A. P. (1985). Perspectives on inquiry: Representation, conversation, and reflection. In M. L. Knapp & G. R. Miller (Eds.), *Handbook of interpersonal communication* (pp. 27–58). Beverly Hills, CA: Sage Publications.

Burke, K. (1984/1935). *Permanence and change* (3rd ed.). Berkeley, CA: University of California Press.

Fishbein, M., & Ajzen, I. (1975). *Belief, attitude, intention, and behavior: An introduction to theory and research*. Reading, MA: Addison-Wesley.

Gergen, K. J. (2000). *An invitation to social construction*. London, England: Sage Publications.

Guba, E. C. (1990). The alternative paradigm dialog. In E.C. Guba (Ed.) *The paradigm dialog* (pp. 17–27). Newbury Park, CA: Sage Publications.

Gunderman, R. B. (2008). *We make a life by what we give*. Bloomington, IN: Indiana University Press.

Klein, D. M., & Jurich, J. A. (1993.) Metatheory and family studies. In P. Boss, W. J. Doherty, R. LaRossa, W. R. Schumm, & S. K. Steinmetz (Eds.), *Sourcebook of family theories and methods: A contextual approach* (pp. 31–67). New York, NY: Springer.

Korzybski, A. (1994/1933). *Science and sanity: An introduction to non-Aristotelian systems and general semantics* (5th ed.). New York, NY: Institute of General Semantics.

Kuhn, T. S. (1970). *The structure of scientific revolutions* (2nd ed.). Chicago, IL: University of Chicago Press.

Lakoff, G., & Johnson, M. (1980). *Metaphors we live by*. Chicago, IL: University of Chicago Press.

Morgan, S. E., Palmgreen, P., Stephenson, M., Hoyle, R., & Lorch, E. (2003). Associations between formal message features and subjective evaluations of the sensation value of anti-drug public service announcements. *Journal of Communication, 53*(3), 512–526.

O'Keefe, D. J. (1975). Logical empiricism and the study of human communication. *Communication Monographs, 42*(3), 169–183.

Phillips, D. C. (1990). Postpositivistic science: Myths and realities. In E.C. Guba (Ed.), *The paradigm dialog* (pp. 31–45). Newbury Park, CA: Sage Publications.

Swoyer, C. (2010). Relativism. In E. N. Zalta (Ed.), *The Stanford encyclopedia of philosophy.* Available from: http://plato.stanford.edu/archives/win2010/entries/relativism/

Taylor, J. B. (2009). *My stroke of insight: A brain scientist's personal journey*. New York, NY: Plume.

INDEX